Lessons from the
GRAND ROUNDS 1

Lessons from the
GRAND ROUNDS 1
A Pediatric Approach

Third Edition

YK Amdekar MD DCH
Senior Faculty
SRCC Children's Hospital, Mumbai
Retired Professor of Pediatrics
Grant Medical College, Sir JJ Group of Hospitals
Mumbai, Maharashtra, India

RD Khare MD DCH
Senior Consultant
Holy Family Hospital, Mumbai
Former Professor
KJ Somaiya Medical College
Mumbai, Maharashtra, India

RR Chokhani MD DCH
Consultant
PD Hinduja Hospital
Mumbai, Maharashtra, India

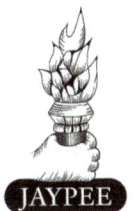

JAYPEE BROTHERS MEDICAL PUBLISHERS
The Health Sciences Publisher
New Delhi | London

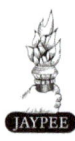
Jaypee Brothers Medical Publishers (P) Ltd

Headquarters
Jaypee Brothers Medical Publishers (P) Ltd
EMCA House, 23/23-B
Ansari Road, Daryaganj
New Delhi 110 002, India
Landline: +91-11-23272143, +91-11-23272703
+91-11-23282021, +91-11-23245672
Email: jaypee@jaypeebrothers.com

Corporate Office
Jaypee Brothers Medical Publishers (P) Ltd
4838/24, Ansari Road, Daryaganj
New Delhi 110 002, India
Phone: +91-11-43574357
Fax: +91-11-43574314
Email: jaypee@jaypeebrothers.com

Overseas Office
JP Medical Ltd
83 Victoria Street, London
SW1H 0HW (UK)
Phone: +44 20 3170 8910
Email: info@jpmedpub.com

EU GPSR Authorised Representative
Logos Europe, 9 rue Nicolas Poussin
17000, La Rochelle, France
Phone: +33 (0) 6 67 93 73 78
E-mail: Contact@logoseurope.eu

Website: www.jaypeebrothers.com
Website: www.jaypeedigital.com

© 2024, Jaypee Brothers Medical Publishers

The views and opinions expressed in this book are solely those of the original contributor(s)/author(s) and do not necessarily represent those of editor(s) or publisher of the book.

All rights reserved. No part of this publication may be reproduced, stored or transmitted in any form or by any means, electronic, mechanical, photocopying, recording or otherwise, without the prior permission in writing of the publishers.

All brand names and product names used in this book are trade names, service marks, trademarks or registered trademarks of their respective owners. The publisher is not associated with any product or vendor mentioned in this book.

Medical knowledge and practice change constantly. This book is designed to provide accurate, authoritative information about the subject matter in question. However, readers are advised to check the most current information available on procedures included and check information from the manufacturer of each product to be administered, to verify the recommended dose, formula, method and duration of administration, adverse effects and contra-indications. It is the responsibility of the practitioner to take all appropriate safety precautions. Neither the publisher nor the author(s)/editor(s) assume any liability for any injury and/or damage to persons or property arising from or related to use of material in this book.

This book is sold on the understanding that the publisher is not engaged in providing professional medical services. If such advice or services are required, the services of a competent medical professional should be sought.

Every effort has been made where necessary to contact holders of copyright to obtain permission to reproduce copyright material. If any have been inadvertently overlooked, the publisher will be pleased to make the necessary arrangements at the first opportunity.

Inquiries for bulk sales may be solicited at: jaypee@jaypeebrothers.com

Lessons from the Grand Rounds 1: A Pediatric Approach

First Edition: 2010
Second Edition: 2018
Third Edition: 2024

ISBN: 978-93-5696-794-6

Dedicated to
*The children who suffered
from whom we learnt a lot.*

Preface to the Third Edition

The continued demand for our book suggests that readers find it useful and identify with the cases discussed—both in content and in style. This has encouraged us to bring out another edition of the same. Since the content matter in our book is largely clinical, not much has "changed"—the clinical approach remains the same. We have added new cases in all the sections. We trust that our readers will find these new additions equally useful.

YK Amdekar
RD Khare
RR Chokhani

Preface to the First Edition

Over the last few years, the science of medicine has rapidly marched forward not only in the field of therapeutics but also in the field of diagnostics. But somewhere along the way, the art of clinical medicine has been left behind. We have moved from an era without many diagnostic aids to an era with a lot of aids (pun unintended). Easy availability of a plethora of investigations and a vast therapeutic armamentarium seems to have made physicians feel that clinical diagnosis is superfluous. However, in the absence of a rationally derived working clinical diagnosis, indiscriminate investigations can be expensive red herrings and polytherapy can be dangerous for the patient and disastrous for the community. Therefore, we firmly believe that these aids are intended to facilitate, and not eliminate, the process of clinical analysis.

We present a collection of cases that try to provide an insight into clinical analysis.

The entire material is derived from unbiased clinical discussions during teaching sessions based on live cases as they actually presented. The analysis of the history would help anticipate physical findings that would be confirmed on physical examination. Similarly, the results of investigations could also be anticipated after physical examination and then confirmed or otherwise. Such a sequential method of clinical analysis is not only effective but is also a self-learning exercise, as errors in clinical interpretation would lead to retrospective brainstorming that enriches the outlook. We wish to share this experience with our friends and colleagues. We do not propose to teach pediatrics or deal with management issues. We only wish to sensitize the readers about the utility of clinical analysis.

While analyzing these cases, the dictum—'if we diagnose common things, we are commonly correct; if we diagnose rare things, we are rarely correct'—has been kept in mind. There are arguments for or against the various common differentials (denoted by a bold print in the text) that should be considered. This is not meant to be an exhaustive list of differentials and there may always be other rarer possibilities given the same/similar situations. However, 'one swallow does not make a summer' and if we were to lookout of the window, we are more likely to see a crow than a golden eagle. Therefore, while discussing the possibilities in any case scenario, the emphasis is on a relative probability as illustrated by the use of terms like 'likely' and 'unlikely'. The inclusion of the odd seemingly exotic case may appear contrary to the above theme; the aim is to focus on the thought process that this particular case illustrates rather than the final diagnosis. Repetition of certain concepts and messages has been deliberately allowed, in the hope that it will serve to reinforce; to us, these are like the ten commandments, we treasure them. Purists may not find 'evidence' in current medical literature in favor of some of the hypotheses put forth by us. However, at this point in time, we believe this is a rational conjecture.

Many disorders present with symptoms that are shared by more than one system. Hence majority of the cases have been listed according to symptoms, largely in an alphabetical order. However, certain symptomatology obviously points to particular system. These cases have been grouped together. For the benefit of the reader, index is given at the end of the book.

These cases represent many but not all pediatric disorders. In particular, emergency cases and neonatology cases have not been included since most of these disorders need immediate management and any further analysis of possible etiology is only after initial stabilization.

As mentioned earlier, the source of these cases are the teaching sessions conducted by us. We sincerely thank all the superspecialists who participated in these sessions from time to time. Some of them also contributed additionally in the compilation of these cases by way of their valuable suggestions and therefore deserve a special mention. These include Vibha Krishnamurthy (Developmental Pediatrician), Mamta Manglani (Hematologist), Kamini Mehta (Nephrologist), Abha Nagral (Hepatologist), Nimesh Nanavati (Rheumatologist), CK Ponde (Cardiologist), Nalini Shah (Endocrinologist), and Vrajesh Udani (Neurologist). We express our heartfelt gratitude to all of them. We also appreciate with gratitude the help rendered by Shri BK Amdekar, Ms Sangita Chokhani and Shri Rajadatta Ranade in various technical areas of production of this book.

YK Amdekar
RD Khare
RR Chokhani

Contents

CLINICAL HEPATOLOGY

CASE 1	Abdominal Distension with Hematemesis for Years	7
CASE 2	Recurrent Hematemesis	11
CASE 3	Abdominal Distension with Breathlessness in an Infant	15
CASE 4	Abdominal Distension with Puffiness of Face	19
CASE 5	Puffiness of Face with Edema Feet	23
CASE 6	Abdominal Distension with Developmental Delay	27
CASE 7	Acute Severe Jaundice	31
CASE 8	Severe Jaundice with High Fever	35
CASE 9	Fluctuating Jaundice	39
CASE 10	Jaundice with Pleural Effusion	43
CASE 11	Progressive Jaundice with Failure to Thrive in an Infant	47
CASE 12	Abdominal Distension, Jaundice, and Irritability in an Infant	51
CASE 13	Recurrent Jaundice in a Child who Remained Healthy	53

CLINICAL PULMONOLOGY

CASE 14	Breathlessness and Fever for a Day	61
CASE 15	Breathlessness and Fever over 5 Days	65
CASE 16	Breathlessness after Few Days of Fever	69
CASE 17	Breathlessness in a Child with Arthritis	73
CASE 18	Sudden Onset of Breathlessness in a 5-year-old	77
CASE 19	Gradually Progressive Breathlessness in an Infant	79
CASE 20	Breathlessness, Palpitations and Chest Pain	83
CASE 21	Fever with Chest Pain	87
CASE 22	Chest Pain with Fever	89

CASE 23	Chest Pain after 2 Weeks of Fever and Cough	93
CASE 24	Hemoptysis in a 10-year-old	97
CASE 25	Cyanosis on Crying in an Infant	101
CASE 26	Recent Onset Cyanosis in a 9-year-old	105
CASE 27	Occasional Choking Episodes in an 8-year-old Child	109
CASE 28	Difficulty in Feeding in an Infant	111

CLINICAL HEMATOLOGY

CASE 29	Ecchymosis in an Infant	117
CASE 30	Ecchymosis in an Older Child	121
CASE 31	Bluish Patches in an 8-year-old Child	125
CASE 32	Ecchymosis with Fever	127
CASE 33	Ecchymosis with Joint Swellings	131
CASE 34	Anemia in a 15-month-old	135
CASE 35	Severe Anemia Noticed Incidentally	139
CASE 36	Generalized Weakness for a Few Months and Recent Facial Asymmetry	143
CASE 37	Fever for 2 Weeks with Constitutional Symptoms	145

PYREXIA

CASE 38	Fever for 2 Months	153
CASE 39	Low Fever, Cough and Failure to Thrive	157
CASE 40	High Fever, Cough and Failure to Thrive	161
CASE 41	Fever for 2 Months: Case 1	165
CASE 42	Fever for 2 Months: Case 2	169
CASE 43	Fever for 3 Months	173
CASE 44	Fever for 6 Months	177
CASE 45	Fever for 12 Months	181
CASE 46	Fever and Cough for a Few Days	183
CASE 47	Fever and Cough with Large Expectoration	187
CASE 48	Fever with "Changing Pneumonia"	191

CASE 49	Fever with Irritability in an Infant	195
CASE 50	Fever with Irritability	199
CASE 51	Fever Followed by Generalized Convulsion	203
CASE 52	Frequent Fever with Inability to Walk	207
CASE 53	Fever, Lethargy and Refusal to Feed	211
CASE 54	Fever with Neck Swelling	215
CASE 55	Fever with Severe Abdominal Pain	219
CASE 56	Prolonged Fever with Jaundice Later in the Illness	223
CASE 57	Fever with Weakness of the Right Side	227
CASE 58	"Osteomyelitis" that would not Get Better or Worse!	231
CASE 59	Fever Off and On, but the Child Remains Healthy!	233
CASE 60	Frequent Wheezing in an Infant	235
CASE 61	Recurrent Hematuria in a 4-year-old	239
CASE 62	Recurrent Hematuria in a 10-year-old	243
CASE 63	Increased Precordial Activity Since Infancy	247
CASE 64	Incidentally Noticed Murmur in an Infant	251
CASE 65	Failure to Gain Height	253
CASE 66	Failure to Gain Height with Onset of Puberty	257
CASE 67	Breast Development in an 8-year-old	263
CASE 68	Pubic Hair Development in a 3½-year-old	267
CASE 69	Excessive Weight Gain in a 10-year-old	271
CASE 70	Progressive Deformity of Lower Limbs	275

CLINICAL RHEUMATOLOGY

CASE 71	Limb Pain with Difficulty in Walking	283
CASE 72	Limb Pain for a Year	287
CASE 73	Joint Pains—Recurrent	289
CASE 74	Joint Pains with Constitutional Symptoms	293
CASE 75	Acute Onset Multiple Large Joint Swellings	297
CASE 76	Joint Stiffness and Pain with Short Stature	299

CLINICAL NEUROLOGY

CASE 77	Developmental Delay Since Birth	307
CASE 78	Regression of Milestones	311
CASE 79	Differential Developmental Delay	315
CASE 80	Delayed Speech in a 2½-year-old	319
CASE 81	Focal Convulsion in a 2-month-old	323
CASE 82	Headache and Vomiting for a Year	327
CASE 83	Gradually Progressive Hemiparesis	331
CASE 84	Paucity of Left Sided Movements for 5 Days	335
CASE 85	Irritability with Refusal to Walk	339
CASE 86	Difficulty in Walking for 5 Years	343
CASE 87	Difficulty in Walking, "Head Nodding" for 8 Days	347
CASE 88	Clumsiness of Gait Since Last 4 Years	351
CASE 89	Fever Followed by Prolonged Seizures	355
CASE 90	Unusual Case of Altered Sensorium	359
CASE 91	Sudden Onset Hemiplegia with Seizures in the Recent Past	361
CASE 92	Irritability and Seizure in an Afebrile Infant	363
Index		*365*

Clinical Hepatology

BACK TO BASICS

Anatomical Diagnosis

It is important to localize the disease to a microanatomical site in the liver. Liver consists of four main components for clinical consideration—liver cell parenchyma, biliary tract, venous channels and the reticuloendothelial cells. Each site leads to characteristic symptoms and signs though at times there may be some overlap.

Hepatocyte disease results in disturbed function—either synthetic or metabolic. However, it must be noted that the liver performs multiple functions; therefore dysfunction can often be selective. In other words, in early liver disease all functions are not equally deranged and there can be isolated manifestations of dysfunction, nevertheless signifying hepatocyte disease. Hypoalbuminemia and hypoprothrombinemia represent synthetic dysfunction. Jaundice and encephalopathy (due to hyperammonemia and/or hypoglycemia) represent metabolic dysfunction. Rarely, bleeding due to vitamin K deficiency or rickets due to vitamin D metabolic defect may be the only manifestation.

Destruction of liver cells results in an increase in ALT (SGPT) and AST (SGOT). Increase in AST is nonspecific as many other tissues share this enzyme.

A child with acute liver cell disease appears sick, while the one with chronic liver disease fails to thrive.

Biliary tract disease is characterized by jaundice, clay colored stools and itching. Generally the jaundice is disproportionately more pronounced as compared to the clinical appearance of sickness. Biochemical changes are characterized by an increase in alkaline phosphatase and gamma GT. The general well-being of the child is maintained till hepatocytes get secondarily affected.

Portal hypertension usually presents as hematemesis and splenomegaly with or without engorged veins over the abdominal wall. The origin (of the venous obstruction and therefore the portal hypertension) may be presinusoidal (splenic or extrahepatic), sinusoidal (hepatocyte disease), or postsinusoidal (hepatic vein or vena caval obstruction). Presence of ascites indicates either liver cell dysfunction or inferior vena cava/hepatic vein obstruction. Often, presence of ascites in portal hypertension represents liver cell failure; increased portal pressure helps to localize the fluid to the peritoneal cavity. In presinusoidal portal hypertension, there is no ascites.

Reticuloendothelial involvement (as in hepatic TB) presents initially with enlarged liver often without any liver cell dysfunction, biliary tract involvement or venous obstruction. RE cell hyperplasia occurs as a reaction to a variety of insults such as infections, immune mediated or hematological disorders. It is worthwhile to note that certain other disorders affecting hepatocytes like storage disorders, and fatty liver as in protein malnutrition, also present with hepatomegaly without any other signs of liver disease.

A disease may involve more than one microanatomical site though it usually begins at one site and then spreads to another.

Hepatobiliary disease is a common denominator of many liver diseases. Such a disease may start as a liver cell disease as in viral hepatitis and subsequently cause cholestasis due to liver cell edema, or the disease may primarily involve the biliary tract as in biliary atresia and subsequently affect the liver cells. It is therefore important to enquire in detail about the origin and progress of symptoms.

Enlarged liver is a common presentation of many liver diseases. Especially in chronic liver disease, a common presenting complaint is that of a generalized abdominal distension which is due to hepatomegaly with or without splenomegaly. Isolated splenomegaly presents as a lump in abdomen rather than abdominal distension. Gradually progressive generalized abdominal distension suggests organomegaly, while that which increases over the first few days but remains static thereafter denotes ascites.

Pathological Diagnosis

The hallmark of a liver disease is an enlarged liver. Liver size is better judged by the *liver span* rather than the extent of palpability of the liver below the costal margin. Normal liver is soft in consistency, whereas a pathological liver is almost always enlarged and may be firm or hard. Enlarged *soft* liver is unusual and may often denote a pushed down liver rather than any liver disease. This is confirmed by the liver span being normal in such cases. Hence, it is always rational to denote the liver size by liver span. It is rare in children for a pathological liver to *shrink* to an extent that it becomes impalpable. In any case, even if it does, the liver functions are so deranged that the diagnosis of liver disease is obvious. A hard liver is characteristic of malignancy or late stages of cirrhosis. Normal liver has a well-defined edge though not sharp. A sharp edge suggests cirrhosis; a rounded edge depicts storage as in a fatty liver. The surface is almost always smooth in children irrespective of the pathology unlike in adults. Tenderness suggests inflammation or venous congestion of short duration. The more severe the tenderness, the more likely it is to be inflammation rather than congestion. Tenderness may not be present in chronic inflammation or congestion.

Normal serum bilirubin in hepatocyte disease indicates that at least 10% of the hepatocytes are intact, as happens in localized infections of the liver (such as liver abscess) or in the early stages of any hepatocyte pathology.

Thus, jaundice is an early manifestation of generalized liver infection as in viral hepatitis and is a late manifestation of liver cell failure in a progressive disease such as cirrhosis.

Jaundice signifies the extent of liver cell disease, serum albumin the chronicity, prothrombin time and its failure to return to normal the seriousness, and increase in ALT and AST the extent of parenchymal destruction. An increase in alkaline phosphatase and GTT denotes cholestasis.

Metabolic disorders due to inborn errors (glycogen and lipid storage disorders, galactosemia, Wilson's disease) present with metabolic disturbances, often associated with multisystem involvement. On the other hand, primary liver diseases (hepatitis) often have isolated liver involvement. It is important to keep in mind that jaundice may be due to hemolysis and does not always denote liver disease.

Etiological Diagnosis

It is a clinical guess, possible only after logical derivation of anatomical and pathological diagnosis. Hence, in the clinical approach to any case, one must follow a sequential attempt at diagnosis.

The following case scenarios represent a wide spectrum of clinical conditions met with in routine practice and offer an insight into clinical analysis.

Clinical Approach to Hepatosplenomegaly

Soft small liver – normal (especially in a young child)
Soft large liver – displaced (pushed down)
Firm or hard liver – always pathological, irrespective of size. (Small, firm, shrunken liver is rare in children).
Palpable spleen – (enlarged more than twice its size) always abnormal, except in infancy
Size of palpable spleen, consistency and duration are proportionate.
Soft palpable spleen is small in size and of recent onset.
Firm splenomegaly denotes chronicity and is usually of moderate or large size. (Spleen in sickle cell disease may be small and firm).

Group Probable Causes

Primary liver disease – hepatobiliary disease/portal hypertension (jaundice/ascites/edema/hematemesis/failure to thrive)

Primary hematological disease – hemolytic anemia/bone marrow infiltration (leukemia/myelofibrosis/myelodysplasia/osteopetrosis) (pallor/bleeding/jaundice)

Systemic infection – Malaria/kala-azar (mainly splenomegaly), typhoid, TB, EB (usually fever)

Primary storage disorder – Gaucher/Niemann-Pick (mainly splenomegaly), MPS (large, progressive organomegaly)

IN TODAY'S AGE OF COMPUTERIZED ANALYSIS AND AUTOMATED ANALYZERS......

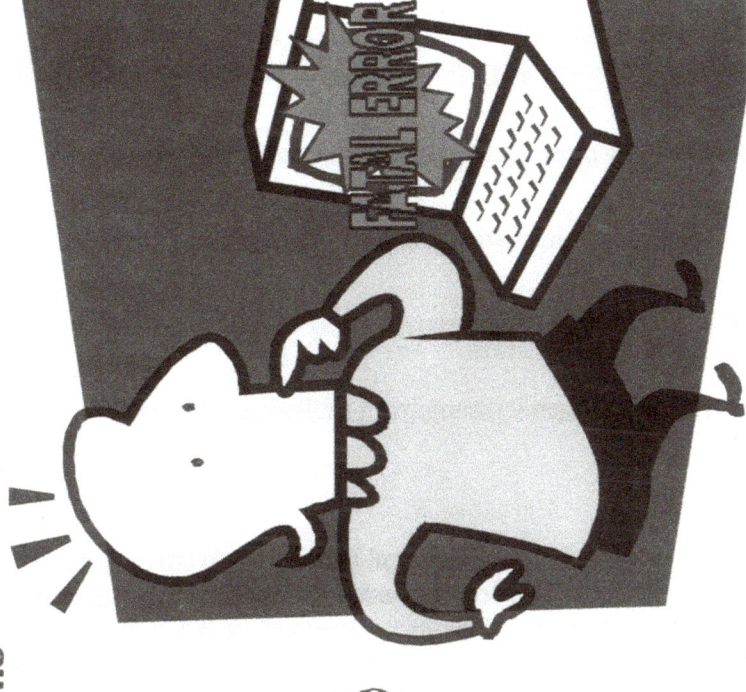
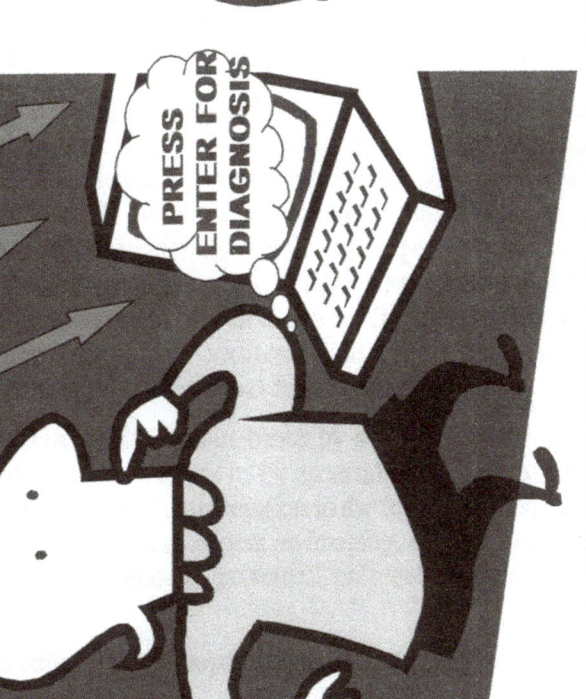

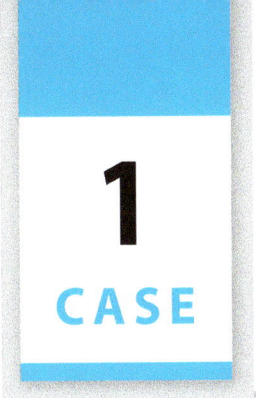

Abdominal Distension with Hematemesis for Years

■ HISTORY

A 15-year-old male child born of 3rd degree consanguineous marriage, presented with the chief complaints of abdominal distension noticed since 4 years of age, episodic epistaxis since 5 years of age, and hematemesis since 9 years of age.

The abdominal distension was progressive; initially localized to upper abdomen but later, involving the entire abdomen. He had been getting spontaneous episodes of epistaxis off and on, which were self-limiting and lasting for 2–3 days. He was hospitalized at 10 years of age following two episodes of massive hematemesis; at that time he was subjected to splenectomy.

He developed jaundice on the 8th postoperative day. It lasted for 15 days.

H/o some intravenous medication given every 15 days since the last 3 years following which there has been a reduction in the abdominal distension.

H/o some vague ankle and knee joint pains, which occurred after starting the medication.

Analysis

This child has a history of a gradual distension of upper abdomen spanning *over years*, suggestive of **organomegaly** in the form of hepatomegaly with or without splenomegaly. Subsequent development of *generalized* abdominal distension may denote development of **ascites** or further progression to a **very large organomegaly**. Recurrent hematemesis over the last few years in this setting suggests portal hypertension. Thus, this child probably had progressive hepatomegaly with portal hypertension and mostly a splenomegaly also. He may or may not have ascites additionally. In other words, he seems to be suffering from slowly progressive **chronic liver disease with portal hypertension**. Epistaxis may have been due to fragile capillary bleeding and therefore unrelated. However, recurrent epistaxis may also represent a bleeding disorder due to thrombocytopenia resulting from hypersplenism, or a coagulopathy arising out of a chronic liver disease.

The exact cause of the chronic liver disease remains to be determined. Common causes of such slowly progressive chronic liver diseases include **HBV or HCV** infections. However, they are often characterized by intermittent jaundice, which has not been reported in this child. History of jaundice in the postoperative period may suggest decompensation of liver function secondary to the stress of surgery. He is being treated with an intravenous medication every 15 days for the last 3 years. At this point, the nature of this treatment modality remains unexplained.

■ PHYSICAL EXAMINATION

Poorly built and nourished child Weight 32 kg Height 141 cm
Vital parameters normal No ecchymosis or purpura
No icterus No KF ring Central cyanosis + Clubbing grade II +
Generalized distension of abdomen, splenectomy scar seen. No ascites
Liver – left lobe palpable, 6 cm, firm with sharp edge, right lobe not palpable
CVS – normal RS – normal Other systems normal

Analysis

At present, this child has evidence of **chronic liver disease** in the form of failure to thrive and a firm enlarged liver. Past history of hematemesis clearly suggests **portal hypertension**, though subsequently it may have resolved following splenectomy. The fact that there is no ascites at present may signify resolution of ascites following treatment, or it may mean that this child never had ascites. Ascites in a liver disease with portal hypertension signifies decompensation of liver function and therefore, would not resolve completely even if portal hypertension was surgically treated. In other words, this child may not have developed ascites at all. Thus, the original generalized abdominal distension reported in this child may have been due to **massive organomegaly** (and **not ascites**). If so, it is possible that splenectomy may have been done not only for control of portal hypertension, but also for massive splenomegaly, which is prone to traumatic complications. Such large organomegaly suggests a possibility of a **storage disorder** as the primary illness.

Central cyanosis and **clubbing** of nails are unusual features in this child. Clubbing of nails without cyanosis is known in chronic liver disease, though not common. Presence of central cyanosis in an otherwise comfortable child suggests **admixture** of venous and arterial blood at some level and it is **not** a **respiratory** problem. As physical examination does **not** reveal any **cardiac** defect, mixing of blood must be occurring at the peripheral level. Portal hypertension in a chronic liver disease is known to develop **hepatopulmonary syndrome**, which is characterized by intrapulmonary vascular dilatation resulting in central cyanosis and clubbing of nails. As this child has a past history suggestive of portal hypertension, cyanosis and clubbing in this child could be explained on the basis of development of hepatopulmonary syndrome. (Ideally it should be referred to as **portopulmonary syndrome** as it is the portal hypertension that leads to such changes in intrapulmonary vasculature and not chronic liver disease, though in a setting of chronic liver disease, portal hypertension causes such changes.)

■ INVESTIGATIONS

Hb –10 gm% CBC- N Platelets – adequate
Serum bilirubin 1.2 mgm% Direct 0.2 mgm% Serum proteins normal
Prothrombin time normal ALT/AST normal Alk. Phos. normal
Serum ceruloplasmin - normal
Liver biopsy suggests Gaucher's disease

Analysis

This child's liver function seems to be normal at present. At this juncture, it is clear that the intravenous therapy every fortnight refers to enzyme replacement therapy that may have prevented further deterioration and stabilized the child's condition. Since, the hematological profile is also normal, the Gaucher's disease seems to be localized to the liver only.

■ FINAL DIAGNOSIS

Type 1 Gaucher's disease.

■ KEY MESSAGES

- Hepatomegaly without hepatocyte dysfunction suggests venous congestion (congestive cardiac failure or venous obstruction), reticuloendothelial hyperplasia (disseminated infections) or storage disorders.
- Presence of portal hypertension in such cases rules out congestive cardiac failure and disseminated infections and may denote venous obstruction or storage disorders.
- Massive hepatomegaly without hepatocyte dysfunction favors a storage disorder.

■ RELEVANT INFORMATION

Gaucher's Disease

Gaucher's disease is a lipid storage disease, characterized by the deposition of glucocerebroside in cells of the macrophage-monocyte system. Deficiency of a specific lysosomal hydrolase, acid beta-glucocerebrosidase, causes the condition. Three clinical subtypes exist and are delineated by the absence or presence of neurologic involvement. Central nervous system (CNS) involvement occurs only in patients with disease types 2 and 3. Type 1 accounts for 99% of the cases. The severity of type 1 Gaucher's disease is extremely variable, such that some patients present in childhood with virtually all the complications of Gaucher's disease, while others are asymptomatic even into the eighth decade. Presumably, the amount of residual enzymatic activity determines the disease subtype and severity.

Children with Gaucher type 1 disease present with chronic fatigue due to anemia. Other common manifestations include hepatosplenomegaly without liver dysfunction, bony pain or pathological fractures and bruises due to thrombocytopenia. In symptomatic patients, splenomegaly is progressive and can be massive. Such children are short. Pulmonary involvement and portal hypertension are also known, but rare.

The diagnosis is confirmed by measurement of acid-beta glucosidase activity in peripheral leukocytes. A finding of <15% of normal activity is diagnostic of the disease. Heterozygotes have half the normal enzyme activity that may overlap with 20% normal children. Molecular diagnosis may be ideal, as it can prognosticate disease progression. ACE (angiotensin converting enzyme) is elevated and so also total acid phosphatase.

Replacement therapy is now available with a recombinant enzyme. The enzyme is typically infused intravenously once a fortnight in a high dose, though small doses thrice a week have also been tried with an equivalent response. The liver and spleen regress considerably within 6 months of treatment, while the hemoglobin and platelet count improve over 6-9 months. Skeletal disease is slow to respond. Other benefits of enzyme replacement therapy include a growth spurt, weight gain and pubertal development. The cost of therapy is prohibitive at present.

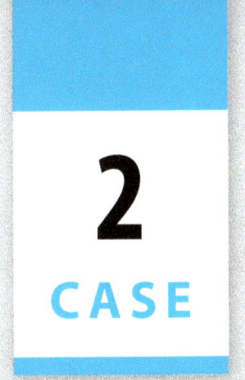

Recurrent Hematemesis

■ HISTORY

An 8-year-old child presented with recurrent hematemesis over the last few months. He was apparently well 8 months ago, when he had his first episode of hematemesis. The bleeding stopped without treatment and he was not investigated then. After another month of normal intervening period, he had another episode of a similar nature.

At that time he was found to be anemic and was given a blood transfusion. Prior to the blood transfusion, he was subjected to some hematological tests, which were reported to be normal. Subsequent episodes of hematemesis were mild, till the last one, which was very severe and at which time he was admitted in a shock state.

He has been a healthy child without any other significant past illnesses.

The antenatal and the neonatal period was uneventful; there was no history of umbilical sepsis or umbilical catheterization.

There was no family history of any significant disease.

Analysis

Recurrent hematemesis is usually suggestive of portal hypertension. In a *healthy* child it is suggestive of **extrahepatic (presinusoidal) portal hypertension**. It is not likely to be **intrahepatic (sinusoidal) portal hypertension** as there are no symptoms of liver disease in the past or at present. Occasionally, a **vascular malformation** in the esophagus may present with recurrent hematemesis. **Bleeding disorders** due to either a coagulation factor deficiency or platelet disorders, do not present with *isolated* recurrent hematemesis without any other bleeding manifestations. **Peptic ulcer disease** is another condition that can explain hematemesis, though large bouts of recurrent hematemesis without any epigastric or retrosternal pain or burning are not a common manifestation in childhood. A single episode of hematemesis may be caused by **severe gastritis** due to a viral infection or **drugs** such as NSAIDs, but recurrent episodes are not likely. So, if it is indeed extrahepatic portal hypertension, its cause may be a malformation of the portal system or portal vein thrombosis which may either be a sequelae of **umbilical sepsis** (there is no such history in this case) or due to a **thrombophilic state**.

PHYSICAL EXAMINATION

Fairly built and nourished — Weight 24 kg — Height 118 cm
Marked pallor — Mild icterus — No edema of feet or puffiness of face
Temp. subnormal — Cold hands and feet
HR 140/min — RR 30/min — BP 70/45 mm — JVP raised
Liver 6 cm +, firm, sharp edge, smooth surface, not tender — Liver span 10 cm
Spleen 5 cm +, firm, not tender — No ascites — No engorged abdominal veins
CNS – drowsy — Plantars down going — No other abnormality

Analysis

Clinical examination reveals a *healthy* child (normal weight and height) with firm hepatomegaly and mild icterus but without other overt signs of liver cell failure such as edema and ascites. This child has presented with shock due to severe hematemesis. History of recurrent hematemesis and presence of splenomegaly points to definite portal hypertension. Thus, this is suggestive of **chronic liver disease with portal hypertension**. Presence of significant pallor with minimal jaundice may also be a typical presentation of hemolytic anemia. However, recurrent hematemesis and firm hepatomegaly rules out such a possibility. Though it is definitely a **chronic liver disease**, the hepatocyte dysfunction is minimal as this child has maintained normal health. The **disparity** between the degree of hepatocyte dysfunction and the portal hypertension suggests that it is unlikely to be primary cirrhosis with sinusoidal portal hypertension. Hence, it may be an **intrahepatic but presinusoidal obstruction,** which is responsible for portal hypertension. Thus, it seems that this disease has started within the liver but outside the hepatocyte and has predominantly obstructed the portal venous system; subsequently it has also involved the hepatocytes to a mild extent. Such a disease is **non-cirrhotic portal fibrosis (congenital hepatic fibrosis)**.

Drowsiness in this child may indicate encephalopathy either due to transient worsening of liver dysfunction or due to the shock state.

INVESTIGATIONS

Hb 4 gm% — WBC 7,000/c.mm — P 65 L 30 E 2 M 3 — ESR 30 mm
Serum bilirubin 2 mgm% — Direct 0.6 mgm% — ALT/AST normal — Alk. phos normal
Serum proteins 6.2 gm% — Albumin 3.2 gm% — Prothrombin time normal
Serum ammonia normal — Serum creatinine normal — Blood sugar normal
Abdominal USG – hepatosplenomegaly with evidence of portal hypertension
— No cavernoma — No ascites — No renal abnormality
Barium esophagogram and endoscopy shows esophageal and gastric varices
Liver biopsy shows non-cirrhotic portal fibrosis.

Analysis

This child has direct hyperbilirubinemia as the direct fraction is >20% of the total bilirubin. However, absence of raised enzymes suggests a mild hepatic dysfunction rather than hepatitis per se. Such a mild hyperbilirubinemia may be seen in congestive liver pathology as in cardiac failure. It may also denote transient hepatocyte dysfunction due to severe blood loss and shock state. Normal serum albumin indicates good liver cell function and thus *chronic liver cell disease* is ruled out. Liver biopsy has proved the diagnosis of non-cirrhotic portal fibrosis.

■ FINAL DIAGNOSIS

Non-cirrhotic portal fibrosis.

■ KEY MESSAGES

- Recurrent hematemesis is a feature of portal hypertension, commonly due to extrahepatic presinusoidal venous obstruction. In children, hematemesis is a rare manifestation of portal hypertension due to cirrhosis, and in fact, may often indicate coagulation factor deficiency due to liver cell failure.
- Normal liver function with portal hypertension rules out cirrhosis.
- Even in the presence of a high indirect bilirubin, if the direct fraction is >20% of the total bilirubin, it is recognized as direct hyperbilirubinemia. Of course, if direct bilirubin is >2 mgm%, it is always direct hyperbilirubinemia.

■ RELEVANT INFORMATION

Non-cirrhotic Portal Fibrosis (Congenital Hepatic Fibrosis)

This is an autosomal recessive disorder, characterized pathologically by diffuse periportal and perilobular fibrosis in broad bands that contain distorted bile duct-like structures, and that often compress or incorporate central or sublobular veins. The duct-like structures may become dilated to the point of microcyst formation but do not communicate with the biliary tract. This condition is often associated with renal abnormalities. About 75% of the patients have renal disease, such as renal tubular ectasia, nephronophthisis, or autosomal recessive polycystic renal disease. It may also be associated with Caroli's disease or choledochal cyst.

Clinical presentation is hepatosplenomegaly with portal hypertension and bleeding varices. Liver functions are usually maintained within normal limits, though rarely they may be minimally deranged.

There is no specific treatment. Management consists of preventing variceal bleeding.

Prognosis is guarded.

CASE 3

Abdominal Distension with Breathlessness in an Infant

■ HISTORY

An 11-month-old male infant born of a non-consanguineous marriage, presented with distension of abdomen since the last 4 months. He was apparently well until 7 months of age, when the parents noticed distension of abdomen, which increased over the first *few days* but thereafter remained static. He continued to feed well and was active without any other significant symptoms. A month later, he developed difficulty in breathing which worsened over the next few days. At about the same time, a further increase in the abdominal distension was also noted. He was diagnosed to have a right-sided pleural effusion and was tapped. Subsequently, he required frequent pleural tapping to relieve his breathlessness.

- No history of jaundice or ecchymosis
- No history of failure to thrive
- Developmental history normal
- No relevant past or family history

Analysis

Distension of abdomen in an otherwise healthy child suggests **organomegaly** or **ascites**. If it were organomegaly, it would commonly be **hepatomegaly with or without splenomegaly** or any other **lump in abdomen**. The association of a pleural effusion with hepatomegaly or any other lump in a healthy asymptomatic infant is extremely unusual. A disseminated infection such as **tuberculosis** does not result in hepatomegaly and pleural effusion at the same time, as the pathogenesis of these two manifestations is different. Therefore, abdominal distension in this infant is likely to be ascites, with or without hepatomegaly, and later he developed a pleural effusion. Though tuberculosis may rarely present as polyserositis, such a manifestation is not seen in *infants*. **Malignancy** does not lead to such symptomatology. In fact, fluid collection in *multiple* body cavities in an acutely sick child (as in **dengue** or **acute pancreatitis**) indicates a third space loss of fluids due to vascular leak. If a similar pathogenesis is extended to a "non sick" setting, it would suggest **lymphatic/venous obstruction** and subsequent leakage as the cause of such a fluid collection. Lymphatic obstruction resulting in ascites leads to malnutrition over time, while a venous obstruction can maintain a healthy nutritional state.

■ PHYSICAL EXAMINATION

Fairly built and nourished	Weight 8.5 kg	Length 73 cm
Temp. normal	Pulse 140/min	RR 45/min
BP - 90/60 mm of Hg	Mild respiratory distress	Neck veins not engorged
Generalized abdominal distension	No edema of feet	

Mildly engorged veins over flanks, flow from below upwards (both above and below umbilicus)
No icterus   No other signs of liver cell failure
Liver 6 cm +, firm, sharp edge, smooth surface, not tender, liver span not delineated
Spleen not palpable   Free fluid in the abdomen +
Respiratory system - right sided pleural effusion +   Other systems normal

Analysis

This apparently *healthy* infant (normal weight and length) has *remained asymptomatic and grown well in spite of progressive abdominal distension* due to hepatomegaly and ascites. (Liver span in this child could not be delineated due to the presence of pleural effusion on the right side. However, 6 cm palpable and firm liver is definitely pathological). This is suggestive of **venous obstruction**. In the absence of hepatic dysfunction, it is not intrahepatic sinusoidal obstruction. Presence of an enlarged firm liver with ascites and absence of splenomegaly rules out extra-hepatic presinusoidal obstruction. Hence, this is likely to be **suprahepatic postsinusoidal** venous obstruction. It may be at the level of hepatic veins or superior vena cava. Absence of engorged neck veins rules out the possibility of superior vena cava obstruction as a part of constrictive pericarditis. Thus, it is likely to be hepatic vein obstruction. Presence of pleural effusion in this child is unusual, though it is known to occur. It results from seepage of ascitic fluid through rents in the diaphragm into the pleural cavity (**hepatic hydrothorax**).

■ INVESTIGATIONS

Hemogram normal	Liver function tests normal Serum albumin 3.8 gm%
Ascitic fluid	– 8 cells all lymphocytes, proteins 1.9 gm% (albumin 1.6 gm%)
Pleural fluid	– 6 cells all lymphocytes, proteins 2.6 gm%
SAAG	– (serum – ascitic albumin gradient) was 2.2
Color Doppler	– non-visualization of the right and central hepatic veins with turbulent flow in the left hepatic vein suggestive of obstruction. Interconnecting veins seen.

Analysis

SAAG >1.1 with a normal serum albumin, suggests **venous obstruction without liver disease**. As the pleural fluid is a mere extension of the ascitic fluid, it is expected to demonstrate similar cellular and biochemical findings. However in this child, the pleural fluid has a higher protein content (falsely suggestive of an exudate; however, the cells are normal). The higher protein content of the pleural fluid is due to the superior ability of the pleura to absorb fluids as compared to the peritoneum. Color Doppler confirmed obstruction of the hepatic veins. Interconnecting veins seen on Doppler study are pathognomonic of Budd-Chiari syndrome.

■ FINAL DIAGNOSIS
Budd-Chiari syndrome.

■ KEY MESSAGES

- Children with hepatic venous obstruction (also extrahepatic portal hypertension and non-cirrhotic portal fibrosis) are not sick.
- Ascites in such children may be accompanied with pleural effusion (hepatic hydrothorax).
- SAAG (serum – ascitic albumin gradient) is a useful indicator of the pathogenesis of ascitic fluid.

■ RELEVANT INFORMATION

SAAG (Serum Ascitic Albumin Gradient)

SAAG is the best single test for classifying ascites into portal hypertension (SAAG >1.1 g/dL and non-portal hypertension (SAAG <1.1 g/dL) groups. Calculated by subtracting ascitic fluid albumin value from the serum albumin value, it correlates directly with portal pressure. Specimens must be collected simultaneously for estimation of albumin. Accuracy of the test in classifying ascites is close to 97%. The terms high albumin gradient and low albumin gradient should replace the terms exudate and transudate in the description of ascites.

As against this, the accuracy of the protein content of the ascitic fluid, to differentiate exudates from transudates is only 50%. The total protein level may be helpful in conjunction with SAAG, but not per se.

Similarly, the cell count is at best suggestive, but not dependable by itself unless grossly abnormal.

SAAG >1.1 g/dL with normal serum protein level – portal hypertension with normal liver (postsinusoidal venous obstruction)

SAAG >1.1 g/dL with low serum protein level – portal hypertension with abnormal liver function (cirrhosis/chronic hepatitis)

SAAG <1.1 g/dL No portal hypertension – infections/malignancy/nephrotic syndrome/pancreatic ascites/chylous ascites.

Budd-Chiari Syndrome

Budd-Chiari syndrome (BCS) refers to the obstruction of hepatic venous blood flow. The site of obstruction may be anywhere from the small central lobar veins of the liver to the proximal inferior vena cava (IVC). Although BCS is frequently caused by thrombosis, extrinsic compression and venous malformations may also cause obstruction. BCS may result in portal hypertension, cirrhosis, and liver failure.

Clinical presentation is variable according to the degree, location, and acuity of the obstruction. Insidious onset of ascites in a healthy child without any liver dysfunction, may be the only feature at the onset. The acute form of the disease presents with severe abdominal pain, hepatomegaly and progressive liver dysfunction. Without treatment, it may evolve into a chronic disease. The chronic form of the disease manifests with portal hypertension with or without associated ascites, splenomegaly, variceal bleeding, cirrhosis, coagulopathy and encephalopathy. The fulminant form of the disease is rare in children. It may manifest with severe abdominal pain, jaundice, hepatomegaly, ascites, acute liver failure and encephalopathy. Early recognition and treatment are essential for survival.

The diagnosis is confirmed by demonstration of the venous block by a color Doppler study. It is at times difficult to define the site of the block on color Doppler study, especially in infants. The use of angiography may be necessary in such cases. Once the venous obstruction is delineated, its cause needs to be ascertained. The USG may show evidence of extrinsic compression if any, caused by a mass lesion in the liver. In the absence of any mass lesion, a congenital malformation in the form of a membrane in one of the hepatic veins may be picked up by angiography. If no mechanical obstruction is evident on imaging, a hypercoagulable state must be ruled out. APLA (antiphospholipid antibody), protein C, protein S or antithrombin 3 should be evaluated.

The treatment consists of angioplasty to relieve the venous obstruction. A hypercoagulable state demands long-term anticoagulant therapy.

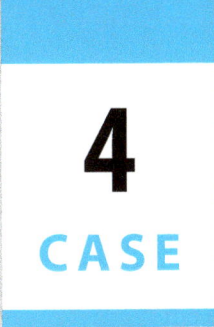

CASE 4

Abdominal Distension with Puffiness of Face

■ HISTORY

A 6-year-old female child presented with a mild puffiness of the face of a few days duration, 8 months ago. The puffiness disappeared with some treatment. This was followed by distension of abdomen. The abdominal distension was generalized and attained a fairly large size over a few days; thereafter it was stationary for the next 8 months.

No history of fever, jaundice or hematemesis.
No history of significant breathlessness or oliguria.
No history of loss of appetite or loss of weight.
She was investigated thoroughly and had received many drugs including anti-TB treatment for the last 6 months without any benefit.

Analysis

The illness started with a mild puffiness of face, which disappeared in a short-time but was followed by a significantly large *generalized* abdominal distension. Though this distension developed over a few days, it remained fairly stationary for the next 8 months in spite of treatment. Abdominal distension could be due to **fluid** in the peritoneal cavity or **massive organomegaly**. Had it been massive organomegaly, it would not have developed within a few days, and further, would not have remained stationary and asymptomatic after such a rapid development. Thus, it is most probably fluid. It can be localized fluid as seen in **large cysts** (ovarian, mesenteric, or pseudopancreatic) or free fluid in the peritoneal cavity (**ascites**). History of puffiness of face reported at the onset of the disease does not corroborate with a localized fluid but supports ascites. As this child has had no other symptoms and has otherwise remained well, ascites is unlikely to be due to **infection or malignancy**. There are no symptoms referable to a **chronic liver, kidney or cardiac disease**. It is unlikely to be nephrotic syndrome because though these children appear otherwise asymptomatic, a large ascites in such cases is associated with generalized edema, which is absent here. Hence, ascites may be due to *mechanical* factors such as **lymphatic or venous obstruction**. Lymphatic obstruction resulting in chylous ascites leads to malnutrition due to loss of fat; since this child has not lost weight, it is more likely to be venous obstruction. Venous obstruction resulting in ascites may be due to obstruction at the level of sinusoids, hepatic vein or inferior vena cava. If the puffiness of face at the onset is to be correlated, it may suggest **superior vena cava obstruction**; in the presence of ascites denoting **inferior vena cava obstruction**, the site of the pathology may be at the **pericardium**. However, as the puffiness of face was quite transient and not associated with any other symptoms at that time, its significance remains unexplained. Thus, the site of venous obstruction cannot be discerned with certainty.

■ PHYSICAL SIGNS

Well nourished child Weight 19 kg Height 108 cm
Looks comfortable Vital parameters normal
No puffiness of face No edema feet No icterus
No lymphadenopathy No pallor No cyanosis
Generalized moderate abdominal distension No engorged veins over the abdomen
Liver 5 cm +, firm, not tender, Liver span 10 cm Spleen not palpable
Free fluid in peritoneal cavity
Neck veins engorged Hepatojugular reflux *absent*
Grade II/VI ejection systolic murmur, best heard at the pulmonary area
P2 loud and widely split, not varying with respiration
Other systems normal.

Analysis

This child has a **large hepatomegaly with ascites**. Though this child has received AKT (albeit without benefit), ascites in tuberculosis is a manifestation of hypersensitivity while hepatosplenomegaly is a result of hematogenous spread of disease. These differing pathogenetic mechanisms indicate different immunological profiles (hypersensitivity being a feature of good immunological status, while hematogenous spread suggesting poor immunity) and are therefore unlikely to coexist in the same patient. Therefore, it is **unlikely** to be **tuberculosis**. Markedly enlarged firm liver with ascites suggests either a liver parenchymal disease such as **cirrhosis** or a congested liver due to **venous obstruction**. Both these conditions closely simulate each other, but an *acute onset of ascites* with hepatomegaly in a *well-nourished* child favors venous obstruction. Absence of portal hypertension as denoted by the absence of splenomegaly, and absence of other signs of liver cell dysfunction rule out cirrhosis. Venous obstruction may be presinusoidal, sinusoidal or postsinusoidal. Presinusoidal obstruction does not present with hepatomegaly or ascites and hence is not considered in this child. Sinusoidal obstruction would usually present with liver dysfunction and is therefore ruled out. Thus, this is mostly a postsinusoidal obstruction. This could be at the level of hepatic veins or the inferior vena cava. Engorged neck veins denote superior vena caval obstruction. In view of a superior vena cava obstruction, this child is more likely to have a inferior vena cava obstruction rather than a hepatic vein obstruction, the common site of venous obstruction being at the level of pericardium. It could be either due to pericardial effusion or constrictive pericarditis. Absence of cardiomegaly on physical examination rules out pericardial effusion and hence it is likely to be **constrictive pericarditis**. Generally constrictive pericarditis is a sequelae of some infection and since there is no such history, this may be **hepatic vein obstruction**. The cardiac findings in this child suggest the possibility of an **ASD**, which is likely to be **unrelated** and an incidental finding.

■ INVESTIGATIONS

CBC normal
LFT normal
Urine normal
Serum albumin 4.5 gm%
Renal function tests normal
Chest X-ray – Heart size normal, prominent pulmonary conus, hyperemic lung fields

Abdominal sonogram – Hepatomegaly and ascites
Color Doppler study – Dilated hepatic vein and inferior vena cava
2D echocardiogram – Demonstrates ASD. No evidence of pericardial pathology

Ascitic fluid – Albumin 2.8 gm% Cells 5 lymphocytes Culture negative
Serum-ascitic albumin gradient (SAAG) 1.7
Transjugular liver biopsy – Venous congestion suggestive of venous obstruction.
CT scan of abdomen – Normal

Analysis

SAAG >1.1 with a normal serum albumin suggests **venous obstruction**. However, imaging studies including color Doppler failed to demonstrate any venous block. As no venous obstruction could be detected, a liver biopsy was carried out which confirmed venous congestion. This reiterated the possibility of a venous obstruction. Hence, a CT scan of the heart was planned in this child, which revealed a thickened pericardium confirming the diagnosis of **constrictive pericarditis**. Generally the site of venous obstruction is detectable on a color Doppler, in which case, liver biopsy is not necessary.

■ FINAL DIAGNOSIS

Constrictive pericarditis with ASD.

■ COMMENTS

It is surprising to note that the association of an ASD with constrictive pericarditis finds a mention in literature. Rarely in ASD, there may be an oozing of RBCs across the wall of the right atrium as a result of a forceful flow of blood from the left to the right atrium. This in turn results in inflammation of the pericardium and leads to constrictive pericarditis.

■ KEY MESSAGES

- Acute onset of ascites with hepatomegaly in a well-nourished child is likely to be due to a mechanical cause such as venous obstruction, without hepatocyte dysfunction.
- High protein in ascitic fluid without a cellular response suggests venous obstruction. SAAG is a good test to analyze the cause of ascites.
- The possibility of a prothrombotic state should be assessed in a case of venous obstruction, if no apparent cause is detected.

■ GENERAL COMMENTS BASED ON THE FIRST-FOUR CASES

Abdominal distension is a common presenting complaint of *diseases related to the liver*. It may due to *hepatomegaly* or *ascites*. Typically, gradually increasing distension over months suggests hepatomegaly, while distension developing over a few days and then remaining static denotes ascites.

Splenomegaly indicates portal hypertension, especially in chronic liver diseases. Hepatomegaly, splenomegaly and ascites may be present in varying combinations. All the three signs together represent cirrhosis (liver dysfunction with portal hypertension).

Hepatomegaly and splenomegaly without ascites suggest a storage disorder or infection related reticuloendothelial hyperplasia. (no liver dysfunction, no portal hypertension)

Hepatomegaly and ascites without splenomegaly denote sinusoidal (with liver dysfunction), or postsinusoidal venous obstruction (without liver dysfunction).

Splenomegaly alone indicates extrahepatic portal hypertension.

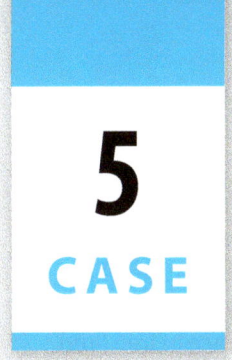

CASE 5

Puffiness of Face with Edema Feet

■ HISTORY

A 9-year-old female child presented with early morning puffiness of face since the last 15 days. She was apparently well 2 weeks ago when she suddenly developed puffiness of face one morning and since then, it had been waxing and waning through the day. A week later, the parents noticed edema of the feet and reduced urine output. However, since she remained comfortable in spite of the edema, she did not seek any treatment for 2 weeks.

No history of hematuria, fever and headache.
No history of any other relevant symptoms.

Analysis

The history suggests edema of an acute onset with oliguria. Such symptoms may result from cardiac, liver or kidney diseases. The chief presenting symptoms of **acute or chronic cardiac failure** are exertional dyspnea or palpitations and edema may be merely an accompanying feature and hence cardiac disease is unlikely in this child. **Acute liver disease** presents with jaundice, generally without edema. **Chronic liver disease** presents with abdominal distension and constitutional symptoms; edema is often mild and not complained of by the patients. Thus, this does not look like a liver disease either. **Nutritional edema** is rare at this age and when present, is secondary to a chronic progressive illness. Oliguria is not a feature of malnutrition, though it may result from a poor intake. Thus, edema in this otherwise well child is likely to be **renal** in origin.

Renal edema signifies a **glomerular** disease. It may be primarily due to reduced glomerular filtration (**nephritis**) or due to proteinuria and hypoproteinemia (**nephrotic syndrome**). Oliguria may be present in both conditions; in nephritis, due to reduced filtration and in nephrotic syndrome, due to a low intravascular volume. The extent of edema does not always help to differentiate between these two diseases, though generalized anasarca is more often seen in nephrotic syndrome. Absence of hematuria may not rule out nephritis, as the hematuria may be microscopic. However, if it is nephritis, it is unlikely to be due to poststreptococcal glomerulonephritis as its symptoms often disappear within 2 weeks. Thus, this child may be suffering from other forms of nephritis or a nephrotic syndrome. The clinical features of both these conditions may overlap; physical examination and investigations might offer further clues to the proper diagnosis. **Tubular** proteinuria is a laboratory finding and does not present with edema.

■ PHYSICAL EXAMINATION

Fairly built and nourished	Weight 30 kg	Height 125 cm
Puffiness of face	Marked edema of feet	Edema of abdominal wall
Pulse 92/min	RR 22/min	BP 122/82 mm of Hg
Temp. normal	JVP not raised	No pyoderma marks
Liver not palpable	Spleen not palpable	Evidence of free fluid +
Other systems normal		

Analysis

Physical examination reveals generalized edema with ascites in a well-grown child who is otherwise comfortable and favors the diagnosis of nephrotic syndrome. It could be **minimal change nephrotic syndrome**, since it is the commonest. However, the onset of the disease (first presentation) at 9 years of age and the blood pressure being on the 95th centile, should caution us about the possibility of it not being a minimal lesion but **other nephropathies**.

■ INVESTIGATIONS

Hb 10.5 gm%	CBC normal	
Urinalysis – proteins +++	RBCs 25–30/hpf	WBCs 6–8/hpf
24 hours urine protein 2.1 gm/dL		
Serum albumin 1.8 gm%	Serum globulin 3.1 gm%	Alpha 2 globulin 1.1 gm%
Serum cholesterol 452 mgm%	BUN 40 mgm%	Serum creatinine 1 mgm%
Tuberculin test negative	HbsAg negative	

Analysis

The proteinuria is definitely in the nephrotic range (>40 mg/m^2/hr). While the other tests are consistent with the diagnosis of nephrotic syndrome, microscopic hematuria coupled with the earlier observations (on age of presentation and blood pressure being on the higher side), raises a suspicion of other nephropathies. A borderline increased blood urea with a normal serum creatinine may reflect a contracted intravascular volume.

■ CASE PROGRESSION

Even though there were some features against it, the possibility of a steroid responsive nephrotic syndrome was considered, and this child was put on 2 mgm/kg/day of Prednisolone. She responded within a week and continued therapy as per the standard protocol for another 3 months.

Subsequently she went to her native place. She suffered 5 relapses during the next 18 months. The second and third relapses occurred immediately on stopping steroids. So the local doctor asked her to continue 15 mg of Prednisolone on alternate days in the morning after achieving remission with the full dose. She was controlled for a few days, but soon relapsed again. She was advised 20 mg Prednisolone on alternate morning. Thereafter, within a few days she developed abdominal pain and distension for which she was referred.

■ PHYSICAL EXAMINATION

Weight 42 kg Height 129 cm (gained 12 kg weight and 4 cm height in 18 months)
Temp. normal Pulse 115/min RR 25/min BP 140/90 mm of Hg
Generalized edema Cushingoid facies
Striae over abdomen and thigh
Ophthalmic examination—bilateral posterior capsular cataract
Abdomen—generalized tenderness, no guarding, free fluid + or rigidity
Resp. system—bilateral pleural effusion Other systems normal

Analysis

This child is not only a frequent relapser but also steroid dependent. There are obvious signs of steroid toxicity. Hypertension could be a part of the side effects of steroids, but could also be due to the disease itself. As long as the child is steroid responsive, one always tries to achieve remission first and then, in steroid dependent disease, the least possible alternate morning dose that can maintain remission is continued. However, if the dose required is high (>0.5 mgm/kg/alternate day), we can anticipate not only a deteriorating response over time, but also chances of developing steroid toxicity. Hence, alternative therapy should have been considered in this child *before* she developed steroid toxicity. This child has now relapsed once again as evident by the generalized edema. In addition, as this child has also presented with abdominal pain and distension, spontaneous bacterial peritonitis must be considered even in the absence of fever and abdominal guarding or rigidity. In fact, control of infection may induce a remission. Renal biopsy is indicated in this child before considering alternate therapy. Renal biopsy was performed which revealed focal glomerulosclerosis.

■ FINAL DIAGNOSIS

Focal glomerulosclerosis.

■ KEY MESSAGES

- If the age of onset of nephrotic syndrome is <1 year or >8 years, it may suggest a lesion other than minimal change, though it must be initially assumed to be steroid responsive and treated accordingly.
- Accompanying symptoms and signs like hematuria and hypertension may suggest other nephropathies.
- Steroid resistant nephrotic syndrome is an indication of renal biopsy before starting other immunosuppressive drugs.

■ RELEVANT INFORMATION

Definitions used in Nephrotic Syndrome

Remission – Urine albumin nil or trace (proteinuria <4 mg/m^2/hr) for 3 consecutive days
Relapse – Urine albumin +++ (proteinuria >40 mg/m^2/hr) for 3 consecutive days

Frequent relapser – 2 or more relapses within 6 months of an initial response or 3 relapses in a year anytime.

Steroid dependent – 2 consecutive relapses when on alternate day steroids, or a relapse within 2 weeks of its discontinuation.

Steroid resistant – Absence of remission despite standard therapy for 6 weeks.

Management of Steroid Responsive Nephrotic Syndrome

First episode – 2 mg of Prednisolone/kg body weight (60 mg/m^2) for 6 weeks followed by 1.5 mg/kg on alternate days for 6 weeks.

(It is ideal to rule out any occult infection such as tuberculosis/hepatitis B by relevant tests before starting steroid therapy).

If resistant – kidney biopsy and further therapy based on histopathology

(It is ideal to refer to a pediatric nephrologist)

In case of relapse – (infection may be the cause of transient relapse and if suspected, should be treated first to expect remission without steroids)

In case of absence of probable infection, start 2 mg/kg of Prednisolone until remission and then 1.5 mg/kg alternate day for 4 weeks

In case of a frequent relapser/steroid dependent – after achieving remission, the lowest dose that can maintain remission (<0.5 mg/kg), on alternate days for 9–18 months.

If not maintained on alternate optimum dose (<0.5 mg/kg), Levamisole or Cyclophosphamide (better refer to a specialist).

CASE 6

Abdominal Distension with Developmental Delay

▐ HISTORY

A 14-month-old male child born of a 3rd degree consanguineous marriage presented with a gradual distension of abdomen noticed since 2 months of age and delayed development. Abdominal distension was noticed to be more in the upper quadrant and had gradually increased to the present size. The child has been feeding well.

- No history of vomiting, jaundice or failure to thrive
- No history of change in bowel pattern or urinary symptoms
- Birth history – full-term normal home delivery, average birth weight
- Developmental history
  - Head holding – 6 months   Turning over – 9 months   Sitting without support –1 year
  - Not standing as yet   Reaching for objects – 1 year   Cooing – 1 year
  - Recognizes parents – 9 months but not strangers
- No history of convulsions or regression of milestones.

Analysis

While **hypotonia** of the abdominal wall may present as abdominal distension, it is often intermittent and not progressive. Abdominal distension due to ascites develops over a few days to remain static thereafter. Further, ascites and delayed development is an unlikely combination. Therefore chronic, gradually *progressive* upper abdominal distension in this case is suggestive of **enlarging liver with or without splenomegaly**. Splenomegaly alone does not present as abdominal distension unless it is very large; even in which case, it presents as a lump in abdomen. There is no evidence of liver dysfunction or biliary tract involvement. Hence, the enlarged liver may either be due to a **storage disorder or reticuloendothelial hyperplasia**.

Splenomegaly, if present, may be due to portal hypertension or share the same pathology as the liver disease.

Developmental delay favors a diagnosis of storage common to both liver and brain.

The other possibility is one of **congenital infection**, which may also present with hepatosplenomegaly and delayed development. However, usually there is a history of intrauterine growth retardation in such cases and the abdominal distension is not progressive. Abdominal distension and delayed development could well be seen in **hypothyroidism**. However, there is no history of constipation, lethargy and/or poor feeding, and the abdominal distension in such cases is not a *presenting complaint* but a finding noted on examination. Thus, this is most likely to be a storage disorder.

■ PHYSICAL EXAMINATION

Poorly built and nourished	Not sick looking	Coarse facies
Weight 6.1 kg	Length 65 cm	US/LS 1.6 to 1
Head ☉ 44 cm	Chest ☉ 40 cm	
Mild pallor +	No icterus	No edema feet
Anterior fontanelle open 1" not bulging, sutures normal		Eyes normal

Abdomen distended more in the upper part
Liver 7 cm, firm, rounded margin, not tender, liver span 10 cm

Spleen 2 cm, firm	No ascites	No engorged abdominal veins
CNS – Generalized hypotonia	Brisk DTR	No localizing signs Fundus N
Developmental examination – Global delay, DQ around 50%		Other systems normal

Analysis

This child has hepatosplenomegaly with global developmental delay and has not grown well. **Congenital infection** may present in this manner. However, one usually expects intrauterine growth retardation (low birth weight) with additional features suggestive of specific infections such as microcephaly (CMV)/hydrocephalus (toxoplasma), purpuric rash, eye involvement, deafness, etc. though their absence does not rule out congenital infections. Appropriate investigations would be necessary to diagnose congenital infections. Though this child is short and is developmentally delayed, **hypothyroidism** is almost ruled out because such significant hepatosplenomegaly cannot be explained, besides the fact that many other typical features are absent. Therefore, in view of the organomegaly being prominent in addition to developmental delay, a storage disorder is more likely. Coarse facies may favor a diagnosis of **mucopolysaccharidoses**.

■ INVESTIGATIONS

Hemogram normal   Liver function tests normal
Urinary mucopolysaccharides elevated
Radiological evidence of MPS

■ FINAL DIAGNOSIS

MPS

■ KEY MESSAGES

- Hepatosplenomegaly without organ dysfunction favors a storage disorder or reticuloendothelial hyperplasia.
- Multisystem involvement and characteristic features differentiate various storage disorders clinically.

■ RELEVANT INFORMATION

Mucopolysaccharidoses and storage disorders are both usually characterized by hepatosplenomegaly. Hence, further differentiation amongst these disorders clinically, is guided by the presence/absence of a few associated findings.

HSmegaly with *mental retardation*
MPS – I   - Hurler
    – II   - Hunter
    – III - Sanfilippo
Sandhoff
GM_1 gangliosidosis
Niemann-Pick type A Fabry's disease
Gaucher type 2

HSmegaly *without mental retardation*
Gaucher type 1
Glycogen storage disorders
MPS – I   - Scheie
    – IV   - Morquio
    – VI   - Maroteaux-Lamy

HSmegaly *with cardiac involvement*
MPS – I   - Hurler
    – II   - Hunter
    – VI   - Maroteaux-Lamy

Glycogen storage disease II (Pompe) (only hepatomegaly)
Sandhoff's disease
Sialidosis

HSmegaly *with coarse facies*
MPS – I   - Hurler
    – II   - Hunter
    – VI   - Maroteaux-Lamy

GM_1 gangliosidosis
Mucolipidosis
Mannosidosis

Corneal clouding
All MPS except MPS III Sanfilippo
GM_1 gangliosidosis
Niemann-Pick (sometimes)
Fabry's disease
Mannosidosis

Cherry red spot
Tay-Sachs
Niemann-Pick
Sandhoff's disease
GM_1 gangliosidosis
Mucolipidosis
Sialidosis

Glycogen Storage Diseases
- Most are characterized by hepatomegaly and hypoglycemia except
- GSD IV – presents as hepatosplenomegaly, progressive cirrhosis, and death by 5 years
- GSD V and GSD VII – present as skeletal muscle involvement only
    GSD per se are not characterized by mental retardation, unless there have been frequent episodes of hypoglycemia and brain damage

Mucopolysaccharidosis
In addition to features mentioned above they are also characterized by skeletal abnormalities.

MPS III Sanfilippo
- Disproportionately severe neurologic involvement and very mild somatic involvement
- Present as hyperactivity

MPS IV and IX
- Present as short stature

MPS V and VIII – no longer used, MPS –VII rarest

Disorders with specific treatment available

Gaucher type 1

Fabry's disease

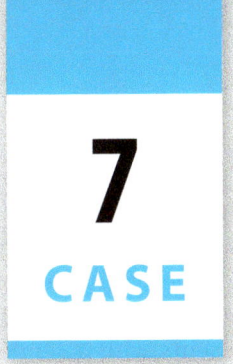

CASE 7

Acute Severe Jaundice

■ HISTORY

An 8-year-old child presented with an acute onset of jaundice, worsening over the next 6 days, followed by drowsiness and melena a day prior to hospitalization. He had mild fever during the present illness for which he had received paracetamol. The urine was dark yellow though the stools were not clay colored. He had been a healthy child without any significant past illnesses.

No relevant family history.

He was born of a 2nd degree consanguineous marriage.

Analysis

An acute onset of jaundice, which is rapidly progressive, denotes **primary liver disease**. When it is quickly followed by drowsiness and an intestinal bleed, it suggests **fulminant hepatocellular failure**. One of the common causes of acute hepatitis in this age group is **viral A hepatitis**. However, by itself it is rarely so fulminant. Occasionally, it may lead to hepatic failure either when it coexists with another liver disease or has been superimposed on a pre-existing liver disease. As this child has been reported to be healthy till the onset of the present illness, a **pre-existing chronic liver disease** is less likely. So it is likely that a **coexisting liver disease** such as viral E or typhoid infection may have been acquired together with the viral A infection, through the same source of contaminated water or food. **Leptospirosis** may be another cause of acute hepatitis. However, this child never had significant fever, so **typhoid** and **leptospirosis** are unlikely. Occasionally, drugs can complicate viral A hepatitis, but there is no history of consumption of any **hepatotoxic drugs** (valproate, rifampicin or pyrizinamide). At this point, one notes that a possibility of **Wilson's disease** cannot be ruled out, as it is known to present with a wide spectrum of clinical manifestations, including acute fulminant hepatic failure as the first presenting feature. A history of consanguinity may strengthen such a possibility.

■ PHYSICAL EXAMINATION

Fairly built and nourished child Weight 24 kg Height 118 cm
Temp normal   Pulse 110/min   RR 30/min   BP 90/55 mm of Hg
Drowsy   No significant pallor   Ecchymotic patches over the skin
Moderate icterus present   No KF ring over the cornea
Liver 6 cm. +, firm, not tender   Liver span 11 cm   Spleen not palpable
No ascites   No engorged abdominal veins
CNS - plantars extensor bilaterally   No localizing signs

Analysis

Hepatomegaly with moderate jaundice and mild splenomegaly suggests **hepatitis**. In view of ecchymotic patches over the skin, drowsiness and extensor plantars, this child has a **fulminant hepatic failure**. The exact cause for the fulminant hepatic failure cannot be ascertained on physical examination. As mentioned above, viral A hepatitis by itself rarely leads to hepatic failure. Viral A hepatitis being an acute inflammatory disease, presents with a tender hepatomegaly and the liver in this child is not tender. Thus, it is unlikely to be viral A hepatitis. Absence of significant fever rules out malaria or typhoid fever as coexisting infections. Further, such infections per se are unlikely to result in fulminant hepatic failure. One needs to quickly investigate for the etiology to consider specific management, especially of a treatable cause such as Wilson's disease.

■ INVESTIGATIONS

Hb 9 gm%
Serum bilirubin 24 mgm% direct 20 mgm%
Serum proteins 6.5 gm% albumin 3.5 gm%
Prothrombin time 35 sec control 12 sec
Serum ammonia elevated
Serum ceruloplasmin low

WBC - normal Platelets adequate
 ALT mildly raised

APTT normal D-dimer normal
Blood sugar normal
Increased excretion of copper in urine

Analysis

This child has evidence of **hepatic failure** as suggested by the increased prothrombin time and an elevated serum ammonia. Mildly raised ALT denotes minimal destruction of liver cells and is against a diagnosis of viral A hepatitis, which presents with a marked rise in ALT. Low serum ceruloplasmin and increased excretion of copper in the urine confirms a diagnosis of **Wilson's disease**. This child has presented as an acute hepatitis and does not have a chronic liver disease, in view of the normal serum albumin.

■ FINAL DIAGNOSIS

Wilson's disease.

■ KEY MESSAGES

- Wilson's disease must be considered in every undiagnosed liver pathology especially >5 years of age.
- Laboratory tests for Wilson's disease need to be evaluated with caution, especially in the setting of fulminant hepatic failure.
- Kayser-Fleischer ring may be absent in children with Wilson's disease; but are always present if there are neurological manifestations of the disease.

RELEVANT INFORMATION

Wilson's Disease

Fetal and neonatal liver normally contains relatively high concentrations of copper and sulfur-rich copper-binding protein (metallothionein). Serum ceruloplasmin and copper levels are relatively low. The mechanisms responsible for copper homeostasis in children reach maturity by 2 years of age. The Wilsonian trait may be expressed only after this time. Therefore, though the disease has been detected in children as young as 3 years, Wilson's disease rarely manifests clinically before 5 years of age.

In Wilson's disease, the distinctive corneal sign is the Kayser-Fleischer ring, a golden brown ring in the peripheral cornea resulting from changes in the Descemet's membrane. Pigmented corneal rings may develop in neonates with cholestatic liver disease. Skin pigmentation and bluish discoloration at the base of fingernails (azure lunulae) have been described in patients with Wilson's disease. Hemolytic anemia and renal involvement are also known.

Most patients with Wilson's disease have decreased ceruloplasmin levels. Serum copper level may be elevated in early Wilson's disease, and urinary copper excretion (usually <40 µg/day) is increased to greater than 100 µg/day and often up to 1,000 µg/day or more. In equivocal cases, the urinary copper output in response to chelation may be of diagnostic help; after an oral dose of d-penicillamine, affected patients excrete 1,200–2,000 µg/day.

Liver biopsy is of value for evaluation of histopathological changes and for measurement of the hepatic copper content (normally <10 µg/gm dry weight). In Wilson's disease, hepatic copper content exceeds 250 µg/g dry weight. In healthy heterozygotes, levels may be intermediate.

Dietary copper intake should be restricted. Examples of copper-containing foods include animal liver or kidneys, shellfish, chocolate, peas, unprocessed wheat, and dried beans.

Prenatal diagnosis based on DNA linkage analysis is currently available.

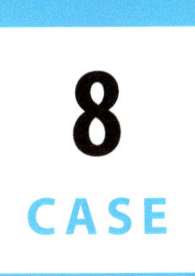

CASE 8

Severe Jaundice with High Fever

■ HISTORY

A 12-year-old child presented with high fever for 5 days followed by a sudden development of severe jaundice and drowsiness. She was well 5 days ago when she started with high fever for which the local doctor treated her. The details of the treatment were not available. Within 2 days of development of jaundice and drowsiness, she was hospitalized for the same. The parents were sure that there was no jaundice during the first 5 days of fever, nor was there any significant anorexia, nausea or vomiting. There was no history of high colored urine or clay colored stools. On direct questioning, there was oliguria, though the parents attributed it to a poor intake over the last 2 days due to drowsiness.

No significant past or family history.

Analysis

Though a common cause of an acute onset of jaundice in the pediatric age group is **viral A hepatitis**, it usually starts with prodromal symptoms of anorexia, nausea and vomiting, followed by the appearance of jaundice which slowly deepens over the next few days. Drowsiness is rare in an uncomplicated viral A hepatitis. Thus, this child is less likely to be suffering from viral A hepatitis. Jaundice in this child has appeared after 5 days of high fever. Hence, it is likely that the primary illness that caused high fever lead to secondary hepatic involvement coming on after a few days of illness, or this is a complication of drugs taken for the primary illness. Febrile illnesses with subsequent liver involvement include **typhoid fever, malaria** and **leptospirosis**. Jaundice in typhoid fever is due to typhoid hepatitis. However, development of sudden and severe jaundice is quite an unusual feature of mere inflammation of the liver cells arising out of such an infection; usually the jaundice develops over a few days and is rarely deep. In clinical analysis, jaundice that develops suddenly is caused either by vascular or allergic (immune) mechanisms or hemolysis. The pathogenesis of jaundice in malaria is complex and can occur through various mechanisms. Most of it is due to hepatitis, but it may also be added upon by hemolysis. At times, it may also be due to acute ischemia of the liver cells due to sludging of parasitized RBCs (vascular mechanism) as seen in complicated **falciparum malaria**. Similarly, severe jaundice can be seen in leptospirosis in the immune phase of the illness. However in this child, a history of a biphasic fever or a severe myalgia in the earlier phase of the illness is lacking. Sudden hemolysis in G6PD deficient individuals following treatment with offending drugs may also lead to sudden jaundice. However, it is rare in females. Oliguria may be due to a poor intake but may also depict renal failure, which is common to both malaria and leptospirosis. Presence of renal failure by itself can also contribute to a sudden rise of bilirubin. The drowsiness may suggest a metabolic complication (hypoglycemia) arising out of hepatic failure, cerebral malaria or a poor intake.

■ PHYSICAL EXAMINATION

Well built and nourished child Weight 37 kg Height 150 cm
Temp 102°F   Pulse 160/min   RR 35/min   BP 90/55 mm of Hg
Markedly pale   Deep icterus   No ecchymosis or purpura
Mild edema feet   JVP raised
Liver 7 cm +, firm, tender, hepatojugular reflux present   Liver span 10 cm
Spleen 4 cm +, firm   No ascites   No engorged abdominal veins
CVS – soft systolic functional murmur
CNS – drowsy   No localizing signs

Analysis

Though a deeply jaundiced child with hepatic failure can bleed and therefore present with significant pallor, such bleeding is obvious and has not been reported in this child. Therefore, sudden development of severe pallor (sudden because this child was absolutely alright before the illness), severe enough to push the child into cardiac failure along with jaundice, suggests **acute hemolysis**. However, even in acute hemolysis jaundice is rarely severe; the severity of the jaundice suggests an additional element of **primary hepatocellular involvement**. Such a combination of acute hemolysis with liver involvement in an infective (febrile) setting suggests malaria. The severity of the illness favors a possibility of **falciparum malaria**. The etiology of the drowsiness and oliguria has to be ascertained by relevant investigations. Microvascular sludging may have lead to an element of renal failure also.

■ INVESTIGATIONS

Hb 4 gm%   WBC 10,000/c. mm   P 60 L 32 E 5 M 3   Platelets 75,000/c. mm
Peripheral smear shows trophozoites of *P. falciparum*   Parasitic index 5%
Serum bilirubin 38 mgm% Direct 28 mgm%   ALT – 180 u/dL
Serum ammonia normal Blood sugar normal   Prothrombin time normal
Serum proteins normal   Serum creatinine 3.5 mgm%   Blood urea 120 mgm%
Serum electrolytes normal

Analysis

This child has a multisystem involvement affecting the liver primarily, but also the brain and the kidney besides causing severe hemolysis. Drowsiness is not due to hepatic encephalopathy in view of the normal serum ammonia, blood glucose and the prothrombin time, but may have resulted from cerebrovascular sludging due to malaria. Renal failure could also be a result of a similar pathology in the renal vasculature. Even though there is hemolysis, the predominant bilirubin in **falciparum malaria** is direct bilirubin due to the involvement of the liver cells.

■ FOLLOW-UP

The patient was treated with IV quinine and supportive therapy including packed cell transfusion. The serum bilirubin came down to 12 mgm% within the next 2 days, drowsiness improved and so also the urine output. The child made a complete recovery within the next 5 days.

Analysis

A quick reduction of the bilirubin from 38 to 12 mgm% is strikingly unusual in hepatitis. It may have occurred in this child due to successful reversal of hepatic vasculopathy and renal failure after anti-malarial therapy.

■ FINAL DIAGNOSIS

Falciparum malaria.

■ KEY MESSAGES

- *Sudden* development of *severe* jaundice is due to ischemia resulting from intravascular sludging by malarial parasites (hepatic vasculopathy) and coexisting renal failure. Acute hemolysis usually leads to a *milder* jaundice.
- Hepatitis may be caused by many infections other than classical viral hepatitis.

■ RELEVANT INFORMATION

Malaria

For clinical purposes, malaria is divided into uncomplicated and complicated (severe) disease. Complicated malaria (mostly due to *P. falciparum*) refers to involvement of organs such as the brain or the liver. Renal failure and respiratory distress syndrome is rare in children as compared to adults.

Usually complications set in after a couple of days of fever, and hence it is important to suspect malaria in the first few days of fever.

Uncomplicated malaria has varied manifestations in different age groups. In neonates and young infants, anemia with hepatosplenomegaly may be the only presentation, often without fever. In toddlers, the disease can manifest with upper respiratory symptoms or diarrhea/vomiting, simulating a viral respiratory or gastrointestinal infection respectively. However, in such cases the respiratory or gastrointestinal symptoms disappear within a couple of days, but the fever persists. As against this, in typical viral infections, the fever is the first to disappear, while the other symptoms persist for a longer period. Convulsions may also be a presenting feature of malaria in this age group. It simulates a simple febrile convulsion. It is different from cerebral malaria. It is only in children >5 years of age that malaria may present with the typical periodic fever with rigors. **Consistent features of malaria at any age are anemia with hepatosplenomegaly and irregular fever**. The child looks quite normal in between episodes of fever. In *P. vivax*, spleen is much more enlarged than the liver, whereas in *P. falciparum* infection, liver is often more enlarged than the spleen.

Demonstration of the malarial parasite in a blood film is the cornerstone of diagnosis. The parasitic index is a denominator of the severity of infection and must be reported in every positive case. However for many technical and scientific reasons, the blood film may be falsely negative. In such cases, one must look for indirect evidences on the peripheral smear examination, such as pigments in white blood cells, neutrophilia with bandemia in a normal to low total white cell count, monocytosis, eosinophilia and thrombocytopenia. Other methods include the Para-sight F test. It is a dipstick method, detecting circulating histidine rich protein-2 by capture assay. It is highly specific for *P. falciparum* and its sensitivity depends upon the parasitic index. It fails to detect *P. vivax*.

Acridine orange QBC method (quantitative buffy coat) involves fluorescent staining of centrifuged capillary blood. Species differentiation is, however, not possible with this test.

The choice of antimalarial drugs depends on the local epidemiology and drug sensitivity pattern. In general, uncomplicated malaria should be treated with chloroquine and complicated malaria with quinine. Quinine is an excellent drug and is very effective, but needs a longer course of therapy. Sulphadoxine-Pyrimethamine combination is not a drug of choice as it is slow acting, which has resulted in resistant malarial strains. Besides it is known to lead to serious side effects such as Stevens-Johnson syndrome. Mefloquine is also a slow acting drug and therefore not ideal for the treatment of an acute attack. It may be good for prophylaxis. Artesunate and Artemether are good drugs, but the final outcome with these drugs is similar to Quinine.

9 CASE

Fluctuating Jaundice

■ HISTORY

A 10-year-old child presented with a low-grade fever for 2 weeks. As there were no other symptoms and she did not look sick, initially she did not seek medical attention. Later as the fever persisted, she was examined by a doctor at the end of 2 weeks of the illness, who noted jaundice. She had a mild elevation of AST/ALT with a mild hyperbilirubinemia and was diagnosed as hepatitis. Viral markers were negative. Thereafter, she improved marginally but was never normal. The jaundice fluctuated over the next 3 months and then worsened recently, for which she was referred.

The parents recalled a history of anorexia and loss of weight for a month – 4 months ago. She was investigated at that time with a routine urinalysis, CBC, chest X-ray and the results of these tests were found to be within normal limits.

No family history of jaundice
No history of consanguinity.

Analysis

This child presented with a low-grade fever for 2 weeks with mild jaundice and mild elevation of liver enzymes. This suggests a mild hepatitis of a *subacute* onset. It may be due to a primary hepatotropic viral infection (commonly **viral A hepatitis**), or a part of disseminated infections such as **CMV** or **leptospirosis**. Further progress in the form of fluctuating jaundice over the next few months, definitely rules out common infections including viral A hepatitis. Fluctuating jaundice may be a feature of **hemolytic anemia** or **chronic liver disease**. Presence of fever and raised enzymes rules out hemolytic anemia. The past history of undiagnosed anorexia and loss of weight for a month may suggest an occult liver disease existing for several months. Thus, this child is most likely to be suffering from a chronic liver disease. Chronic liver disease may be chronic hepatitis (**HBV**), metabolic disease (**Wilson's disease**) or an immune mediated inflammatory disease (**autoimmune hepatitis**).

■ PHYSICAL SIGNS

Average build, poorly nourished Weight 21 kg Height 130 cm
Sick looking Icterus ++ No Kayser-Fleischer ring
Moderate pallor No edema feet or puffiness of face
Moderate abdominal distension, no engorged veins over the abdominal wall

Liver 7 cm +, firm, sharp edge, smooth surface, not tender   Liver span 11 cm
Spleen 4 cm + firm   No ascites   No other signs of liver cell failure
Other systems normal

Analysis

Significant firm non-tender hepatomegaly with moderate icterus in a sick looking poorly nourished child confirms **chronic liver disease**. It may be either **chronic hepatitis** or **cirrhosis**. Both these conditions may be clinically indistinguishable and chronic hepatitis may lead to cirrhosis. Splenomegaly in this child may denote portal hypertension (favoring cirrhosis) or reticuloendothelial hyperplasia (suggestive of hepatitis). However, presence of moderate jaundice without ascites and other signs of liver cell failure are against cirrhosis. Jaundice is a late feature of cirrhosis and suggests decompensation and hence is almost always accompanied with ascites. Hence, this is likely to be a slowly progressive chronic hepatitis with a fluctuating course. The etiology of such a disease cannot be clinically guessed. It is unlikely to be a viral infection as viral markers are reported to be negative. It may represent **autoimmune hepatitis** or **Wilson's disease**. Absence of Kayser-Fleischer ring does not rule out Wilson's disease.

■ INVESTIGATIONS

Hb 8 gm%   Macrocytic normochromic anemia
WBC and platelets normal   ESR 80 mm
Urine – bile salts and pigments + ve   Serum bilirubin 22 mgm%   Direct 20.5 mgm%
ALT/AST mildly raised   Alk Phos mildly raised
S. Protein 7 gm%   Albumin 2.5 gm%   Globulin 4.5 gm   Gamma-globulin 3.1 gm%
Prothrombin time normal   Serum ammonia normal   Serum creatinine normal
Serum ceruloplasmin normal   HbsAg –ve   HCV – ve   Slit lamp - Kayser-Fleischer
                                                                         ring negative
ANA 1:40 +ve   SMA +ve   LKM antibody –ve

Analysis

Moderately elevated direct bilirubinemia with minimally raised enzymes and hypoalbuminemia suggests a chronic hepatitis. Increased gamma-globulins and a positive ANA and SMA favor **type 1 autoimmune hepatitis**. The mild elevation of alkaline phosphatase is unusual, though it may be explained by a **coexisting sclerosing cholangitis** or it may originate from other tissues and may not be related to liver disease.

■ FINAL DIAGNOSIS

Liver biopsy confirmed Type 1 autoimmune hepatitis.

■ KEY MESSAGES

- Chronic hepatitis with high gamma-globulin favors autoimmune hepatitis.
- Every undiagnosed liver disease must be investigated for Wilson's disease, especially beyond 5 years of age.

■ RELEVANT INFORMATION

Autoimmune Hepatitis

Autoimmune hepatitis is a progressive inflammatory disease of the liver that occurs more commonly in girls and young women. The exact etiology is not known but it is postulated that some environmental factors may incite an autoimmune response towards the liver. Such trigger factors may be viruses, chemicals or unknown agents. The resultant chronic hepatitis eventually leads to fibrosis and cirrhosis. It is also known to progress into hepatocellular carcinoma, but not as frequently as liver disease resulting from hepatitis B viral infection.

The clinical features and the course of autoimmune hepatitis are extremely variable. It may present with a widespectrum of symptoms and signs, that include a substantial number of asymptomatic patients and some who have an acute, even fulminant onset. In 25–30% of patients, particularly children, the illness may mimic acute viral hepatitis.

Autoimmune hepatitis is a clinical diagnosis based upon certain diagnostic criteria; no single test confirms the diagnosis. Diagnostic criteria with scoring systems have been developed for adults and modified slightly for children. Important positive features include the female gender, primary elevation in transaminases and not alkaline phosphatase, elevated gamma-globulin levels, the presence of autoantibodies (most commonly antinuclear, smooth muscle, or liver kidney microsome), and characteristic histologic findings. Important negative features include the absence of viral markers (hepatitis B, C, D infection) and absence of a history of exposure to drugs or blood products.

Most patients have hypergammaglobulinemia. A characteristic pattern of antibodies defines specific subgroups. Antineutrophil cytoplasmic antibodies may be seen more commonly in autoimmune cholangiopathy. Autoantibodies are rare in healthy children so that titers as low as 1:40 should be considered significant. Up to 20% of patients with apparent autoimmune hepatitis may not have autoantibodies at presentation.

Other autoimmune diseases that these patients may suffer from include idiopathic thrombocytopenic purpura, glomerulonephritis, pulmonary fibrosis, ulcerative colitis, insulin dependent diabetes mellitus, vitiligo and Graves' disease.

The initial response to therapy is generally prompt, with a greater than 75% rate of remission. However, of those who respond, 50% patients suffer a relapse, which is treated with similar medicines and few of them may need long-term steroids for maintenance. A few of them may develop cirrhosis.

CASE 10

Jaundice with Pleural Effusion

■ HISTORY

A 6-year-old boy presented with nausea, vomiting, and loss of appetite along with mild fever, over 2–3 days. This was followed by jaundice. He was diagnosed to have viral hepatitis A that was proved by a positive HAV IgM. He was given symptomatic treatment and he started feeling better over the next 3–4 days; his appetite started returning to normal.

Two days later, he was brought to the hospital because he had developed breathlessness over the last few hours.

Prior to this illness, he was an absolutely normal healthy child.
No h/o palpitations, cough, or fever.
No h/o similar disease in the past.
No h/o frequent cough in the past.
No h/o atopy in the family.

Analysis

The description of the initial illness is quite consistent with a **hepatotropic viral infection** like hepatitis A, so let's first analyze the second part of the illness, and then correlate the two.

In general, acute onset breathlessness may result from respiratory, cardiac or metabolic disease. Since this child was absolutely alright prior to this illness, any chronic illness is ruled out. In the absence of palpitations and cough, acute **cardiac** disease is **unlikely**. A metabolic disorder that can present with "breathlessness" at this age is diabetic ketoacidosis, though usually the presenting complaints are different and such children actually have tachypnea that is noticed by the physician. Further, there is no history of polyuria, polidypsia or polyphagia, the breathlessness developed rapidly over a few hours, and even though he was vomiting earlier in the illness, he had started feeling better before the development of breathlessness. Hence, **diabetes** can be **ruled out**. It means this breathlessness must be due to respiratory disease. Absence of cough goes against an airway disease; in addition, this child does not have any past history of repeated cough to suggest hyper-reactive airway disease or asthma. Absence of fever rules out lung parenchymal involvement as the cause of breathlessness. So, it is likely to be a **pleural disease** – either an **effusion** or a **pneumothorax**. A spontaneous pneumothorax can occur as a result of a rupture of a subpleural bulla in a previously asymptomatic child. However, it usually manifests as breathlessness only if it is rapidly progressive (tension pneumothorax) in which case the history is likely to be further hyperacute. Of course, this may amount to splitting of hair as to over how much time the breathlessness developed. Similarly, a pleural effusion can develop over a few hours and cause breathlessness. When an effusion develops over few hours, it suggests an allergic disorder rather than an infection. Thus, this could be an **immune mediated pleural disease** with an effusion.

Now we need to **correlate** the initial **hepatitis with** the subsequent **breathlessness**. This breathlessness could theoretically be the result of dissemination of the original viral infection causing hepatitis. However, this child had already started recovering from his hepatitis. Further, the initial presentation of such viral infections which tend to disseminate to other organs would not be like that of classic viral hepatitis as was in this case.

If the breathlessness represents a pneumothorax, it is totally unrelated to the earlier illness.

Finally, if the breathlessness represents an effusion, one of the common causes of such a disease is tuberculosis. In that case, we will have to dissociate the hepatitis and consider two unrelated pathologies. However, it is a dictum to try and ascribe all events to a single disease and hence we must consider it to be an **immune reaction to hepatitis A infection**.

■ PHYSICAL EXAMINATION

Weight 20 kg   Height 112 cm   Not sick looking
Mild respiratory distress   RR 35/min   HR 100/min
Temp 99°F   BP 100/60 mm Hg   Mild icterus

Respiratory System

Impaired note on the right side below the 5th intercostal space both anteriorly and posteriorly, with diminished vesicular breath sounds and no foreign sounds.

Liver 3 cm nontender. Other systems normal.

Analysis

The physical signs denote a **pleural effusion** with mild respiratory distress and mild fever. As this effusion has developed acutely without fluid collection or edema at any other site, it is an exudate. The child is not sick looking, and never had high fever, hence it is obviously **not an empyema**. Thus, our earlier analysis of an immune mediated pleural effusion stands. Mild icterus and mild hepatomegaly persist, which is expected to resolve over time; this clinical picture is consistent with a recovering hepatitis. Thus, this is a child with **recovering hepatitis** who has developed an **immune mediated pleural effusion**.

■ INVESTIGATIONS

CBC normal   ESR 60 mm   Mt –ve
S. bilirubin 2.8 mg (D 1.8 mg)   ALT 850 IU   AST 230 IU
Alk phos normal   IgM HAV +ve

Pleural fluid — clear, colorless, CBNAAT-ve, 120 cells, P 80% L 20%, Proteins 100 mg, Sugar 60 mg.
Chest X-ray — pleural effusion on right side, no lung lesion

Analysis

The test results have confirmed the diagnosis of hepatitis A disease and when correlated clinically, are consistent with recovering hepatitis. The analysis of the pleural fluid suggests an exudate; however, a negative Mantoux and CBNATT have ruled out tuberculosis as a cause of pleural effusion. Thus at this stage, the pleural effusion may be presumed to be due to an immune reaction to hepatitis A infection.

■ FURTHER PROGRESS

Considering it to be an immune mediated pleural effusion due to HAV infection, the child was not treated with any drugs and observed for further evolution. In the next 5 days, the pleural effusion resolved completely.

■ FINAL DIAGNOSIS

Immune mediated pleural effusion due to HAV infection.

■ KEY MESSAGE

As a rule, all symptoms and physical signs during any illness must be considered to be due to a single disease though there may be rare exceptions. Thus, in this child, development of pleural effusion should be correlated with confirmed hepatitis A disease rather than searching for another unrelated disease. Immune response does occur following various infections and presents in the form of pleural effusion, arthropathy, skin rash and at times other organ involvement. Most of the times, such an immune response is self-limiting, once the primary infection recovers. Steroids are rarely necessary only in case of life threatening immune complications. In this case, the Mantoux test was negative. Just in case it would have been positive, it would have been difficult to conclude one way or the other. Even then, the prudent action would have been to wait and watch, because steroids would have been unindicated and ATT would have had to be modified suitably.

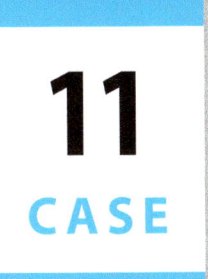

CASE 11: Progressive Jaundice with Failure to Thrive in an Infant

■ HISTORY

A 6-month-old infant presented with jaundice since the age of 3 months and failure to thrive. Born after full term normal delivery with a weight of 2.5 kg, he was exclusively breast-fed and did apparently well during the first 3 months, though the weight gain was less than expected. Thereafter, parents noticed high colored urine though the stools continued to be yellow. With the passage of time, the jaundice increased, the infant started vomiting off and on and started feeding poorly. He became very irritable and would often refuse feeds. He was the first child of his parents.

No h/o any antenatal complaints in the mother.
No h/o similar disease in the family.
No h/o consanguinity.

Analysis

This infant has progressive jaundice due to **hepatocyte disease** and not primary biliary tract disease as evident by high colored urine suggesting direct hyperbilirubinemia and failure to thrive denoting hepatocyte involvement. A low normal birth weight and subsequent failure to thrive may suggest a **congenital infection**. However, if so, the jaundice should have manifest shortly after birth. It is unlikely that the parents did not notice the jaundice for the first 3 months, and it is also unlikely that the jaundice was minimal for the first 3 months and then started progressing only after 3 months. This is **unlikely** to be due to **acquired infection** as no hepatotropic viral infection presents at this age for the first time. Systemic infections may present with jaundice due to hepatocyte involvement but would have other systemic manifestations and other organ affection as in case of CMV infection. Immune mediated disorders do not present so early in life. **Storage disorders** present with abdominal distension before organ dysfunction comes up and hence are not possible in this child. Thus, this is most likely to be an **inborn error of metabolism**. Amongst disorders of carbohydrate metabolism, galactosemia and glycogen storage disease type IV can be considered. **Galactosemia** may be **less likely** since there are no other symptoms like vomiting, seizures, etc. Disorders of lipid metabolism do not usually present with jaundice. So, the other **likely** possibility is that this may be due to a **defect in protein metabolism**.

■ PHYSICAL EXAMINATION

Irritable, wasting, poor muscle mass

Weight 4 kg	Length 62 cm	Head C. 40 cm
Temp 100°F	HR 140/min	RR 40/min deep and rapid
Signs of rickets +	Moderate pallor	
Icterus ++	No ecchymosis	

Abdomen distended, liver 4 F+, span 8 cm, firm, not tender
Spleen 3 F+, firm, not tender　　　　　　　　　Ascites +
Other systems normal

Analysis

The findings are suggestive of chronic progressive liver disease—**cirrhosis with portal hypertension in liver cell failure**. Presence of rickets in a severely malnourished infant suggests renal rickets due to **renal tubular dysfunction**. Thus, this infant has a progressive hepatocyte and renal tubular disorder starting early in life and worsening relentlessly. Therefore, **tyrosinemia** could be a strong possibility.

■ INVESTIGATIONS

Hb 8 gm%	WBC 5200	P54 L40 M4 E2
Platelets 1.2 L/cmm	S. bil. 18 mg% (D 12 mg%)	ALT 210 IU
AST 120 IU	INR 2.3	Alk phos 820 IU
S. albumin 2.9 gm%	Serum Ca 8.5 mg%, P 5.2 mg%	S. creatinine 2.2 mg%
Urinalysis — protein ++	Urinary protein-creatinine ratio 1.5	

Arterial blood gas (ABG) — compensated metabolic acidosis
X-ray wrist — evidence of active rickets
Abdominal USG — enlarged liver with coarse echotexture, enlarged spleen, evidence of portal hypertension, both kidneys are enlarged.

Analysis

Liver function tests reveal significant hepatocyte damage and liver cell failure as denoted by increased INR. Renal function tests support active rickets and ABG reveals metabolic acidosis. High serum creatinine indicates renal failure.

　　Metabolic tests confirmed the diagnosis of tyrosinemia.

■ FINAL DIAGNOSIS

Tyrosinemia with liver and kidney involvement.

KEY MESSAGE

Direct hyperbilirubinemia is due to either hepatocyte or biliary tract involvement. Generally, jaundice in biliary tract disease is severe as compared to the health status, while in hepatocyte disease, the child is disproportionately sicker as compared to the degree of jaundice. There are broadly three groups of hepatocyte diseases – infective, metabolic and immunological. Infections may be either caused by hepatotropic viruses such as viral A to E or by other infections that are primarily extrahepatic and then subsequently spread to hepatocytes, such as typhoid or malaria. Metabolic disorders are usually inborn and inherited. Immunological disorders are usually seen in older children as happens in immune mediated complications in leptospirosis. Jaundice presenting in the immediate newborn period has various differentials, but jaundice presenting in early infancy (but after the immediate newborn period) is mostly due to metabolic defects.

CASE 12

Abdominal Distension, Jaundice, and Irritability in an Infant

■ HISTORY

A 4-month-old infant was presented with an upper abdominal distension for a month, high-colored urine for 2 weeks, and irritability for a week. Born full-term normal delivery (FTND), exclusively breastfed, he was well prior to the onset of this disease.

Analysis

Upper abdominal distension suggests most likely hepatomegaly. The subsequent appearance of high-colored urine indicates conjugated bilirubinemia. Irritability on such a background may denote itching due to deposition of the bile acids and therefore, cholestasis. In view of hepatomegaly, this is likely to be **intrahepatic cholestasis**, not primary biliary obstruction. As the onset of this disease is later than neonatal age, this is not neonatal hepatitis. **Infection** and **sepsis** are ruled out as the illness is not acute but slowly progressive. There is no history of (H/o) any drug administration so drug-induced hepatitis is ruled out. An **autoimmune** process is not common at this age and one of them—sclerosing cholangitis starts as a primary biliary tract disease. Thus, we may conclude that this is most likely to be a genetically determined progressive hepatitis—**progressive familial intrahepatic cholestasis (PFIC)**.

■ PHYSICAL EXAMINATION

The infant looked chronically sick and irritable

Wt 4.2 kg (birth weight 2.5 kg)	Length 60 cm	HC 41 cm
Liver 3F+, firm, span 9 cm	Spleen 1F+	No ascites
Other systems normal		

Analysis

These findings suggest a chronic progressive liver disease as evidenced by failure to thrive and probable portal hypertension in the form of splenomegaly, but without liver cell failure. It favors the diagnosis of progressive intrahepatic cholestasis.

■ INVESTIGATIONS

Hb 9 g%	WBC 9,000/cmm	P 45 L 50 M 2 E 3	PC 1.8 L/cmm
S bilirubin 6.2 mg%	D 4.9 mg%	ALT 320 U/L	AST 210 U/L
S proteins 4.9 g%	Alb 2.8 g%	Alk phos 780 U/L	GGT 30 U/L
			Prothrombin Time N

Ultrasound (USG) showed hepatomegaly

Analysis

High-direct bilirubin, high ALT, and low-serum albumin indicate a chronic hepatocyte disease that is most likely cholestasis. When alkaline phosphatase is elevated in the presence of a normal GGT, it may be due to causes other than liver disease, such as rickets. This child may have been growing well before the onset of this disease and may have developed vitamin D deficiency rickets which did not progress further due to malnutrition. However, PFIC type 1 and 2 are known to have a normal GGT (but elevated alkaline phosphatase), while type 3 presents with high GGT because of accompanying cholangitis.

■ FINAL DIAGNOSIS

Progressive familial intrahepatic cholestasis type 1 (proved by a genetic study).

■ KEY MESSAGES

> Cholestasis presents with itching and jaundice. Jaundice is milder in primary hepatocyte disease, but the general health of the patient is comparatively poor; as against this, jaundice is more severe in primary biliary tract disease, but the general health is relatively maintained, especially in the initial days.

■ RELEVANT INFORMATION

Cholestasis is a condition where bile cannot flow from the liver into the duodenum. It is either caused by obstruction to bile flow (biliary atresia) or metabolic disorders causing disturbances in the formation and transport of bile. Bile formation begins in the bile canaliculi that are situated in between two hepatocytes, from where the bile moves into the ductules onto the bile ducts, on to the right and left hepatic ducts, on to a common hepatic duct that joins the cystic duct coming from the gallbladder to form the common bile duct that enters the duodenum at the ampulla of Vater. In cholestasis, bile accumulates in the hepatocytes. Cholestasis may be intrahepatic (hepatitis due to infection, metabolic disorders, genetic defects, autoimmune disorders, and drug-induced hepatitis) or extrahepatic (biliary atresia and biliary hypoplasia—Alagille syndrome, primary sclerosing cholangitis, bacterial cholangitis, cholelithiasis, choledochal, cyst, and other tumors). Manifestations vary as per severity. Jaundice with itching is the classic symptom, but itching may precede jaundice occasionally and may be wrongly interpreted as a primary skin disease.

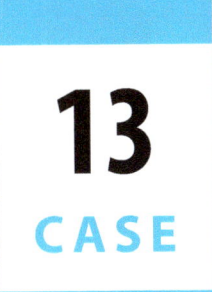

CASE 13

Recurrent Jaundice in a Child who Remained Healthy

■ HISTORY

A 10-year-old healthy child presented with jaundice with high-colored urine and itching for the last 3 days. Past history of (H/o) similar disease—three times in the last year. Each episode would last for a few days and resolve by itself. The intervening period would be normal.

Analysis

Jaundice with high-colored urine and itching denotes cholestasis. It may be either intrahepatic or extrahepatic. **Extrahepatic cholestasis** is unlikely to be recurrent and self-limiting. Hence this is most likely to be **intrahepatic cholestasis**. **Chronic infections** do not present with cholestasis as the initial symptom. A vascular pathology such as **sickle cell disease** with hepatopathy is unlikely to present with such jaundice as the only recurring symptom without any other complaints. **Metabolic disorders** may present with cholestasis and rarely such cholestasis may be recurrent, but these disorders are usually not self-limiting. A normal intervening period between recurrent episodes in this child indicates a recurrent and not a persistent disorder. A persistent disorder with recurrent symptoms is accompanied by deteriorating health. Since this child has remained healthy over this 1 year, this is likely to be a benign recurrent cholestasis. **Autoimmune** disorders or **genetic defects** are likely in this child. We would need further investigations to label the final diagnosis.

■ PHYSICAL EXAMINATION

Comfortable	Wt 30 kg	Ht 138 cm	Mild icterus
Liver 3 cm, not tender, span 13 cm		Spleen not palpable	
No ascites	No other abnormalities		

Analysis

Usually, a healthy child with mild jaundice and mild hepatomegaly suggests acute hepatitis. Considering the history, acute or chronic infections, metabolic, or vascular disorders are unlikely in this child. Autoimmune hepatitis is a possibility that needs to be ruled out by investigations; however, the points against it are that it may not resolve without treatment (as did happen in this child) and that it may be accompanied by the affection of other organs over time. Thus, an isolated genetic defect is a stronger possibility in this child.

■ INVESTIGATIONS

Complete blood count (CBC): Normal
S bilirubin 4.2 mg%   D 3.1 mg%   ALT 180 IU   AST 100 IU
Alkaline phosphatase 490 U/L   GGT normal
S proteins 6.2 g/dL   Alb 3.8 g/dL
Viral markers negative   S ceruloplasmin N
Anti-LKM, anti-SM antibodies, ANA: All negative

Analysis

Direct hyperbilirubinemia with a mild rise in ALT and AST and increased alkaline phosphatase with normal serum proteins indicates acute cholestatic hepatitis, but the GGT is normal. This rule out the extrahepatic causes of obstruction. These investigations also rule out infections, autoimmune hepatitis, and Wilson's disease; hence, it may be a genetic defect.

■ FINAL DIAGNOSIS

Benign recurrent intrahepatic cholestasis (BRIC) (confirmed by genetic studies).

■ KEY MESSAGES

> When acquired etiologies such as infections and drug-induced diseases are ruled out, genetic disorders (metabolic and other genetic defects) and immune-mediated disorders need to be considered. Due to the overlap between many of these conditions, it is necessary to order relevant tests to arrive at the final diagnosis.

■ RELEVANT INFORMATION

Though the majority of cholestatic disorders are progressive and need therapeutic intervention, BRIC is a benign disorder. Diagnostic criteria of BRIC include short-lasting (usually 2 weeks) jaundice with itching, separated by jaundice-free intervals of a few months, laboratory evidence of cholestasis (with GGT normal or mildly raised), liver biopsy showing centrilobular cholestasis and ruling out any biliary tract abnormality [USG, magnetic resonance cholangiopancreatography (MRCP), or endoscopic retrograde cholangiopancreatography (ERCP)]. There is no specific treatment. Supportive therapy includes supplementation of fat-soluble vitamins and use of cholestyramine, an opioid antagonist, or ursodeoxycholic acid (UDCA) for control of pruritus. Rifampicin has been used to reduce itching and shorten the episode and so also plasmapheresis and endoscopic biliary drainage.

HIT or MISS

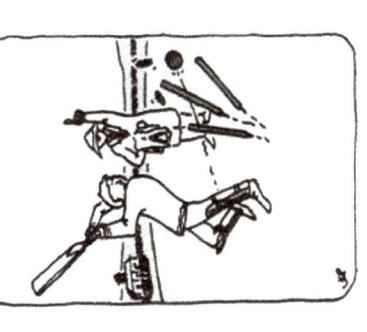

If we follow the order of

History, it's Inference, & then few Tests if needed,

we are quite likely to HIT the right diagnosis

BUT

If we almost start with

Management, then Investigate, & not look at Symptoms, Signs

we might MISS the right diagnosis

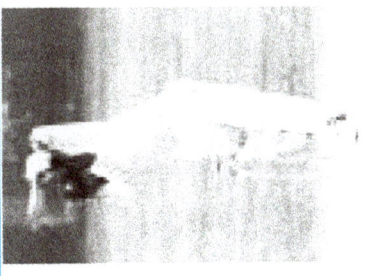

Clinical Pulmonology

BACK TO BASICS

Symptoms and physical signs often overlap in pulmonary and cardiac diseases. Cough, breathlessness, chest pain and fever are symptoms common to both systems. Palpitations signify a cardiac disease. It is important to localize the disease primarily to one or the other system, though rarely a disease of one system may subsequently affect the other system also. The onset, duration and the progress of symptoms may help in distinguishing a pulmonary from a cardiac disease and physical examination would confirm the affected system.

For clinical purposes, the pulmonary system can be divided into the airways, the lung parenchyma (alveoli), the pleura and the interstitium. Though diseases may affect more than one part of the system, specific characteristics help in localization of the disease.

Significant cough denotes an airway disease. Cough, though present, is not a predominant symptom in lung parenchymal (alveolar), interstitial or pleural disease. Dry hacking cough suggests pharyngeal affection, while a barking cough with hoarseness is a feature of laryngeal involvement. Cough with expectoration (wet cough) indicates lower airway disease as in bronchitis. Often young children are unable to expectorate and a wet cough may simulate a dry cough, though the parents report a rattling sound in the chest indicative of a wet cough. Diseases of smaller airways such as bronchioles, present with predominant tachypnea and minimal cough. Nocturnal episodic cough is a feature of hyper-reactive airways (asthma and wheeze associated viral respiratory infection). **This is the commonest cause of severe and recurrent cough in office practice**. It does not need investigations for infections such as tuberculosis nor justifies antibiotic therapy. Postnasal discharge and mouth breathing due to enlarged adenoids lead to a similar cough, which however, needs antibiotic treatment.

Breathlessness denotes a generalized airway disease (asthma, bronchiolitis), interstitial lung disease or a severe, acute localized disease (pneumonia or pleural effusion). An airway disease leading to breathlessness is acute and/or recurrent, while an interstitial disease is often slowly progressive.

Chest pain localizes the disease to the pleura and is commonly a manifestation of pleuropneumonia or an early stage of pleuritis prior to the collection of fluid. *Fever* most commonly indicates an acute infection. Absence of fever may almost rule out an acute infection. Though a chronic infection may present without fever, there may be intermittent episodes of fever, mimicking a *recurrent* infection.

The sound produced during the phases of respiration offers a clue to the anatomy and the pathology of the disease. Stridor indicates upper airway obstruction, wheeze denotes lower airway expiratory obstruction, and grunt an attempt at increasing end-expiratory pressure to prevent alveolar collapse (natural PEEP) as in a pneumonia.

Chest retractions suggest respiratory distress. Isolated suprasternal retraction indicates an extrathoracic upper airway inspiratory obstruction. Subcostal retraction alone, denotes a lower airway expiratory obstruction. Predominant intercostal retractions signify alveolar disease as in a pneumonia. The severity and extent of chest retractions increase proportionately to the severity of the disease. Chest retractions are also seen in a malnourished child due to a compliant chest wall.

Tachypnea needs a cautious interpretation. When present in pulmonary diseases, it is often accompanied *with respiratory distress* as evident by the use of accessory muscles of respiration and chest retractions. Marked tachypnea *without respiratory distress* may signify *metabolic acidosis*. The breathing is deep and rapid in such cases and the absence of abnormal auscultatory findings point to such a possibility. *Loss of voice* with tachypnea ("silent" tachypnea) indicates respiratory muscle paralysis which may be seen in Guillain-Barré syndrome.

Physical examination of the chest should localize the disease to the airways, alveoli, pleura or the mediastinum, based on the surface anatomy. This is clinically depicted as a *lobar, pleural or non-lobar non-pleural distribution* of abnormal signs. A disease affecting the upper lobe of the lung results in physical signs restricted to the upper half of the chest anteriorly, middle lobe affection to the lower half of the chest anteriorly and lower lobe affection mainly to the posterior side of the chest. Thus, a *lobar distribution* of abnormal signs indicates a lung parenchymal disease (lobar pneumonia). Abnormal physical signs are not restricted to a lobar pattern in pleural diseases, but are found on the anterior, lateral as well as the posterior side of the chest, below a particular intercostal space (*pleural distribution* as in an effusion). However, physical signs of a small pleural effusion may be restricted to a few lower intercostal spaces posteriorly only. Chest signs not consistent with a lobar or a pleural distribution (*non-lobar non-pleural distribution*) indicate a space-occupying lesion (encysted pleural effusion, a lung cyst or an abscess, mediastinal mass).

Recurrent symptoms are common in pulmonary disorders, seen most often in hyper-reactive airway disease such as *asthma* or *wheeze associated viral infection*. However, recurrent respiratory infections are also not uncommon. It is important to differentiate recurrent viral from recurrent bacterial infections, as the management of these two conditions differs significantly. The first step is to localize the respiratory infection to either the upper or the lower respiratory tract, or both. A bacterial infection is localized to a part of either the upper or the lower respiratory tract (Acute tonsillitis has no lung involvement and a pneumonia presents without any symptoms or signs of upper respiratory tract involvement. Similarly, neither of them have a running nose.)

A viral infection is generalized and affects the upper as well as the lower respiratory tract. *Recurrent viral infection* is a rule in infants and toddlers. It does not need investigations or antibiotic therapy. *Recurrent bacterial infection* demands further investigations to assess the underlying abnormality leading to such a recurrence of infection. Recurrent bacterial upper respiratory infections are due to *adenoiditis* in early childhood and *sinusitis/tonsillitis* in older children. Recurrent bacterial lower respiratory infections are invariably due to a serious underlying abnormality such as *immune deficiency, ciliary dyskinesia* or *cystic fibrosis*.

Tuberculosis may mimic recurrent disease as its symptoms are often seen "off and on". However, the diagnosis of tuberculosis should be based on reasonable proof, and before starting anti-TB treatment, its justification must be documented Empirical trial with anti-TB drugs is rarely recommended.

■ APPROACH TO RECURRENT/PERSISTENT COUGH

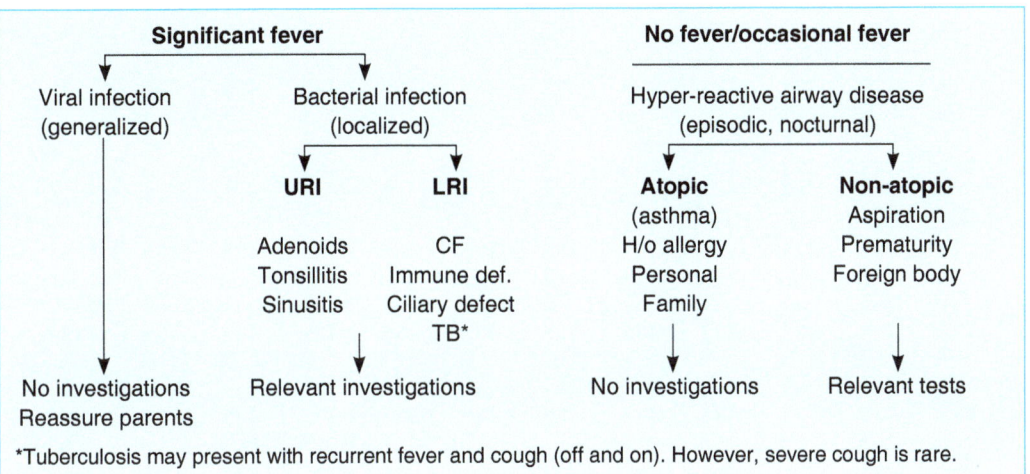

*Tuberculosis may present with recurrent fever and cough (off and on). However, severe cough is rare.

CASE 14

Breathlessness and Fever for a Day

■ HISTORY

A 10-year-old child presented with an acute onset of high fever for a day and respiratory distress of a few hours duration. He was apparently healthy and had no significant prior illness. The rest of the history was not contributory.

He was rushed to a doctor who found the following on examination:

Febrile, temp. 103°F	Chest examination on **Right** side	**Left** side
Pulse 120/min. RR 50/min	Diminished movements all over	Normal
Respiratory distress	Trachea and apex beat shifted to left	
Alae nasi working	Impaired note on percussion below 3rd space	
No chest retraction	Breath sounds absent below 3rd space	
No grunting	TVF and VR diminished in above area	
No stridor	Localized bronchial breathing posteriorly	
No wheeze	above the area of impaired note	

He was investigated and results were as follows:

Chest X-ray confirmed pleural effusion on right side

WBC 14,000/c.mm.	P 76%, L 18%, E 4%, M 2%	ESR 80 mm
Pleural fluid was tapped.	It was a clear fluid	
WBC 200/c.mm	P 80% L 20% Proteins 250 mgm%	
Gram staining –ve	Fluid was sent for culture.	

Considering it to be an empyema, an intercostal drain was inserted, and IV Ampicillin and Cefotaxime was started. The breathlessness quickly disappeared on tapping. However, in spite of a proper drainage and antibiotics for a week, the fever continued. Suspecting drug resistance, the antibiotics were changed to Vancomycin and Amikacin, but there was still no response at the end of another week. At this stage, the child was referred for further management.

Analysis

Persistence of fever in this child, diagnosed as empyema, may be due to *improper drainage* of pus, *drug resistance, immunocompromised host* or a *wrong diagnosis*. This child continued to have a good drainage, which quickly relieved his breathlessness. Drug resistance in community-acquired infections is rare. As this child has so far been a healthy child without any significant prior illness, an immunocompromised state is unlikely. Thus, the failure of treatment in this child has mostly resulted from a wrong diagnosis.

An acute onset (within 24 hours) of a pleural effusion in a healthy child is likely to be either immune mediated (**TB, dengue, collagen vascular disease**) or **traumatic** (hemorrhagic effusion). An intrathoracic **malignancy** may present with a hemorrhagic effusion, but in such a case, the child would be very sick for at least a few days prior to the onset of the illness. Fever suggests inflammation and may be present in any of these conditions. In this child, the presence of fever with a neutrophilic leukocytosis led to the diagnosis of an acute bacterial infection and hence he was treated as an empyema. However, an empyema is a complication of an acute bacterial pneumonia and would develop only after a few days of untreated or a poorly treated pneumonia. Thus, an empyema would not present on the first day of the illness. *This fact was missed and led to a wrong diagnosis.*

Neutrophilic leukocytosis is not specific to acute bacterial infections but indicates acute inflammation due to any cause. In fact, severe and persistent neutrophilic leukocytosis is seen in collagen vascular disorders. Eosinopenia is a feature of acute infections – bacterial or viral. As this child had 4% eosinophils, it was against an acute infection.

Dengue fever would have presented with shock and a capillary leak syndrome (third space loss), with polyserositis and edema, typically at the end of defervescence of fever. Hence, it is unlikely in this child. It is unusual for collagen vascular diseases to present with a large isolated pleural effusion without any other manifestations. Thus, it is most likely to be tuberculosis. Acute onset pleural effusion in tuberculosis is classically seen in healthy older children with good immunity and hypersensitivity.

This child improved on anti-TB therapy over the next 2 weeks. Steroids are not necessary for such a patient; he did improve (as expected) even without steroids.

■ KEY MESSAGES

- Acute onset of pleural effusion is either due to **allergy** (TB), **trauma** (hemothorax) or a **vascular** cause (capillary leak syndrome as in Dengue fever).
- Empyema is a complication of bacterial pneumonia and hence develops over a few days.
- Neutrophilic leukocytosis is a feature of any acute stress and is not specific to bacterial infections. Eosinopenia is indicative of an acute bacterial or viral infection.
- If two sets of antibiotics fail, a change of diagnosis is relevant rather than a further change of antibiotics.

■ RELEVANT INFORMATION

Immunological Considerations

A functional equilibrium between the efficacy of cell-mediated immunity (necessary for eradication of the pathogen) and delayed-type hypersensitivity reaction (contributing to tissue destruction) are observed in infected individuals.

Hypothetical Model based on Immune Response

It is clear from the above discussion that the outcome of infection in tuberculosis depends upon the immune response of the host, in terms of the degree of cell mediated immunity and hypersensitivity, relative to each other. This immune response is affected by multiple variables in relation to the host as well as the bacteria. Age, nutrition, vaccination status and previous exposure to mycobacteria play a significant role in the ultimate host response. The number of bacteria and their virulence also decide the outcome to some extent. Drug therapy modifies the response mostly in favor of the host. A hypothetical model can be constructed for a simplified understanding of the clinical consequences of this interplay, based on a model similar to that of leprosy.

Immunity (Protective)	Hypersensitivity (Destructive)	Pathological outcome
++	−	Primary infection − no disease
++	+	Primary complex (localized lymph node disease)
++	++	Pleural effusion (unidentifiable subpleural focus)
+	+	Progressive primary complex
+	++	Chronic pulmonary cavitatory disease
+/−	++	TBM
+/−	−	Disseminated disease
−	−	Miliary TB

It is clear that there would be an overlap of immune response resulting in changing pathology. Decrease in protective immunity may lead to progression of local pathology as in progressive primary complex or dissemination to distant organs as in miliary TB.

Hypersensitivity response may promote destructive pathology as in cavitatory pulmonary disease or TB meningitis.

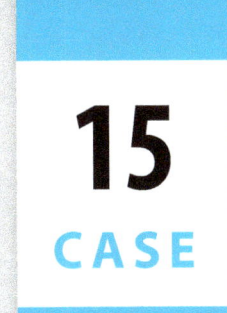

CASE 15

Breathlessness and Fever over 5 Days

■ HISTORY

A 12-year-old child presented with high fever for 5 days and increasing breathlessness for the last 2 days prior to admission to the hospital. He had been apparently healthy prior to the onset of high fever. Fever continued to be high in spite of treatment by the local doctor. He started feeling breathless 3 days after the onset of fever; it increased rapidly over the next 2 days to necessitate hospitalization.

No history of cough.   No history of palpitation.   No history of chest pain

No past history of breathlessness or any other significant illness.

No family history of asthma.

Analysis

An acute onset of breathlessness may suggest a respiratory, cardiac or a metabolic disease. Cardiac diseases may present with high fever for the first few days, followed by breathlessness as in acute **rheumatic carditis**. However, breathlessness in such cases rarely deteriorates so fast. Acute **viral myocarditis** presents with breathlessness at the *onset* of the illness. Acute **pyogenic pericarditis** with effusion is likely to present with high fever and increasing breathlessness, but severe chest pain is the hallmark of such a disease. Hence, this child is unlikely to be suffering from a cardiac disease. **Diabetic ketoacidosis** may present as breathlessness and may be triggered by an acute infection presenting as fever at the onset of the disease. Respiratory conditions leading to acute breathlessness include asthma, pneumonia or pleural diseases such as effusion or pneumothorax. It is unlikely to be **asthma** as it presents without fever and significant cough is a predominant symptom. Besides, there is no personal or family history of asthma or atopy. **Pneumothorax** results from rupture of noninfective alveoli as in asthma, histiocytosis or a lung cyst and hence is also unlikely. This patient may therefore either have a **pneumonia** or a **pleural effusion**. Pneumonia in such a healthy older child is often localized to a lobe and less likely to result in progressive breathlessness unless it is an **expanding or a necrotizing pneumonia** (staphylococcal or *Klebsiella pneumonia*) or it complicates into an empyema. So it is quite likely that this child may have developed an **empyema**. Pleural effusion due to **tuberculosis** is also a possibility.

■ PHYSICAL EXAMINATION

General examination	Chest exam. **Right** side	**Left** side anteriorly
Well-built and nourished child	Bulging of chest wall	First two spaces
Anxious and sick looking child	No movements at all	Impaired note
Wt 42 kg Ht 148 cm	Trachea shifted to left	Absent air entry
Temp. 103°F HR 140/min		**Other areas**
RR 50/min. Resp. distress ++	TVF and VR absent all over	Apex beat not
No chest retractions	Dull note all over	localized, otherwise
No grunting	Absent breath sounds all over	normal
CVS - heart borders cannot be delineated	Heart sounds distant	No murmur
No signs of cardiac failure	No engorged neck veins	No free fluid
Liver 2 cm + soft, not tender	Spleen not palpable	CNS - Normal

Analysis

This child obviously has signs of a massive **pleural effusion on the right side**. Such a massive pleural effusion is seen in **tuberculosis** or **malignancy**. Empyema is never massive and is accompanied with signs of a pneumonia. Further it is rare in a 12-year-old healthy child. However, the chest signs are not restricted to the right side only but have partly extended to the left side also. An impaired note on percussion and absent breath sounds on the **left side anteriorly** suggest a localizing lesion. It may be either **atelectasis** or an **encysted fluid**. Consolidation results in bronchial breath sounds and crepitations. However, the absence of such classical signs of consolidation may be due to an accompanying collapse, as is commonly seen in tuberculosis. Thus, it could also be a **consolidation with collapse**. Generally, a pleural effusion is associated with a lung lesion on the same side which is often hidden by the overlying fluid, but not a lesion on the other side. Such left sided physical findings are difficult to explain in the presence of a right-sided massive pleural effusion. As the heart borders could not be delineated and the heart sounds are distant, one needs to consider a **pericardial effusion**. Pleural effusion and pericardial effusion may go together in polyserositis. However, absence of engorged neck veins and hepatomegaly is against a pericardial effusion. Thus at this stage, it is difficult to judge the nature of the disease that has spread to the left side in addition to the pleural effusion on the right side. There is a possibility that the **left sided lesion** may be **unrelated** and may represent a pre-existing occult congenital defect such as **sequestration** or **cystadenomatoid malformation**.

■ INVESTIGATIONS

Hb 6 gm%   Normocytic normochromic anemia
WBC 18,000/c.mm   P 76% L 18% E 2% M 4%   Platelets 4.5 lacs/c.mm
ESR 120 mm   ABG normal   Mt test negative
Chest X-ray - massive effusion on the right side with mediastinal shift to the left
No evidence of pericardial effusion
Pleural tap - hemorrhagic fluid

Analysis

Severe anemia and a high ESR suggest an acute destructive inflammatory pathology. Neutrophilic leukocytosis with a normal eosinophil count does not favor an infection, but instead, indicates an acute stress to the bone marrow. A high platelet count could be in response to bleeding (hemothorax). Hemorrhagic pleural effusion may occur in malignancy, tuberculosis, acute pancreatitis or result from trauma. There is neither a history of trauma, nor any severe abdominal pain to suggest acute pancreatitis. Thus, it may be a malignancy or tuberculosis. In tuberculous pleural effusion, tuberculin test is invariably positive as such a disease is seen in an immunocompetent and sensitized child. Hence, a search for a malignancy is mandatory in this case. This malignant lesion must be intrathoracic, and hence has led to the pleural effusion. If the chest X-ray has failed to demonstrate any other lesion, it is likely that it is hidden under the massive pleural fluid. Hence, a CT scan of the chest is indicated for further evaluation.

■ FURTHER INVESTIGATIONS

CT scan of the chest showed a large solid mass extending to the left thorax along with a massive pleural effusion on the right side.

The pleural fluid tested positive for malignant cells.

Analysis

The abnormal left sided physical findings are now clearly explained as due to a space occupying lesion extending to the left upper zone. Unless the hemorrhagic nature of the effusion was known, it would have been difficult to guess such a pathology. Such problems are rare.

Operative intervention and biopsy proved it to be a malignant pleuroendothelioma.

■ FINAL DIAGNOSIS

Malignant pleuroendothelioma.

■ KEY MESSAGES

- Massive hemorrhagic pleural effusion is mostly malignant, though rarely it may be tuberculous.
- Children with an acute onset of a malignancy, look anxious and sick unlike those suffering from acute manifestations of tuberculosis.
- A plain X-ray of the chest (PA view) may fail to demonstrate the underlying lung lesion in presence of a massive pleural effusion, and hence, a CT scan of the chest is required.

CASE 16

Breathlessness after Few Days of Fever

■ HISTORY

An 8-year-old healthy child had moderate fever for 4 days and a mild cough.
   No other significant symptoms
   Past history not contributory
   He was treated with amoxicillin hypothetically. The fever was controlled within 2 days.
   After remaining afebrile for 3 days, the fever returned in spite of continuation of amoxicillin. The next day, he developed acute respiratory distress.
   He was hospitalized for the same and the doctor found the following on examination.

Sick looking	Mild respiratory distress		
Temp. 101°F	HR 120/min.	RR 45/min.	BP 70/50 mm
No chest retractions	No cyanosis	No clubbing	
Facial puffiness +	No edema feet		
Signs of pleural effusion on the right side		Free fluid in peritoneal cavity +	
No cardiomegaly	No signs of cardiac failure	Other systems were normal.	

   He was investigated and the results were as follows.
   Hb 16 gm%   WBC 8,000/c.mm   P 75% L 18% E 4% M 3%   ESR 80 mm
   Chest X-ray – moderate pleural effusion
   Abdominal USG – ascites

   The pleural fluid was tapped
   Pleural fluid - 100 cells, 90% lymphocytes   Proteins 200 mgm%

After pleural tapping, his breathlessness was relieved and he was comfortable. The antibiotics were changed to IV Cefotaxime and Amikacin. After 2 days, he started getting breathless again and the pleural fluid was found to have increased again. At this stage, anti-TB drugs were introduced, but as the child was deteriorating in his general condition, he was referred for further management.

■ ANALYSIS OF HISTORY AS NOTED FROM PREVIOUS RECORDS

This child started with a trivial upper respiratory infection and settled within the next 2 days. It suggests either a response to the antibiotic or a self-limiting viral infection. In spite of the antibiotic therapy being continued, fever recurred after the child was afebrile for 2 days. Initial "improvement" on amoxicillin but subsequent deterioration while on the same treatment quite definitely rules out a bacterial infection. Biphasic fever is often seen in viral infections. However in common viral infections, the second phase of fever is shorter and milder than the first phase, and the patient recovers completely within 1–2 days. In this child, the second phase of fever led to respiratory distress, and is, therefore, not the self-limiting second phase of infection.

Sudden development of acute respiratory distress may occur with pulmonary diseases such as **pneumothorax, pleural effusion** or **pulmonary embolism**. Absence of palpitations and the sudden development of breathlessness is unlikely to be due to a **cardiac disease**. Pneumothorax is a mechanical complication in patients with asthma, emphysema or a lung cyst and is not accompanied with fever. Pulmonary embolism is a rare complication of bacterial endocarditis in a child with a heart defect, and hence, unlikely in this child. Thus, a pleural effusion is the most probable.

It cannot be an **empyema**, as the child had initially recovered from the fever. An acute development of a pleural effusion does favor an immune mediated response, as in **tuberculosis** or **dengue fever**. Pleural effusion in tuberculosis presents with a continuous high fever at the onset of the illness. As the fever had abated in this child after 2 days, tuberculosis is less likely. Biphasic fever may favor the diagnosis of dengue fever with a capillary leak syndrome (third space loss).

ANALYSIS OF PHYSICAL EXAMINATION AS NOTED FROM PREVIOUS RECORDS

The presence of a pleural effusion, ascites and facial puffiness suggests a collection of fluid in multiple sites. Moreover, this child is in decompensated shock, as is evident by the low blood pressure. This is suggestive of a poor intravascular volume due to loss of fluids in the third space. That is why he looks sick even though he has only a mild respiratory distress. This favors a diagnosis of capillary leak syndrome, a common cause being **dengue fever**. Pleural effusion in tuberculosis is mostly an isolated manifestation; though polyserositis is known, it is rare. The facial edema and the shock state are also against tuberculosis.

ANALYSIS OF PROGRESS AND TREATMENT AS NOTED FROM PREVIOUS RECORDS

Starting this child on IV antibiotics was irrational, as empyema was never a possibility. The neutrophilic response may have prompted such a therapy. However, it is well-known that neutrophilia is a response to any acute stress and is not pathognomonic of acute bacterial infection.

Tuberculosis is also not in question as mentioned above. Anti-TB therapy was instituted probably on the basis of lymphocytosis in the pleural fluid. What was ignored was the collection of fluid at multiple sites, in a child who was in shock. Hb 16 gm% indicates a contraction of the intravascular volume and should have also led to the correct diagnosis.

PHYSICAL EXAMINATION AT THE REFERRAL CENTER

Sick looking	Severe respiratory distress		Facial edema +	
Cold and clammy extremities	HR 145/min	RR 50/min	BP 65/45 mm	
Abdominal distension	Liver 2 cm +	liver span 7 cm	Spleen not palpable	
Signs of bilateral pleural effusion and ascites				
Other systems normal				

■ INVESTIGATIONS

Hb 16 gm%   WBC 5,300/c.mm   Differential count N   Platelets 65,000/c.mm
Chest X-ray – bilateral pleural effusion   Abdominal USG – ascites
IgM and IgG dengue antibodies were positive in high titers.

Analysis

Bilateral pleural effusion, ascites, facial edema and shock represent a capillary leak syndrome with third space loss of fluids. 16 gm% hemoglobin signifies hemoconcentration due to a contracted intravascular volume. IgM dengue antibody confirms a recent dengue infection; IgG denotes a previously sensitized child due to dengue infection in the past. This is the classical serology of dengue shock syndrome.

The child was resuscitated with large amounts of intravenous fluids and he improved over the next 2 days. The pleural effusion and the ascites regressed, and he recovered completely.

■ FINAL DIAGNOSIS

Dengue shock syndrome.

■ KEY MESSAGES

- Biphasic fever with the second phase manifesting with severe symptoms, and often involving multiple systems, is an immune mediated response to an infection in a previously sensitized host.
- Such an immune mediated response needs symptomatic treatment at the earliest to maintain homeostatic balance and normal tissue perfusion.
- Tuberculosis rarely causes polyserositis and there is no compromise of intravascular volume in such cases with the exception of pericardial effusion, which presents with cardiac tamponade.

■ RELEVANT INFORMATION

Dengue illnesses have a varied clinical presentation. Majority of children suffer from a mild undifferentiated illness with a self-limiting fever lasting for 5–7 days with or without a macular skin rash and respiratory symptoms. Some of them have a classical "break bone" fever with severe myalgia. Less than 10% patients manifest dengue hemorrhagic fever (DHF) (hemoconcentration and thrombocytopenia). It is only 1 in 200 patients who may present with severe and serious Dengue shock syndrome (DSS).

It is the body's immune mechanisms rather than the virulence of the virus that is responsible for the clinical symptomatology. The second attack of dengue fever leads to an interaction with pre-existing non-neutralizing antibodies to develop an immune mediated vasculopathy and abnormal hemostasis. Positive Hess's test along with increasing PCV and reducing platelet count is diagnostic of DHF. The vasculopathy presents as third space loss (pleural effusion, ascites). If untreated, it may evolve into DSS. Thus, DSS is a subset of DHF. Such immune mediated complications occur around the time of defervescence, and are especially seen in well-nourished children.

Maintaining intravascular volume with adequate fluids is the key to the management of DHF and DSS. Vasculopathy resulting in third space loss is self-limiting and on recovery, may lead to congestion and overhydration as the fluid returns to the intravascular compartment. Thus, this disease goes through three distinct phases – febrile (first phase), shock (generally at the time of defervescence) and congestion (recovery phase). A careful evaluation of all the phases is mandatory, as the management is quite different.

CASE 17

Breathlessness in a Child with Arthritis

■ HISTORY

A 10-year-old male child presented with fever and joint pain and swelling, off and on for the last 3 years, and breathlessness for the last 10 days.

He was apparently well 3 years ago when he developed high fever of an acute onset, which was followed by pain in both the knee joints. He was treated with symptomatic therapy and was relieved after 2 weeks. He continued to suffer similar attacks of joint pain and swelling, affecting both the large and the small joints. Each attack left behind some swelling and restriction of movements in the involved joints. The pain was at its worst on getting up in the morning and was partially better thereafter. He had taken prolonged anti-inflammatory drug therapy but no other treatment. He was also prescribed oral steroids in two of the episodes, which were very severe and were not relieved by anti-inflammatory drugs alone.

He developed breathlessness of a gradual onset, over the last 10 days prior to hospitalization. He was not breathless at rest but was uncomfortable on exertion, though he continued his daily routine activities.

No history of skin rash, alopecia, mouth ulcers, nail abnormalities.
No history of breathlessness in the past.
No relevant past or family history.

Analysis

This child obviously has a history of a chronic recurrent arthritis affecting both small and large joints over the last 3 years, without complete remission. It suggests a possibility of **juvenile chronic arthritis**. Other systemic inflammatory disorders would not have restricted themselves to joint involvement alone. The recent development of *breathlessness* in this systemic inflammatory disease may indicate **pulmonary** or **cardiac** involvement. Pulmonary involvement in rheumatological disorders may be in the form of pleural, alveolar or interstitial lung disease. Pleural disease presents either as pleuritis with chest pain or a small pleural effusion, whereas a localized pneumonia due to vasculitis is the feature of alveolar disease. Both pleural and alveolar diseases do not result in breathlessness and are hence unlikely. Interstitial lung disease usually occurs slowly over many years and hence may not be considered in this child. Further, pulmonary involvement may be typically seen in scleroderma or SLE; absence of a history of Raynaud's phenomenon and other skin manifestations nearly rule them out. Cardiac involvement is known in many systemic inflammatory disorders but it is often in the form of pericardial involvement, which does not give rise to breathlessness and in fact may present as chest pain. Though a pericardial effusion with cardiac tamponade could present as severe breathlessness, it is rare, and there are other associated symptoms such as edema. These disorders do not commonly involve the endocardium or the myocardium to give rise to breathlessness. Hypertension may be another cause of cardiac affection in some systemic inflammatory disorders, but is unlikely in juvenile chronic arthritis. As this child is suffering for the last 3 years, he is likely to have an anemia of chronic inflammation and occasionally breathlessness may be due to **severe anemia**.

■ PHYSICAL EXAMINATION

Poorly built and nourished	Weight 20 kg	Height 122 cm
Temp normal	Pulse 120/min	RR 30/min
BP 90/50 mm of Hg	Moderate pallor
No clubbing of nails	No lymphadenopathy

Joint swelling, pain and restriction of movements involving both wrists, knees, ankles, small joints of the hand and spine, in various stages of inflammation.
Deformities of the involved joints and wasting of muscles around the knee joints.
CVS - heart size normal	Heart sounds normal	Soft systolic murmur
Other systems normal

Analysis

This child has a chronic (as suggested by the deformities and the muscle wasting), persistent, active arthritis affecting multiple small and large joints due to an inflammatory disorder, with significant pallor. There is no evidence of any other organ involvement; specifically the respiratory and cardiovascular systems appear clinically normal. It favors a diagnosis of juvenile chronic arthritis with significant anemia. In this case, the anemia is more likely to be due to chronic inflammation, rather than it being a primary hematological disorder. Joint involvement is seen in **hemophilia** or **sickle cell disease**. Though chronic arthritis may be a manifestation of hemophilia, it generally involves only the large joints (mainly the knee joints). There would also be a history of a bleeding disorder. Sickle cell disease may mimic rheumatological disorders, though the joint involvement occurs as an acute crisis and is mainly restricted to the small joints or the bones. Leukemia and scurvy may also result in anemia and bony involvement, but both are acute conditions. Thus, anemia in this child is unlikely to be a primary hematological disorder. In the absence of any clinical evidence of a respiratory or a cardiac disease, the breathlessness must be due to significant anemia, the soft systolic murmur being functional. As reported, this child was merely uncomfortable on exertion and not acutely breathless. This signifies *easy fatiguability* rather than breathlessness.

■ INVESTIGATIONS

Hb 6 gm%	Peripheral smear - normocytic, normochromic
MCV - 76 fL	MCH - 32 pg	MCHC - 33%
WBC 28,000/c.mm	P 82% L 15% E 3%	Platelets 4.8 lacs	ESR 65 mm
Serum Iron - 34 µg/dL		TIBC - 200 µg/dL
ANA -ve	RA -ve
X-ray chest - N	PFT - N	Echocardiogram - N

Analysis

The indices and the serum iron studies suggest an anemia of chronic inflammation. The diagnosis of juvenile chronic arthritis is clinical; the leukocytosis, thrombocytosis and a high ESR are known to be associated with this condition and support the diagnosis.

■ COMMENT

A prolonged course of the illness, with several relapses and deforming arthritis is the end result of a poorly managed disease. Since this child did not receive any disease-modifying drugs but was treated only with anti-inflammatory medications, the disease was never controlled but only temporarily suppressed, and it got worse with every relapse.

■ KEY MESSAGES

- Systemic inflammatory disease is diagnosed by an evolving clinical pattern and not by laboratory tests; they just support the clinical diagnosis (or otherwise).
- It may take 6 months or more at times for the disease to evolve for a definite diagnosis.
- Once the disease is diagnosed as juvenile chronic arthritis, it is mandatory to treat with disease-modifying drugs at an early stage of the disease to prevent deformities.
- Methotrexate is the drug of choice in juvenile chronic arthritis and it is a fairly safe drug in the dosages used to treat this condition, though many pediatricians may be reluctant to use it for the fear of side effects.

■ RELEVANT INFORMATION

Pulmonary Manifestations of Rheumatological Diseases

In juvenile chronic arthritis, pulmonary involvement may take several forms including pleural effusion, interstitial fibrosis, nodular lesions (Caplan's syndrome) and bronchiolitis obliterans-organizing pneumonia.

Pulmonary involvement of SLE includes acute and chronic diseases. Pleurisy with chest pain with or without effusion is the commonest feature of acute involvement. Acute lupus pneumonia may present with acute breathlessness and so also chronic interstitial lung disease; however both are rare. Diffuse alveolar hemorrhage is an acute life-threatening process seen in acute lupus. Pulmonary embolism may present with acute dyspnea. Pulmonary hypertension without underlying lung disease may rarely occur. In all these rheumatological disorders, a primary infection may present as a pulmonary disease and must be promptly recognized and treated.

Pulmonary nodules and cavitatory pulmonary lesions may be the manifestations of Wegener's granulomatosis, a disease that is characterized by histologic evidence of granulomatous inflammation. Patients with clinical evidence of ANCA positive small vessel vasculitis, who lack granulomatous inflammation, are classified as having microscopic polyangiitis (MPA).

CASE 18: Sudden Onset of Breathlessness in a 5-year-old

■ HISTORY

A 5-year-child presented with sudden onset of breathlessness He was apparently well prior to this event. There is no history of cough, palpitation or fever. There is no significant past personal or family history. His growth and development has been normal.

Analysis

Sudden onset breathlessness can be due to a mechanical cause such as an inhaled foreign body or pneumothorax, or a vascular cause such as pulmonary embolism or myocardial infarction. However, **pulmonary embolism** and **myocardial infarction** present with sudden collapse more than breathlessness and are therefore unlikely; besides both are extremely rare. **Inhaled foreign body** is less likely at this age, and can only cause breathlessness when lodged in the trachea/major bronchus, when it would lead to a bad cough along with stridor. So, one may not consider it in this child. Though an **asthmatic attack** can start acutely, one needs to appreciate the subtle difference between an "acute" onset and a "hyperacute" onset – in asthma, the breathlessness does not start "suddenly" in a minute or two, as happened in this case. Besides, in asthma, usually there is history of associated significant cough or wheezing or a similar history in the past. Hence, an acute attack of asthma seems to be unlikely. **Metabolic acidosis** may mimic breathlessness but is not sudden and so ruled out. **Pneumothorax** is possible though it seems to have occurred in an otherwise normal child. It suggests the presence of an underlying abnormality in the lung that may have suddenly given way to give rise to an air leak resulting in sudden pneumothorax. This could be a congenital malformation of the lung that has been asymptomatic such as a lung cyst or emphysematous bullae. This could also be the result of an acquired condition such as an infection or tumor that may have lead to air retention and has now suddenly burst. However, there are no symptoms to suggest any preexisting disease. Thus, this child has mostly developed a pneumothorax, and the cause seems to be a **pre-existent silent lung abnormality**.

■ PHYSICAL EXAMINATION

Acutely breathless
Weight 20 kg
RR 50/min
General examination normal
Resp. system — Trachea and cardiac apex shifted to left
No chest retractions
Height 106 cm
BP normal
Temp. normal
HR 122/min

R side — reduced movements, TVF and VR decreased, hyper-resonant note no foreign sounds.
L side — normal
Other systems normal

Analysis

Chest examination confirms the presence of a pneumothorax but without any clue to the cause of the pneumothorax. The clinical signs do not suggest emphysema as the distribution of signs is pleural rather than lobar. Pleural distribution of signs means the presence of signs below a particular intercostal space all over the chest – anterior, lateral and posterior, on the affected side. As discussed earlier, the cause of the pneumothorax could be a pre-existing lung abnormality that has remained asymptomatic. Once such a pre-existing defect or disease bursts to leak air, it cannot be picked up by physical examination. So, this child needs further investigations, though at times, even imaging may not pick it up.

■ INVESTIGATIONS

CBC normal
Chest X-ray — Pneumothorax on right side, small areas of pneumomediastinum, suggestion of few miliary shadows scattered on both sides
CT scan of chest — small nodules scattered over both sides
Biopsy of lung nodule suggestive of Langerhans's histiocytosis, no evidence of tuberculosis

Analysis

Diagnosis is confirmed by histopathology.

■ FINAL DIAGNOSIS

Langerhans's histiocytosis with pneumothorax.

■ KEY MESSAGES

- In children sudden onset of breathlessness is usually mechanical though occasionally, vascular obstruction may also result in breathlessness; however, in that case there is concomitant shock due to myocardial dysfunction.
- Some defects or diseases may remain apparently silent and the first manifestation may be a sudden complication. Physical examination would often fail to identify such a defect or disease but investigations or imaging usually helps.

CASE 19

Gradually Progressive Breathlessness in an Infant

■ HISTORY

A 3-month-old infant presented with gradual increasing breathlessness over the last 1 month. He was well till the age of 2 months when his mother noticed that he was breathing somewhat faster than usual. This gradually progressed over a month and he started finding it difficult to feed. He was reluctant to suck at the breast and mother had to offer expressed breast milk with a spoon. He would also not sleep well and was irritable. He was growing well till the age of 2 months (gained 2 kg since birth) but did not gain weight in the third month. On direct questioning, mother gave history of dry cough in the infant. There was no history of sweating while feeding or any other complaints. No significant birth or family history.

Analysis

This infant has gradually progressive breathlessness that started at 2 months of age. An infant with a metabolic disorder is less likely to be absolutely normal and gaining weight for the first 2 months; besides, the "breathlessness" would not be progressive. Hence, it could be cardiac or respiratory disease. **Congenital heart defects** present with breathlessness on exertion as denoted by suck-rest-suck cycle. It means that infant starts feeding actively but stops in between feeds to rest and recover from breathlessness and then start sucking again. This infant is *reluctant to suck* at the breast and mother had to feed expressed breast milk with a spoon. So, this infant's **breathlessness** is present **even at rest** and is not just getting aggravated by exertion. Besides, infants with congenital heart defects would also present with other symptoms like wet cough and excessive sweating. Finally, they present early and progress fast. Hence, breathlessness in this infant is likely to be of respiratory origin. **Congenital lobar emphysema** would present with symptoms starting in first few weeks of life and as this infant was well for the first 2 months, it is unlikely. **Interstitial lung disease** is rare at this age and may present with gradually increasing breathlessness almost since birth as happens in chronic lung disease resulting from severe lung damage at birth. Gradually increasing breathlessness may indicate a space occupying lesion and dry cough denotes external compressive pressure over airways. Thus, it suggests probable **mediastinal tumor**. History cannot guess etiology and it would need further investigations.

■ PHYSICAL EXAMINATION

Breathless infant but not so uncomfortable

HR 120/min	RR 50/min	Temp. normal
Weight 4.7 kg	Length 58 cm	Head Cir 40 cm
BP normal	No cyanosis	No clubbing of nails
Minimal intercostal retractions	No lymphadenopathy	No signs of rickets

Chest examination — Movements decreased on right side anteriorly in lower half, TVF and VR decreased, no evidence of mediastinal shift, hyper-resonant note on percussion and decreased breath sounds in same area, no foreign sounds

Other areas on right side and the left side are normal
Other systems normal

Analysis

This infant is breathless but not so uncomfortable. It suggests a chronic slowly progressive disease that has made the infant get adapted to the breathlessness to some extent. Minimal intercostal retraction indicates lung parenchymal involvement. Since the signs are restricted to the anterior lower half of the chest, it suggests a lobar distribution (right middle lobe). Hyper-resonant percussion note suggests emphysema. This is not a pneumothorax as the signs are not pleural in distribution. Thus, findings confirm **right middle lobe emphysema**. A common cause of such a finding is congenital lobar emphysema. However as this infant was normal till 2 months of age (weight gain of 2 kg and absence of any symptoms), congenital lobar emphysema seems less likely. It is possible that the mother had not noticed mild symptoms early in life, but the good weight gain suggests that there may not have been any early symptoms. So, it could be an **acquired disease** in the form of a space occupying lesion compressing on a bronchus. The recent irritability and poor weight gain in last 1 month may suggest chronic inflammation, and thus, the lesion could be a large hilar lymph node secondary to tuberculosis that has compressed the right middle lobe bronchus producing localized lobar emphysema. However, other etiologies cannot be ruled out.

■ INVESTIGATIONS

Chest X-ray - Moderate sized mass at right hilum with air retention in right middle lobe, no other abnormality
Mt test +ve
Gastric aspirate was negative for AFB
Contact study in family members –ve

Analysis

Circumstantial evidence strongly suggests tuberculosis as a positive Mt test in an infant is in favor of active tuberculosis. A hilar mass suggests an enlarged lymph node. Thus, the diagnosis of a tuberculous primary complex is reasonably sure. The gastric aspirate being negative for AFB does not go against the diagnosis.

FINAL DIAGNOSIS

Tuberculous primary complex with right middle lobe emphysema due to external compression produced by hilar lymphadenopathy.

KEY MESSAGE

Mother's observation is rarely wrong. Though signs of lobar emphysema at this age are usually due to a congenital lesion, this infant certainly was normal in the first 2 months. Hence, disease did start manifesting sometime in third month as suggested by history and it fits in typically with the incubation period of tuberculosis. This infant must have come in contact at birth – may be with one of the staff members of the hospital where he was delivered and hence family screening was negative. It is important to screen family members more so in case of infants as it may help prove the diagnosis and also treat the contact properly.

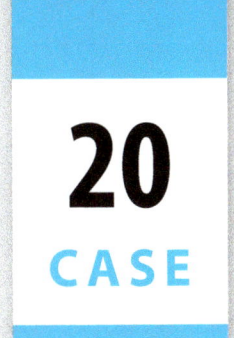

CASE 20

Breathlessness, Palpitations and Chest Pain

■ HISTORY

An 11-year-old male child complained of breathlessness on exertion for the last 2 years, and palpitations and chest pain for the last 6 months. The breathlessness had been gradually progressive, and of late, he was breathless even on accustomed exertion. The palpitations were initially noted only on exertion, but lately even at rest. He had never noticed any irregularity of rhythm during the palpitations. The chest pain had been episodic and was localized to the retrosternal area. It was precipitated by exertion and relieved by rest.

One month back, he developed fever and edema feet and deteriorated over 2–3 days, for which he required hospitalization and since then, he has been on regular medications.

Analysis

Exertional dyspnea, over a period of time, can be **respiratory** or **cardiac** in origin. Distinction between the two can often be made by the rate of progression and the associated symptoms. In this case, palpitations suggest a cardiac disease. In this context, exertional dyspnea signifies an (early) inability of the cardiac output to meet the oxygen requirements of the body without an increase in the pulmonary capillary wedge pressure (PCWP). In other words, it signifies an early, but gradual, failure of left ventricular function. Palpitations signify forceful ventricular contractions due to a volume overload. Therefore, these symptoms signify a volume overload of the left ventricle resulting in gradual LV dysfunction. This could be a result of congenital heart disease, cardiomyopathy (both dilated or hypertrophic) or rheumatic valvular heart disease.

Amongst **congenital heart diseases** (acyanotic), the commonest lesions are the left to right shunts. Their natural history is that of either infancy or early childhood presentation, or subsequent asymptomatic detection. *Symptomatic* presentation at an older age is unlikely to be in the form of LV dysfunction alone; symptoms of pulmonary hypertension and therefore right-sided failure would follow.

Chest pain may be pericardial or ischemic. The nature of chest pain in this child suggests that it is ischemic or anginal pain. It is a not a feature of left to right shunts. While **cardiomyopathy** may present as an insidious onset, slowly progressive LV dysfunction, chest pain is unlikely in dilated cardiomyopathy.

So even though there is no history suggestive of rheumatic fever in the past, one has to keep in mind a **valvular heart disease of rheumatic origin**. Regurgitant lesions of the mitral and aortic valves usually cause volume overload of the left ventricle. Though **mitral regurgitation** is the commonest lesion, presence of chest pain suggests aortic involvement (since coronary perfusion is mainly in diastole, the diastolic runoff in aortic regurgitation leads to coronary ischemia). Therefore, there has to be **aortic regurgitation**, either as the dominant lesion or coexisting with mitral regurgitation.

The episode that occurred a month ago suggests congestive cardiac failure. If this child has rheumatic valvular heart disease, sudden deterioration of cardiac function can be usually triggered by a fresh attack of rheumatic carditis or bacterial endocarditis or arrhythmias. Since the patient has not noticed any irregularity during the palpitations, arrhythmia seems less likely.

■ PHYSICAL EXAMINATION

Poorly built and nourished	Weight 25 kg	Height 128 cm
Comfortable at rest	Steroid facies	
Pulse – 90/min regular, brisk	RR – 28/min	BP – 110/50 mm
JVP – Normal No edema	No cyanosis	Joints normal

CVS – Mild precordial bulge
Apex beat – in the left 5th intercostal space outside the mid clavicular line, forceful and ill sustained, well localized

Systolic thrill at apex	S1 N S2 narrowly split	P2 loud, S3 at apex

Grd IV/VI holosystolic murmur, radiating to the axilla at the apex
Grd II/VI mid diastolic murmur at the apex.
Grd II/VI high pitched early diastolic murmur at aortic area

Liver 1 cm soft not tender	Spleen not palpable	Other systems normal

Analysis

The brisk pulse confirms a hyperdynamic circulation. The wide pulse pressure (a low diastolic) suggests, amongst valvular lesions, a regurgitant lesion. A well-localized apex impulse, which is forceful but ill sustained, suggests a left ventricular hypertrophy, which is probably due to volume overload. (As against this, a forceful and well-sustained apex impulse suggests a pressure overload, while a diffuse not very well-localized apex suggests right ventricular hypertrophy). The apical thrill, and the apical murmur (specifically its character, and the direction of radiation) suggest turbulence of blood flow across the mitral valve during systole, thereby indicating **mitral regurgitation**. Congenital left to right shunts and cardiomyopathy are other lesions that can cause a volume overload of the left ventricle. However, the only shunt that may occasionally be confused with a mitral regurgitation is a ventricular septal defect. The murmur in a VSD is more prominent parasternally than at the apex, and it would not radiate in this manner. Similarly, the nature of the apical findings rule out a cardiomyopathy also. The aortic murmur suggests **additional aortic valve involvement**. The mid diastolic murmur suggests an excessive flow across the mitral valve rather than mechanical mitral stenosis, because there is no presystolic accentuation. Also, S3 at the apex suggests rapid ventricular filling which is usually not possible in the presence of significant mitral stenosis. So we have a dominant MR with a mild AR, without MS. The loud P2 and the narrow split suggest development of **pulmonary hypertension**. Clinically, it may not be easy to differentiate congenital from rheumatic MR, but the presentation of progressive symptoms at 11 years of age and the associated AR favor a **rheumatic etiology**. The history suggestive of cardiac failure 1 month ago, was possibly due to acute carditis. Bacterial endocarditis often presents with high fever and the cardiac failure is difficult to control. Also, the steroid facies denotes that the attending physician made a diagnosis of rheumatic carditis at that time.

At present there is **no** evidence of **active carditis**.

INVESTIGATIONS

Hb 10 gm%   WBC 7,500/c.mm   P 62 % L 35% E 1% M 2%   ESR 45 mm
ASO negative
Chest X-ray - cardiomegaly, LA and LV enlarged
ECG bifid P waves, evidence of LVH
No signs of rheumatic activity on ECG
Echocardiogram – evidence of mitral and aortic regurgitant lesion.
No evidence of bacterial endocarditis.

Analysis

Cardiomegaly with left atrial and ventricular enlargement seen on the chest X-ray denotes a left sided lesion. The bifid P waves in the ECG confirm left atrial hypertrophy; together with left ventricular hypertrophy it favors a left sided valvular lesion such as a mitral and/or an aortic lesion. The echocardiogram confirms the valvular lesions and establishes the absence of active carditis or bacterial endocarditis.

A negative ASO titer is not against a diagnosis of rheumatic valvular disease, as these antibodies can disappear 6 months after an acute attack of rheumatic fever. Anti-DNAse B antibodies last for a longer period and may prove the past streptococcal infection.

FINAL DIAGNOSIS

Rheumatic mitral and aortic regurgitation with left ventricular hypertrophy and pulmonary hypertension, without cardiac failure, in normal sinus rhythm, without active carditis or bacterial endocarditis.

KEY MESSAGES

- Symptoms in cardiac disease result from disturbed physiology and may be shared by many different defects.
- Physical signs denote abnormalities in volume, pressure and blood flow across heart chambers and valves and their functional competence.
- While echocardiogram has revolutionized investigatory modalities in cardiac diseases, chest X-ray and ECG do offer selective information that may not be available with an echocardiogram.

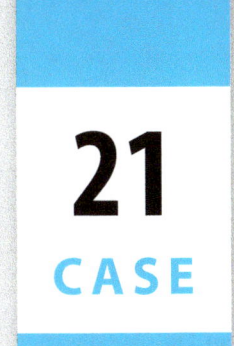

CASE 21

Fever with Chest Pain

■ HISTORY

An 11-year-old male child presented with fever and sudden onset of chest pain for the last 3 days. The fever was high and continuous. The pain in the chest was retrosternal and also in the epigastrium. He preferred to sit up, leaning forwards, the position in which he found some relief. The pain was continuous and was not aggravated by deep breathing or any other factors. It was so severe that he was in agony and could not sleep. It was not relieved even by potent analgesics. He also had intermittent, projectile, non-bilious vomiting.

No history of cough or breathlessness
No other complaints
No relevant past or family history.

Analysis

Retrosternal pain may arise from the esophagus, trachea or pericardium, or it may be an extension of epigastric pain. Typically, epigastric pain may arise from the stomach or liver. **Esophagitis** and **gastritis**, though the most common causes of retrosternal and epigastric pain in children, do not present with fever. The pain in hepatitis is never retrosternal. **Bacterial tracheitis** results in stridor, acute breathlessness and cough. Therefore, this pain seems to originate from the pericardium and could be due to **pericarditis**. As this child feels somewhat relieved when he leans forwards in the sitting posture, it strongly suggests a space-occupying lesion in the mediastinum. In the context of pericarditis, such a space-occupying lesion would be a **pericardial effusion**. It may result from tuberculosis or an acute bacterial infection. It may also be a manifestation of collagen vascular diseases. A pericardial effusion that is caused by **tuberculosis** may lead to pain only in the early stage of the disease (prior to the development of effusion), akin to what happens in a pleural effusion. Agonizing pain and the high fever, not relieved by analgesics/antipyretics may denote a collection of pus, suggesting **purulent pericarditis** or in other words, pericardial empyema. **Collagen vascular disease** is also a possibility, though there are no other symptoms such as a skin rash or joint involvement. It is well-known that collagen vascular diseases may not necessarily present with all their typical symptoms and signs at a given point in time; they may develop sequentially. However, there is no past history of any such pointers in this child.

Intermittent non-bilious vomiting can be a reflex response to any severe inflammatory pathology and may not help in localizing the disease.

■ PHYSICAL EXAMINATION

Fairly built and nourished
Prefers to sit leaning forwards
Temp. 103°F   Pulse 160/min
JVP – raised with prominent "a" waves
CVS – No precordial bulge
Weight 34 kg   Height 142 cm
Looks acutely ill and in agonizing pain
RR 24/min   BP – 90/60 mm
No edema feet or puffiness of face
Apical impulse is diffuse and not localized

Apex beat is in the 5th left intercostal space 1" outside the midclavicular line, diffuse
Left border of the heart does not correspond to and is beyond the apex beat.
Right border of the heart is retrosternal.
Heart sounds are soft and distant.   No gallop or murmur.
Respiratory system normal
Liver 4 cm +, firm, not tender   Spleen not palpable   No free fluid
Other systems normal

Analysis

In view of the enlarged heart (heart borders beyond the apex beat), soft and distant heart sounds, engorged jugular veins and hepatomegaly in a child with high fever and severe retrosternal pain, a diagnosis of a pericardial empyema is almost certain.

■ INVESTIGATIONS

Hb 10 gm%   WBC 24,000/c.mm   P 85% L 13%   E 0% M 2%
Chest X-ray showed cardiomegaly suggestive of a pericardial effusion
Echocardiogram revealed pericardial fluid with multiple loculations and septae suggestive of pus.

■ KEY MESSAGES

- Relief of discomfort by leaning forward in the sitting position suggests a space-occupying lesion in the mediastinum of a solid consistency, like a tumor or organized pus.
- Persistent fever and severe pain indicate acute severe inflammation; if this is caused by infection, it is likely to be a bacterial infection that suppurates.
- Pericardial empyema is a medical emergency. It must be drained with an in situ drainage left in place for a minimum of 48 hours.

CASE 22: Chest Pain with Fever

■ HISTORY

A 9-year-old child presented with chest pain on the right side aggravated by deep breathing, and moderate fever, mild cough and occasional vomiting for 3 days prior to admission. She was treated with some medications the details of which are not known. The chest pain disappeared after 3 days, but the fever persisted.

Analysis

An acute onset of chest pain localized to the right side, along with fever and cough suggests pleural inflammation. It could represent a primary pleural disease or secondary pleural involvement due to either a pneumonia or liver inflammation. As the pain disappeared after 3 days, it is likely that either the child developed an effusion or it could suggest recovery of the primary pathology. Since the child continued to run fever, disappearance of pain does not signify recovery but the development of a **pleural effusion**. Such an effusion is likely to be infective (**tuberculosis** or **empyema** with an underlying pneumonia) or due to **collagen vascular disease**. Vomiting in this child is not significant as it was never the main presenting symptom. Vomiting is often a nonspecific symptom of any acute toxic condition such as a pneumonia.

■ PHYSICAL EXAMINATION

General examination	Chest examination **Right** side	**Left** side
Average build, poorly nourished	3rd, 4th and 5th intercostal space	Normal
Wt 17 kg Ht 125 cm	In axilla and posteriorly	
Temp. 102°F	Impaired note on percussion	
HR 115/min RR 25/min	TVF and VR reduced	
No clubbing No cyanosis	Breath sounds diminished	
No respiratory distress	No foreign sounds	
No chest retractions	Other areas normal	
Other systems normal		

Analysis

Anatomical localization of the disease in such cases is determined by the distribution of chest signs on physical examination. *Lobar distribution* refers to signs restricted to the surface anatomy of a lobe of a lung. A lesion of the *upper lobe* produces signs in the upper half of the chest anteriorly, while that of the *middle lobe* produces signs in the lower half of the chest anteriorly. Similarly, *lower lobe* lesions produce signs mainly on the posterior aspect of the chest. *Pleural distribution* refers to signs distributed equally anteriorly, laterally and posteriorly below a particular intercostal space. A small amount of pleural fluid may produce signs only at the base posteriorly.

In this child the abnormal chest signs are localized to a few intercostal spaces laterally and posteriorly on the right side. As this distribution of signs is neither lobar nor pleural, it is likely to be a **localized pleural or a segmental parenchymal** disease.

Diminished breath sounds without foreign sounds favor a pleural disease. However, parenchymal diseases such as a cavity without communication with a bronchus, or atelectasis with an obstructed bronchus may also produce similar findings. A localized pleural pathology may be in the form of an **encysted pleural effusion** or a **thickened pleura**. Since, this child is running high fever indicative of an active disease, it is unlikely to be thickened pleura, which is a sequelae and not an active disease. Encysted pleural effusion is a possibility. Localized segmental parenchymal disease may be **atelectasis** or a **cavity**. Since there is a history of chest pain suggesting pleural involvement, such a localized parenchymal lesion is likely to be a complication of an acute pleuropneumonia. Atelectasis is not an accompaniment of acute pleuropneumonia and hence is unlikely. (A tubercular pneumonia may be accompanied with a collapse due to pressure by the enlarged mediastinal lymph nodes). Cavitatory lesions include **tuberculosis, lung abscess** or a **congenital cyst**. The short duration of the illness and the absence of accompanying fibrosis rules out tuberculosis. A lung abscess is a complication of an acute pleuropneumonia and is likely in this child. A congenital cyst, if infected, would present in a similar way.

■ INVESTIGATIONS

Hb 11 gm%   WBC 18,000/c.mm   P 82% L 16% E 0% M 2%
Chest X-ray PA view - cavity with thick irregular walls in the right lower zone
No fluid level seen
No pleural effusion or thickened pleura

Analysis

Hemogram is suggestive of an acute bacterial infection in view of the marked neutrophilic leukocytosis with eosinopenia. Thus, the cavity seen on the chest X-ray is likely to be a lung abscess. The thick irregular walls of the cavity favor an acute inflammatory pathology. Absence of a fluid level in the cavity indicates that the cavity has no communication with a bronchus. That is the reason why this child did not demonstrate bronchial breathing and crepitations on physical examination.

■ FINAL DIAGNOSIS

Lung abscess.

■ KEY MESSAGES

- Impaired note on percussion of the chest with absent or diminished breath sounds on auscultation, without foreign sounds suggest either pleural or mediastinal disease. However, such signs may also be mimicked by a parenchymal disease if the lung lesion has no communication with a bronchus.
- Non-lobar and non-pleural distribution of signs in the chest suggests a space-occupying lesion in the pleural cavity (encysted pleural effusion), in the lung parenchyma (lung abscess) or in the mediastinum (tumor arising from any of the mediastinal structures). Clinical distinction between these lesions is difficult and the diagnosis is possible only with imaging studies.

CASE 23

Chest Pain after 2 Weeks of Fever and Cough

■ HISTORY

A 12-year-old male child presented with a history of mild to moderate fever and mild cough for the last 1 month. He developed pain on the right side of the chest 15 days ago which was aggravated by deep breathing. He took some treatment without any relief; the details were not available. Thereafter, he developed high fever for a day and was mildly breathless for which he sought admission to a hospital.

Analysis

Mild to moderate fever and mild cough for a month suggests a *chronic infective process* involving the lung parenchyma. A common cause of such a chronic infection is tuberculosis. However, a partially treated acute bacterial infection may have a prolonged course and may mimic tuberculosis. Chest pain indicates extension of the parenchymal disease to the pleura. Thus, this child has a low-grade infective **pleuropneumonia** on the right side of the chest. Thereafter, he developed mild breathlessness suddenly, which suggests a complication of the pleuropneumonia. It could be in the form of an **empyema** or a pyopneumothorax (if the underlying disease is pyogenic) or **effusion** or **pneumothorax** due to tuberculosis. Simultaneous development of high fever along with the breathlessness may suggest an acute inflammation. This may be due to the sudden development of an empyema or it may be mediated by hypersensitivity in tuberculosis.

■ PHYSICAL EXAMINATION

Comfortable child	Looks sick	Acute on chronic malnutrition
Weight 16 kg	Height 122 cm	Temp. normal
Pulse 95/min	RR 24/min	BP 100/65 mm
No clubbing	No cyanosis	No lymphadenopathy

Resp. system – Impaired note at the base posteriorly, on the right side of the chest
Tidal percussion suggestive of suprahepatic disease over the lower 3 intercostal spaces

Diminished breath sounds	Vesicular breathing	No foreign sounds or pleural rub

Other systems normal

Analysis

The physical examination reveals a malnourished child. Impaired note and diminished breath sounds at the base posteriorly, and absence of foreign sounds suggest a localized **atelectasis** or a **cavity** with an obstructed bronchus or a **small pleural effusion**. If it is a small pleural effusion, it may be a **bacterial empyema**, a **tubercular empyema** or a **tubercular effusion**. Bacterial empyema is a complication of a pneumonia and therefore, the physical signs of the underlying pneumonia would have been prominent. So, it cannot be a bacterial empyema. In terms of physical signs, a tubercular empyema mimics a bacterial empyema and hence, is not possible in this child. Thus, it may be a tubercular pleural effusion. A *typical pleural effusion* is an acute onset hypersensitivity reaction, resulting in a large collection of pleural fluid in a healthy, sensitized child. As this child is malnourished, sensitization may result in a milder reaction, leading to a small pleural effusion. Hence, it is likely to be a tubercular effusion in this child. However, the history suggested a primary parenchymal pathology with subsequent extension to the pleura (**pleuropneumonia**). So, if it is a pleural effusion, it must have been a complication of a primary pneumonia.

If the physical signs indicate a probable atelectasis, it is unlikely to complicate into a pleural lesion by itself. Hence, it must have been a *collapse with consolidation*, in which the physical signs of consolidation may have been masked due to the accompanying collapse. Such a lesion is likely to be due to tuberculosis. (Enlarged mediastinal lymph nodes in tuberculosis lead to a collapse and extension of the tubercular infection into the lung parenchyma results in consolidation). This child must have started with a **tubercular pneumonia** and later developed a **small pleural effusion**.

If these physical signs indicate a localized cavity, it would have resulted from an acute bacterial pleuropneumonia developing into a **lung abscess**.

■ INVESTIGATIONS

Hb 10 gm% WBC 8,500/c.mm P 45% L 48% E 4% M 3%
ESR 75 mm Mt test 10 mm +ve
Chest X-ray showed a small pleural effusion with right middle lobe consolidation.
Pleural tap was performed: the pleural fluid showed a total cell count of 150 cells/c.mm, mostly lymphocytes, proteins 2.5 gm%.

Analysis

The chest X-ray confirms a small pleural effusion with a pneumonia. The pleural fluid shows a mild inflammatory response and rules out empyema. A positive tuberculin test in this malnourished child may favor a diagnosis of tuberculosis. The high ESR indicates an active disease. WBC counts rule out an acute bacterial infection.

■ FINAL DIAGNOSIS

TB pneumonia with a small pleural effusion.

■ COMMENTS

As this child developed a pleural effusion after a month of illness, it indicates a sensitized host but with a milder and a delayed allergic pleural reaction. This kind of a milder allergic response is known in sensitized but malnourished children. Had he been a well-nourished child, he would have developed a sudden onset of high fever and a large effusion leading to acute severe breathlessness. Instead, this malnourished child developed a small pleural effusion and that too late in the course of the illness. However, had he been a non-sensitized child, he would not have developed an allergic reaction at all and would have presented with a pleural rub without an effusion, indicating dry pleuritis. Thus, evolution of tubercular pleuropneumonia depends upon the sensitization status of the host, and the capability of an allergic response, based mainly on the nutritional state.

■ KEY MESSAGES

- Tubercular pleural effusion presents with a wide spectrum of symptoms and physical signs, in terms of both the duration and the degree of symptoms.
- Allergic hypersensitivity reaction in tuberculosis is proportionate to the nutritional state. A well-nourished child mounts an acute, large reaction over a short-time, while a poorly nourished child develops a small response over a long-time.
- Empyema is a complication of bacterial pneumonia and must give rise to clinical and radiological signs of the underlying parenchymal lesion. A tubercular empyema mimics an acute bacterial empyema to a large extent; though the clinical signs of a pneumonia may not be obvious, the radiological signs clearly depict the underlying lung lesion. In a typical tubercular pleural effusion, the underlying lung appears normal both clinically and radiologically as it results from a hypersensitivity reaction to a small subpleural tubercular focus that is unidentifiable.

CASE 24

Hemoptysis in a 10-year-old

■ HISTORY

A 10-year-old male child presented with hemoptysis on 3 different occasions over the last 3 weeks. He brought out a cup full of fresh blood with a bout of cough on the last occasion.

On direct questioning, there was a history of reduced effort tolerance over the last 6 months, and cough off and on.

No history of fever
No history of breathlessness
No history of edema feet or puffiness of face
No past history of joint pain or swelling
No major illness in the past
No history of TB contact.
Family history not contributory.

Analysis

It is important to differentiate hemoptysis from hematemesis. The differentiation may not always be easy. Between the two, hematemesis is the more frequently encountered symptom in children and is commonly due to portal hypertension. This child brought out fresh blood with a bout of cough and hence it is definitely hemoptysis.

Hemoptysis may not be an uncommon symptom in adults, but it is rare in children. In adults, it may commonly be due to cavitatory lung disease or bronchiectasis, less common causes being mitral stenosis, pulmonary hemosiderosis or systemic vasculitis. However, in children, since hemoptysis itself is a rare symptom, all the aforementioned causes are equally rare as a cause of hemoptysis.

A reduced effort tolerance over the last few months suggests gradually decompensating cardiac or pulmonary function. A pulmonary disease with a gradual decompensation is usually a slowly progressive interstitial lung disease. **Pulmonary hemosiderosis** is one such disease that can also cause hemoptysis and therefore needs to be considered. On the other hand, though a **cavitatory disease** or **bronchiectasis** can cause hemoptysis, they are localized diseases that may maintain pulmonary function within normal limits till very late in the disease. Therefore, they will not present with breathlessness; besides, fever and cough would be the predominant associated symptoms in these patients.

When slowly progressive breathlessness is due to a cardiac disease, it suggests gradually developing pulmonary venous hypertension, which is known to cause hemoptysis. Such a disease is classically **mitral stenosis of rheumatic origin**. Though there is no past history suggestive of rheumatic fever in this child, it is possible that the initial attack went unnoticed.

■ PHYSICAL EXAMINATION

Poorly built and nourished child   Comfortable, not sick looking
Wt 27 kg   Ht 124 cm
P 85/min, regular, collapsing nature, all peripheral pulses well felt
RR 25/min   BP 95/45 mm of Hg (Rt upper limb)   Temp. normal
Mild pallor   No clubbing   No cyanosis   No lymphadenopathy
Bones and joints normal
CVS—No precordial bulge
Apex beat localized to 5th left intercostal space just outside midclavicular line, hyperdynamic in nature
Left heart border coincides with cardiac impulse, right border retrosternal
M1 loud, P2 loud and split normally
Mid-diastolic murmur at mitral area
No signs of cardiac failure
Other systems normal.

Analysis

The typical signs of mitral stenosis are evident (Loud M1 and P2 with a mid-diastolic murmur). Mild cardiomegaly (apex just outside the midclavicular line in the left 5th intercostal space) with a hyperdynamic apex and a wide pulse pressure, suggest that it is not an isolated mitral stenosis but there is likely to be a regurgitant lesion as well. In fact in mitral stenosis, one would have expected a normal pulse pressure. So one would expect either mitral regurgitation or aortic regurgitation. As mitral regurgitation would have been obvious with a pansystolic murmur, this child is likely to have an aortic regurgitation, wherein the short early diastolic murmur may be difficult to appreciate, especially if the lesion is mild. Thus, though the major physical signs denote a mitral stenosis, there are subtle signs suggesting an aortic regurgitation.

If this child would have been significantly decompensated, he would have had a tachycardia. A normal heart rate either suggests a subtle decompensation which is not evident at rest, or the patient could be on some treatment.

■ INVESTIGATIONS

Chest X-ray showed signs of pulmonary edema.

ECG revealed right ventricular and left atrial hypertrophy with minimal right ventricular strain.

Echocardiogram confirmed the diagnosis of mitral stenosis with aortic regurgitation.

KEY MESSAGES

- Though rare in children, gradually worsening pulmonary venous hypertension results in hemoptysis.
- Cardiomegaly and wide pulse pressure in a child with mitral stenosis indicates an accompanying regurgitant lesion, even in the absence of any other signs.

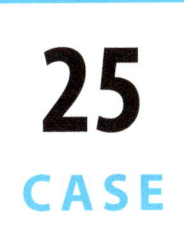

CASE 25

Cyanosis on Crying in an Infant

■ HISTORY

A 3-month-old infant presented with a bluish discoloration of the lips on crying, noticed since the last 2 weeks. He was born of a non-consanguineous marriage after a full-term normal vaginal delivery and the perinatal period was uneventful. He weighed 3 kg at birth. He was put on direct breastfeeds and had gained adequate weight over the first-2 months. There were no complaints until the parents noticed cyanosis on crying.

No history of suck-rest-suck cycle.
No history of sweating.
No history of cough or breathlessness.
No other relevant history.

Analysis

Central cyanosis is commonly due to **respiratory** or **cardiac** diseases. Rarely it may be due to abnormal hemoglobins. Cyanosis in a respiratory disease, is a manifestation of respiratory failure due to a severe disease and is not episodic. On the other hand, cyanosis in a heart disease may be present even with compensated heart function. Therefore, it is likely that this is a heart defect and not cyanosis due to a respiratory disease. Acyanotic congenital heart diseases present with cyanosis only on reversal of the shunt, which usually occurs after a variable but long, symptomatic course and hence is not possible in this child. **Cyanotic congenital heart diseases** can be clinically divided into *two groups*, those with *increased pulmonary blood flow* and those with *normal or decreased pulmonary blood flow*. The *first group* can be further divided into *two subgroups* - those with *abnormal ventriculo-arterial connections* (transposition of great vessels, which usually present with deep cyanosis shortly after birth) and the other subgroup where there is *obligatory complete mixing of blood* (common atrium or ventricle or truncus arteriosus, which usually present with symptoms of failure and subtle but persistent cyanosis). Since, there are no symptoms to suggest cardiac failure or increased pulmonary blood flow and the cyanosis is neither deep nor persistent, it is likely that we are dealing with cyanotic conditions with decreased pulmonary blood flow. Such lesions are characterized by an obstruction to the pulmonary outflow tract coupled with a shunt at some level. It is worthwhile to note at this point that, only an obstruction to the pulmonary outflow tract *without* a shunt as in pulmonary stenosis, is not primarily a cyanotic malformation (except pulmonary atresia, which presents as a neonatal emergency with severe cyanosis and shock). Cyanosis only on crying suggests a transient right to left shunting of blood in a shunt, which is otherwise balanced. A balanced shunt means equal pressures on both the right and the left side of the defect, which can only happen in a large non-restrictive defect. In this situation an "imbalance" can be created due to decreased systemic vascular resistance during crying. In the face of a fixed obstruction to the RV outflow tract, this leads to an extra shunting of blood across the defect, from the right to the left. This is typically known as **Fallot's physiology**, which is classically seen in **Fallot's tetralogy**, but also in some other complex malformations which behave similarly (**DORV with VSD and PS**). Infants with a **long QT interval** may also present with cyanosis on crying; they appear normal at other times and clinical examination does not reveal any abnormality.

■ PHYSICAL EXAMINATION

Fairly built and nourished   Weight 5.2 kg   Length 59 cm   Head Ⓞ 40 cm
Temp. normal   Pulse 110/min   RR 28/min
Central cyanosis present, worsened on crying   No clubbing of nails
No pallor   No edema   No respiratory distress

CVS – no precordial bulge
Apex beat localized to left 4th intercostal space inside the midclavicular line, normal
No thrill but epigastric pulsations felt (at the tip of the finger)
Ejection systolic murmur Gr 3/6 best heard at pulmonary area, but also heard parasternally in the 3rd and 4th space
S1 normal P2 single   No signs of cardiac failure
Liver 2 cm +, soft   Spleen not palpable   Other systems normal

Analysis

Presence of central cyanosis without clubbing of nails suggests recent development of cyanosis, as clubbing would take sometime to develop. Cardiac findings suggest a *silent precordium* without cardiomegaly. Epigastric pulsations suggest right ventricular hypertrophy. The site and the ejection systolic character of the murmur suggest an obstruction at the right ventricular outflow level. However, there has to be a shunt in this situation to explain cyanosis. In the absence of any murmur attributable to a shunt, it is likely that the shunt is non-restrictive and therefore large. Since there is no turbulence across the shunt, there is no murmur. Thus, the findings denote a right ventricular outflow tract obstruction with right ventricular hypertrophy and a large non-restrictive shunt, all of which are consistent with the hemodynamics of a Fallot's physiology, the most common lesion being **tetralogy of Fallot**.

■ INVESTIGATIONS

Hb 15 gm%   WBC normal
Chest X-ray showed oligemic lung fields and a normal heart size
ECG - right ventricular hypertrophy
2D echo confirmed the diagnosis of Fallot's tetralogy.

■ FINAL DIAGNOSIS

Fallot's tetralogy.

■ KEY MESSAGES

- Normal clinical findings at birth and early infancy do not rule out a congenital heart defect.
- Ideally, P2 should be split by D3 of life once pulmonary vascular resistance decreases. Such a finding rules out severe pulmonary stenotic defects but it is not easy to be sure about a split P2 in a neonate, particularly in the presence of a tachycardia.
- Similarly, persistence of left parasternal heave beyond D3 of life indicates right ventricular hypertrophy, a clinical sign that is not too easy to evaluate.

CASE 26

Recent Onset Cyanosis in a 9-year-old

■ HISTORY

A 9-year-old child presented with moderate fever and cough for 3 days to the physician. No other significant symptoms.

On routine physical examination, the doctor noticed mild cyanosis, and his other findings were as follows:

Poorly built and nourished	Weight 15 kg	Height 102 cm	
Temp. 100°F	Pulse 110/min	RR 40/min	BP 100/60 mm
Central cyanosis +	No clubbing		
No respiratory distress	No chest retraction		

RS– Chest bilaterally symmetrical, normal breath sounds, no foreign sounds
CVS – normal heart size and sounds, no murmur, no signs of cardiac failure
Other systems normal.

In view of the central cyanosis, he was referred to a cardiologist for further investigations. Results of the tests were as follows:

Hb 15.5 gm%	Microcytosis +	Hypochromia +
WBC 8,000/c.mm	P 62% L 34% E 4%	
Chest X-ray normal	No cardiomegaly	ECG normal 2 D Echo normal

Since no obvious cardiac abnormality could be detected, a diagnosis of pulmonary A-V fistula was considered on the basis of central cyanosis and he was further investigated.

Cardiac catheterization, angiography and radionuclide scan ruled out such a possibility. At this stage, the child was referred for an opinion.

■ PHYSICAL EXAMINATION

The physical findings were confirmed to be the same, i.e., the only positive findings were a mild central cyanosis, mild tachypnea (RR 40/min) and significant growth retardation (weight age 3 years and height age 4.5 years).

Analysis

Accidental detection of central cyanosis is mostly **cardiac** in origin, though at times it could be due to abnormal hemoglobin. **Hemoglobinopathies** that cause cyanosis can be hereditary or acquired. Hereditary disorders like **HbM** disease usually manifest early in life, though occasionally they can manifest later. **Acquired methemoglobinemia** (a result of exposure to toxic substances) is more common in infancy than in older children. In a hemoglobinopathy, except cyanosis, the children are not very symptomatic and they thrive well unlike this child. Cyanosis due to **cyanotic congenital heart disease** is often detected early in childhood. Conditions like an Ebstein's anomaly or a "pink" Fallot may occasionally be detected so late. However, they do not present with such a marked failure to thrive. Similarly, though a child with a total anomalous pulmonary venous drainage may present late, a completely asymptomatic infancy almost rules it out. It is also important to note that such cardiac anomalies exist since birth irrespective of the age of clinical presentation and hence in such patients, central cyanosis is accompanied with clubbing of nails. This child had no clubbing in spite of central cyanosis suggesting that the cyanosis must have begun rather recently. When acyanotic congenital heart diseases present with cyanosis due to **eisenmengerization** and reversal of shunt, it is preceded by a highly symptomatic period in early childhood, which is not so in this case. Hence, it is most unlikely to be a cardiac disease.

Central cyanosis in a **pulmonary disease** indicates respiratory failure. It is usually seen as a late manifestation in acute lung diseases. However, in **chronic slowly progressive respiratory diseases**, the initial respiratory dysfunction may manifest as exertional dyspnea, which may be missed in a routine history, and a subtle onset of respiratory failure may occasionally present as mild cyanosis with minimal distress at rest. In a child of this age, the respiratory rate of 40/min at rest is definitely abnormal. He may have been well compensated till recently, has recently started decompensating and hence has developed a mild cyanosis lately. It will take a few months for clubbing to develop.

On leading questions, it was clear that over the last 3 years, this child was reluctant to play and would get unduly tired on walking. However, the parents did not consider it serious enough to seek medical attention. This suggests a slowly progressive chronic lung disease. It has also reflected in his stunting of growth and under nutrition.

In the absence of cough, airway disease can be ruled out. Hypoxia (as denoted by cyanosis) suggests desaturation and in the absence of an airway disease, points to an alveolar or interstitial pathology. Since, there are no parenchymal signs on clinical examination, alveolar disease is unlikely. **Interstitial lung diseases** are known to present with relatively minimal physical signs (fine crepitations) in comparison to the functional derangement. Hence, absence of abnormal physical findings on chest examination and a normal plain chest X-ray may not rule out such a diagnosis.

■ INVESTIGATIONS

CT scan of chest showed evidence of interstitial lung disease.
Lung biopsy indicated probability of allergic alveolitis.

■ FINAL DIAGNOSIS

Interstitial lung disease.

KEY MESSAGES

- Central cyanosis without clubbing of nails indicates *recently developed* cardiac or pulmonary cyanosis, or abnormal hemoglobins.
- When the presenting symptoms are of a short duration and apparently acute, and the physical findings suggest a chronic disease, it is mandatory to enquire a detailed history to bring out occult symptoms.
- Slowly progressive symptoms are often not complained of by the patients and need to be found out on direct leading questions.
- Physical examination of the chest and the plain chest X-ray may be apparently normal in interstitial lung diseases. CT scan of the chest would confirm such a disease.

CASE 27

Occasional Choking Episodes in an 8-year-old Child

■ HISTORY

An 8-year-old child presented with a history of occasional choking episodes while drinking; there was no problem while eating solid food. He remained well between episodes. The first episode occurred around 4 years of age. During such an episode, he would cough violently which would last for a variable period but resolve by itself. He has also had two episodes of lower respiratory tract infection (LRTI) after an episode of choking which required hospitalization and antibiotic therapy. On direct questioning, choking occurs as soon as he swallows, without significant vomiting, and there is no burning sensation in the upper chest.

Analysis

Choking episodes while drinking suggest aspiration into the airways; difficulty in swallowing solid food would indicate dysphagia. **Swallowing incoordination** is less likely in this child as there is no evidence of a neurological disorder in the form of delayed development or lower cranial nerve paresis. Moreover, such episodes in this child are infrequent with normal intervening periods. **Gastroesophageal reflux disease (GERD)** at this age is secondary to a disorder such as achalasia or chalasia. The absence of a burning sensation rules out esophagitis that usually accompanies GERD. **Esophageal obstruction** due to extrinsic compression such as a vascular ring may not be episodic and would also present with vomiting and cough. A **functional** disorder may be present erratically, but this child has had two episodes of LRTI needing hospitalization, and so such a probability is unlikely. The fact that such episodes occur infrequently but then lead to significant consequences, suggests a defect that seems to be sporadic in presentation. There is no clue as to its exact nature after analyzing the history and we may expect a surprise.

■ PHYSICAL EXAMINATION

He looked comfortable without any abnormal physical findings. When asked to drink water, he suddenly choked with a bout of cough.

Analysis

It was clear that something was leading to aspiration that required investigations. The site of the problem appeared to be close to the proximal part of the food pipe (esophagus) beyond the oropharynx. Physical examination could not show this hidden cause and figuring it out would need invasive investigations.

■ INVESTIGATIONS

Routine tests were normal as expected. Cine-esophagoscopy failed to demonstrate any defect. Thereafter, a bronchoscopy was done that picked up an H-type of tracheoesophageal fistula.

■ FINAL DIAGNOSIS

H-type tracheoesophageal fistula.

■ KEY MESSAGES

Difficulty in swallowing solid food but not liquids, suggests esophageal obstruction, while difficulty in swallowing liquids but not solids indicate a neurological disorder or an anatomical defect. Aspiration of ingested liquid can be suspected clinically, but it is not easy to prove the cause of aspiration. Common causes such as GERD and palatopharyngeal incoordination are not easy to confirm even with the help of several tests. Tracheoesophageal fistula must be suspected early and confirmed radiologically or through bronchoscopy.

■ RELEVANT INFORMATION

Tracheoesophageal fistula is often suspected in neonate. If the esophageal end of the fistula is at a higher level than the tracheal end, aspiration results in acute respiratory distress with severe hypoxia. If the tracheal end is at a higher level, air can accumulate in the stomach and these babies are present with abdominal distension. Such a neonate may also present with respiratory distress in which bag-mask ventilation must be avoided. However, in the case of H type of fistula, if both ends are at the same level, aspiration episodes may be delayed and also less frequent. Further, the length of the esophagus and trachea may not increase in the same proportion during the period of growth and hence, such a defect may present anytime later in childhood.

CASE 28

Difficulty in Feeding in an Infant

■ HISTORY

A 3-month-old infant born after a full-term normal delivery, presented with feeding difficulty and irritability noticed a month ago. The feeding difficulty had worsened over the month, and he had now developed fast breathing and sweating. He used to feed well and had gained adequate weight in the first 6 weeks, but thereafter he started faltering in weight.

Analysis

The complaint of "feeding difficulty" needs to be probed further. The first step is to assess whether the infant wants to feed or not, it may be that he has a **poor appetite**. Once anorexia is ruled out, "feeding difficulty" could mean **pain** due to mouth ulcers (oral thrush), breathlessness due to **cardiac** or **respiratory** disease or swallowing incoordination due to a **neurological** disorder. On direct questioning, the feeding difficulty turned out to be due to fast breathing. In this case, the irritability could be due to hypoxia. The next step is to differentiate between primary cardiac and respiratory disease. **Congenital lobar emphysema** can present in a similar way, but the symptoms should have come up in the first few weeks soon after the birth. Of course, it is possible that the initial fast breathing, being mild, may have been missed. Sweating may suggest a cardiac disease and one must find out whether there was also a typical suck-rest-suck cycle; it would favor a cardiac disorder. **Congenital acyanotic heart disease** with a left to right shunt would have presented with cough (along with fast breathing), while severe stenotic lesions would have presented with acute onset cardiac failure; mild stenotic lesions would not have presented so early; thus, it is most probably a **myocardial disease**. In view of the progression of symptoms over a month, it is unlikely to be an acquired disorder, such as acute viral myocarditis. **Cardiomyopathy** can have a variable age of onset depending on its etiology and therefore must considered. Another probability at this age is a congenital lesion that causes ischemia and subsequent dysfunction of the myocardium, like an **anomalous origin of the left coronary artery from the pulmonary artery (ALCAPA)**.

■ PHYSICAL EXAMINATION

Infant looked sick
Wt 4.2 kg (birth weight 2.5 kg)   Length 57 cm   HC 39 cm
HR 140/m   RR 30/m   BP 58/38 mm Hg
Precordial pulsations, Apex Beat outside MCL in 5th ICS, systolic murmur at mitral area, P2 N
Liver 3F+, span 8 cm   Spleen not palpable
Other systems are normal.

Analysis

This infant has failed to thrive. He has gained 1.7 kg in weight and around 7 cm in length (assuming a normal length at birth). This suggests that the onset of the disease was not at or soon after birth but a bit later. The infant has signs of cardiomegaly with cardiac failure. The precordial pulsations and the systolic murmur at the apex may suggest a regurgitant lesion at the mitral valve, but the murmur is not conducted to the axilla. Besides, a congenital valvular lesion is unlikely to be so fastly progressive. Hence, these signs may be due to an enlarged heart itself. Hence findings favor a myocardial disease like a dilated cardiomyopathy which could be either genetic in origin or could be secondary to other causes, one of them being ischemic myocardial damage due to ALCAPA.

■ INVESTIGATIONS

CBC, ESR normal
2D echocardiogram confirmed enlarged heart with mitral valve regurgitation
Angiography confirmed ALCAPA

■ FINAL DIAGNOSIS

Anomalous origin of Left Coronary Artery from Pulmonary Artery (ALCAPA)
Surgical correction of the defect led to a complete cure

■ KEY MESSAGES

> Myocardial disorders must be kept in mind when a child presents with cardiac disease. The myocardium is affected by generalized muscle disorders [Duchenne muscular dystrophy (DMD)], vascular diseases (Kawasaki disease), metabolic diseases (mitochondrial disorders), electrolyte disturbances (hypocalcemia, hypokalemia, or hyperkalemia), infections, sepsis, etc., besides acute viral infection.

■ RELEVANT INFORMATION

The anomalous origin of the left coronary artery from the pulmonary artery results in poor perfusion of the left-sided myocardium and mitral valve as they are perfused by relatively desaturated blood under low pressure. Low-pressure results in the backflow of blood into the pulmonary artery and worsens hypoperfusion of the left ventricle and the mitral valve. Thus, the initial symptoms may be transient while feeding or crying, but thereafter, as the myocardial ischemia and mitral valve insufficiency increase, the infant presents with congestive cardiac failure with tachypnea, irritability, and poor feeding, classically around 2–3 months of age. The irritability and crying episodes may be mistaken as intestinal colic if approached casually. This condition is amenable to surgical correction and thereafter the infant could lead a normal life. So, this condition should always be kept in mind when faced with myocardial affection in early life.

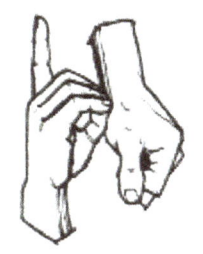
The origin

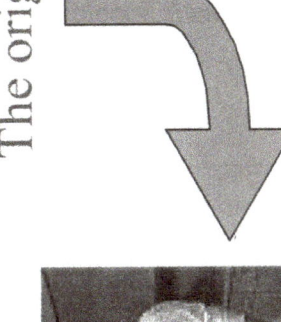
The progress

History of Medicine

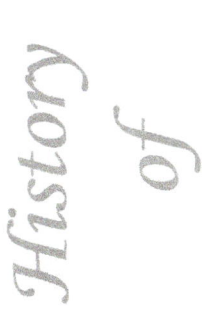

Where do we go from here

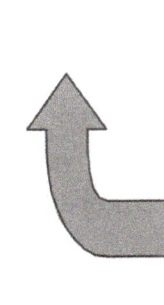
The dependence

History repeats itself?....Looks like it does!

Clinical Hematology

BACK TO BASICS

Anemia

Anemia is best assessed as pallor visualized on the ventral surface of the palm. The degree of pallor is difficult to judge on physical examination. Clinically, anemia can be classified as follows.

	Deficiency	Hemolysis	Hemorrhage	Marrow disease
Onset	Chronic	Mostly chronic Rarely acute	Manifest- acute Occult - chronic	Mostly acute Rarely chronic
Occurrence	Acquired	Mostly congenital	Acquired	Acquired
Liver/spleen	None	+/- in acute ++ in chronic	None	None in aplasia ++ in leukemia
Platelets	Reduced in B12 def. Increased in iron def.	Normal Reduced in Hypersplenism	Increased	Reduced
Leucocytes	Normal	Increased (normoblasts counted)	Normal	Reduced in aplasia Increased in Leukemia

Examination of the peripheral blood smear and evaluation of the mean corpuscular volume (MCV) and the red cell distribution width (RDW) helps in diagnosing the cause of anemia.

MCV low		MCV normal		MCV high	
RDW Normal	RDW High	RDW Normal	RDW High	RDW Normal	RDW High
Thal trait Chr. disease	Iron def. Thal major	Chr. disease Spherocytosis Hemorrhage	Mixed def. Sideroblastic anemia	Aplasia	B12 def Folate def.

■ BLEEDING DISORDER

Platelet disorder - superficial bleed, purpura, spontaneous
Coagulation defect - Deep bleed - hematoma/hemarthrosis, provoked

SCREENING TESTS

Platelet count	PT	PTT	Disease
Reduced	Normal	Normal	ITP/aplastic anemia/leukemia
Reduced	Increased	Increased	DIC
Normal	Increased	Normal	Liver disease/Vit K deficiency
Normal	Normal	Increased	Coagulation defect
Normal	Increased	Increased	Advanced liver failure
Normal	Normal	Normal	Factor XIII def/vascular purpura/Battered baby syndrome/fictitious

PERIPHERAL BLOOD SMEAR EXAMINATION

This is the most useful part of blood examination in hematology. It helps identify the cause of anemia by recognizing the abnormal cell morphology. The following are examples of abnormal cell morphology:

Schistocytes or fragmented cells (microangiopathic hemolytic anemia)
Spherocytes (hereditary spherocytosis – uniform in size and density,
   autoimmune hemolytic anemia – varying size and density)
Sickle shaped cells (sickle cell disease)
Target cells (hemolytic anemia)
Stippled red blood cells (nonspecific but may suggest lead poisoning)
Increased polychromasia (reticulocytosis)
Ghost or bite cells (G6PD deficiency)

It is important to note that normal red cell morphology does not rule out hematological disease.

CASE 29

Ecchymosis in an Infant

■ HISTORY

A 2-month-old male child presented with ecchymotic patches over the skin noticed since the last 2 days. There were no other symptoms. He had been feeding and growing well.

- No history of bleeding from any other site
- Born after full term normal delivery
- Antenatal and perinatal history normal
- No history of fever or drug ingestion
- Birth weight 3.2 kg
- Exclusively breastfed

He was administered vit K injection on D1 as a routine prophylaxis.

Analysis

Ecchymotic patches may represent platelet, coagulation or a vascular disorder. If petechiae are present, they definitely indicate a platelet or a vascular disorder, but their absence does not necessarily rule out these disorders. Platelet disorders that are usually seen at this age are the ones that are seen in sick infants as in **disseminated intravascular coagulation, sepsis** or **purpura fulminans**. Less commonly seen are congenital disorders like **platelet functional disorders** or bone marrow failure syndromes, which may evolve over time and therefore the infant may not necessarily appear sick at the time of presentation. These could be in the form of isolated thrombocytopenia as in congenital **a megakaryocytic thrombocytopenia**, or as a part of pancytopenia as in **Fanconi's anemia**. An acquired platelet disorder like **idiopathic thrombocytopenic purpura** is rare in early infancy. A congenital vascular disorder may be a part of a connective tissue disorder such as **Ehlers-Danlos syndrome,** which is a heterogeneous group of disorders with varied clinical presentations. However, these infants are usually normal at birth and gradually develop various clinical features over time. A coagulation disorder is usually characterized by deep bleeds, which are generally induced by injury, though some **congenital coagulation disorders** may present even at birth such as factor XIII deficiency or a severe form of hemophilia. **Vitamin K deficiency** can also manifest at birth or within a couple of days thereafter, or it may manifest as late as 2–3 months of age, often with an intracranial bleed. However, this child has been administered vitamin K at birth, and he was born after a full term, therefore vitamin K deficiency is most unlikely. An **acquired disorder of coagulation** system may result from chronic diarrhea, prolonged antibiotic therapy or liver dysfunction. In the absence of diarrhea and antibiotic therapy in this infant, it may be a **liver disease** though there are no other symptoms of liver disease such as jaundice or clay colored stools. Finally, a **battered baby syndrome** may be kept in mind, especially if there is no clue towards any organic disease on physical examination and investigations.

■ PHYSICAL EXAMINATION

Comfortable	Not sick looking	
Weight 4.4 kg	Length 57 cm	Head O 39 cm
Temp. normal	HR 110/min	RR 30/min
No pallor	No cyanosis	No icterus
Ecchymotic patches scattered over the skin		No purpuric spots

No marks of any physical injury
No mucosal bleeds or bleeding from any other site
No hyperelasticity of skin and subcutaneous tissue

Liver 2 cm + soft, not tender   Spleen just palpable
Other systems normal

Analysis

Besides ecchymotic patches on the skin, the only other abnormal finding is a suboptimum weight gain. This infant has gained 1.2 kg in a 2 month period on exclusive breastfeeding. Failure of adequate weight gain while on exclusive breastfeeding may suggest **inadequate feeding** or occult organ dysfunction. However, there is no history of excessive crying or a demand for frequent or prolonged feeds to suggest inadequate feeding. Thus, it is likely to be **occult organ dysfunction**; in view of the ecchymosis, it may be either of the liver or the bone marrow. Since congenital **bone marrow aplasia** can evolve over time, it cannot be ruled out. Liver diseases at this age could be broadly divided into **neonatal hepatitis** or **biliary atresia**. While neonatal hepatitis usually presents with jaundice, it may occasionally manifest with an isolated disturbance of a single liver function; other hepatic dysfunctions may follow over time. However, biochemical evidence of liver dysfunction would be obvious in such a case. On the other hand, while biliary obstruction may lead to vitamin K deficiency and ecchymosis due to poor absorption of fat-soluble vitamins, it would essentially present with jaundice, high colored urine and clay colored stools. Ecchymosis is a late manifestation of biliary obstruction. Hence, biliary obstruction is ruled out in this infant.

Since, there is no evidence of any physical injury anywhere, it is unlikely to be a battered baby.

■ INVESTIGATIONS

Hb 11 gm%	WBC normal	Platelet count normal
PT 25 sec control 12 sec	PTT normal	
Serum bilirubin 4 mgm%	Direct 1.2 mgm%	
ALT/AST moderately increased		Gamma GT mildly increased
Serum proteins 6 gm%	Albumin 3.5 gm%	Alk. phos mildly increased

Abdominal USG – enlarged liver, patent biliary tract
Viral serology negative   Torch titers negative

Analysis

Direct bilirubinemia with raised liver enzymes suggests neonatal hepatitis. Primary biliary disease is ruled out by demonstration of a patent biliary tract on abdominal USG.

Liver biopsy is necessary to confirm the diagnosis of neonatal hepatitis.

Viral serology including Torch titers are negative; however viral serology is difficult to interpret and hence viral infections cannot be ruled out. Further investigations may also be necessary to rule out metabolic disorders or other rare conditions such as alpha 1 antitrypsin deficiency.

■ FINAL DIAGNOSIS

Neonatal hepatitis.

■ KEY MESSAGES

- Icterus may not be evident in neonates and young infants until the serum bilirubin rises to > 5 mgm%.
- A liver disease may manifest initially with an isolated disturbance of a single function, though biochemical tests would prove disturbances in other functions as well. While jaundice obviously points to a possible liver disease, isolated symptoms such as behavior disturbance, edema, hematemesis or ecchymosis may be the only initial manifestation, before rest of the symptoms and signs appear.

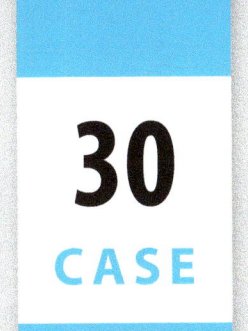

CASE 30

Ecchymosis in an Older Child

■ HISTORY

A 7-year-old male child born of nonconsanguineous parents presented with spontaneous bluish green patches noticed all over the body since the last 20 days. He was reported to be a healthy child till the onset of this problem. New patches appeared over the first 1 week and then stopped. Thereafter, the old ones have been changing color.

- No history of bleeding from any other site
- No history of fever
- No history of any recent illness, drug consumption or vaccination
- No history of similar illness in the past
- No history of excessive bleeding after trauma in the past
- No relevant past or family history.

Analysis

Spontaneously appearing bluish green patches, which change color over time, suggest ecchymosis. A **fixed drug eruption** can be mistaken for ecchymosis as it is also a colored patch on the skin. However, it is blackish in color and fades over a long-time. It is due to a drug reaction and is self-limiting. Ecchymosis may result from platelet, vascular or a coagulation disorder. If petechiae are present, they definitely indicate a platelet or a vascular disorder, but its absence does not necessarily rule it out. Coagulation disorders usually lead to deep bleeds like muscle or visceral hematomas, or joint bleeds. However, ecchymosis may be the only manifestation of a coagulation disorder as well. Thus in this child, ecchymosis may represent any of the bleeding disorders, congenital or acquired. While the absence of any past or family history favors an acquired disease, a congenital disease cannot be ruled out completely. But if we consider a **congenital coagulation disorder**, since it is presenting for the first time at 7 years of age, it favors a mild deficiency of one of the coagulation factors, and therefore should have developed symptoms *only after trauma* (however mild) and *not spontaneously*. On the other hand, a severe deficiency would have presented earlier in life. Therefore, it is less likely to be a congenital coagulation disorder. If it is an **acquired coagulation factor defect**, it may result from vitamin K deficiency due to chronic diarrhea, prolonged antibiotic therapy or liver disease. There is no history of diarrhea or prolonged antibiotic therapy in this child. Liver disease may rarely present with ecchymosis as the only initial manifestation but not at this age. **Congenital vascular disorders** are uncommon; an **acquired vascular disorder** is a part of a systemic vasculitis in which other organs may be involved and the child is not well (e.g., Henoch-Schönlein purpura), and thus is also unlikely.

Therefore, if it is a platelet disorder, since majority of the clinically encountered platelet disorders are acquired (and there is no past or family history), this child may have an **acquired platelet disorder**. These could be due to decreased production as in a **bone marrow disease** or increased destruction of platelets as in idiopathic thrombocytopenic purpura (**ITP**) or **hypersplenism**. (Most functional platelet disorders are congenital). As this child is otherwise asymptomatic, it is more likely to be idiopathic thrombocytopenic purpura (ITP).

■ PHYSICAL EXAMINATION

Fairly built and nourished child "Well" child (not sick looking)
Weight 24 kg   Height 116 cm
Temp. normal   HR 90/min   RR 24/min   BP 95/65 mm
Ecchymotic patches of various sizes scattered over the skin   Few petechial spots
No pallor   No bony tenderness
No evidence of bleeding from any other site
Systemic examination normal

Analysis

As mentioned earlier, petechiae always signify a **platelet** or a **vascular** defect. Petechiae predominate, and ecchymotic spots are relatively less widespread in vascular purpura. Often these are *palpable purpura*. A platelet function disorder like **von Willebrand's** disease cannot be ruled out completely, but usually gum bleeds and epistaxis are common associated manifestations. A bone marrow disease is almost ruled out, as this child does not look "sick", and is also not anemic. In the absence of splenomegaly, hypersplenism is ruled out.

Absence of a history of preceding viral infection, recent drug intake or vaccination does not rule out an immune thrombocytopenia (**ITP**).

■ INVESTIGATIONS

Hb 11 gm %   TLC 10,200   N 63 E 3 L 34
PS – microcytic hypochromic anemia
Platelets significantly reduced on smear, platelet clumps seen, megaplatelets seen
Pl count – 35,000/cmm
Bone marrow aspiration normal.

Analysis

Isolated thrombocytopenia without anemia or leukopenia almost rules out a bone marrow disease. Though the cause of thrombocytopenia is not apparent on these investigations, increased production of platelets (in response to peripheral destruction) is confirmed by the presence of megaplatelets on the peripheral smear, indicating a normally responsive bone marrow.

Immune mediated thrombocytopenia may be diagnosed by assessing platelet antibodies, though it is not routinely indicated in clinically suspected self-limiting ITP.

FINAL DIAGNOSIS

Idiopathic thrombocytopenic purpura.

KEY MESSAGE

Majority of the clinically encountered platelet disorders are acquired, while majority of the clinically encountered coagulation disorders are congenital.

RELEVANT INFORMATION

- Platelet count as determined by coulter counter should always be correlated with the adequacy of platelets on smear. A rough platelet count can be estimated by number of platelets per oil emulsion field (average of 20 fields)   X 10,000
- Megaplatelets (giant platelets) on peripheral smear indicate rapid turnover of platelets and therefore increased marrow production. It therefore rules out bone marrow disease and favors peripheral destruction.
- Platelet clumps rule out a platelet function disorder.
- If steroid treatment is contemplated in ITP, a bone marrow examination is a prerequisite to rule out leukemia.
- "Purpura" is a general term describing a bleeding disorder. Petechiae are intradermal bleeds up to 3 mm in size. Ecchymosis are larger than 3 mm and are subcutaneous bleeds.
- Petechiae do not blanch on pressure while mosquito bites do. In spider nevi, if a pin head is used to compress the central arteriole, the feeder vessels will blanch. Spider nevi are uncommon in pediatrics.
- Common drugs leading to petechiae are aspirin, antiepileptics, antihistamines, cephalosporins, quinine.

CASE 31

Bluish Patches in an 8-year-old Child

■ HISTORY

An 8-year-old male child presented with spontaneously occurring recurrent bluish patches over the skin for the last 2 weeks. There were no other symptoms, nor any bleeding from any other site. There was no history of any preceding illness or any drug intake. There was no significant past or personal history, nor any family history of a bleeding disorder. He had grown normally and studied in 3rd standard.

Analysis

Spontaneously occurring bluish patches on the skin may indicate a fixed drug reaction, or ecchymosis that can be caused by a platelet, vascular or a coagulation factor disorder. Congenital **coagulation factor deficiency is unlikely** as it usually presents with bleeding in deep structures triggered by trauma and not as isolated ecchymosis. Acquired coagulation factor defects arise from liver diseases or vitamin K deficiency as a result of intestinal malabsorption or prolonged antibiotic use. There is no history suggestive of any such events in this child.

Since the history does not suggest any petechial spots, it is unlikely to be immune thrombocytopenic purpura **(ITP)**. However, **thrombasthenia** and **vascular disorders**, are possible. Though these are congenital disorders, they can present at a later age like this, and in children who are previously healthy. These are insidious in onset and hence may present only with ecchymosis, unlike ITP which is acute and therefore usually manifests with petechiae as well.

It is unlikely to be **child abuse** because such lesions are painful; besides, an 8-year-old is likely to resist and also report such incidents.

■ PHYSICAL EXAMINATION

Comfortable child	Weight 28 kg	Height 123 cm
Temp normal	Pulse 82/min	RR 20/min
Ecchymosis +	No purpura	No pallor
No lymphadenopathy	Bones and joints normal	Liver just palpable, soft
Spleen not palpable	Other systems normal	

Analysis

A comfortable healthy child with isolated ecchymotic spots without purpura, pallor and hepatosplenomegaly favors a diagnosis of platelet function disorder, as other disorders seem to be ruled out.

■ INVESTIGATIONS

Hb 12 gm%
Platelets 2.4 Lakh/c.mm
Platelet function tests normal
PT normal

WBC 6,500/c.mm
Peripheral smear normal
Thrombin test normal
aPTT normal

P 62 L 36 E 2

Analysis

The above-mentioned tests are normal and therefore do not explain the cause of the bleeding disorder in this child. Child abuse is unlikely as this is not the form of abuse at this age and he would have complained about it. So most likely this child is inflicting injuries on himself to achieve some purpose.

■ FINAL DIAGNOSIS

Munchausen syndrome by proxy.

■ KEY MESSAGE

Bluish patches on skin in a healthy 8-year-old child rules out coagulation factor defect while platelet disorders are more likely. Amongst all common bleeding disorders, platelet function abnormality is the least common, but was nevertheless considered in this child because other platelet disorders seemed less likely. However, when tests ruled them out, one had to think "out of box". Details of social history would help arrive at possibility of self-inflicted injuries that would further necessitate psychological evaluation.

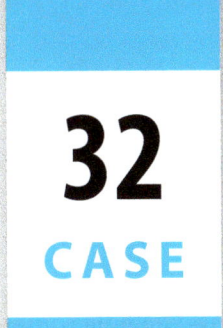

CASE 32

Ecchymosis with Fever

■ HISTORY

An 8-year-old female child presented with fever for a month and spontaneous bruises over different parts of the body for the last 20 days. The fever was moderate to high and was continuous. There was no bleeding from any other sites. When the patient was taken to a district hospital 15 days ago, the parents were told that she was quite pale and would require a blood transfusion. She was investigated and treated with some medicines, though for some reason (which the parents were unable to explain) she was not transfused. Since she did not feel better even after 2 weeks of treatment, she was referred to a tertiary center. The details of the treatment were not available.

No history of any drug consumption prior to the onset of this illness.
No past history of a similar disorder
No family history of a bleeding disorder

Analysis

This febrile child has presented with anemia and bruises over the skin. This *seems to* suggest a suppression of all the three cell lines due to a **bone marrow disorder**. *Bicytopenia* is definitely evident clinically (anemia and bruises), and it should always be *considered as pancytopenia* and investigated accordingly. However, in such cases fever may or may not represent affection of the WBC series; it may often be due to the primary disease itself and not due to infection resulting from leukopenia. Disorders affecting two or three cell lines could be either infiltrative diseases (like **leukemia, myelodysplasia** or **myelofibrosis**) or **marrow aplasia** (due to viral infections or drugs). Though an **HIV** infection may occasionally present with isolated thrombocytopenia almost mimicking an ITP, it is unusual to present with marrow aplasia alone, i.e., it would manifest with involvement of multiple systems.

■ PHYSICAL EXAMINATION

Poorly built and nourished
Weight 15 kg
Temp. 102°F
Severe pallor
Insignificant cervical lymph nodes, small, discrete
Bones and joints normal

Looks "sick"
Height 103 cm
Pulse 130/min
Petechiae and ecchymosis present
No bony tenderness

RR 35/min

No other lymphadenopathy
No skin pigmentation

Hypertrophy of gums, not bleeding on pressure, no dental caries
Liver just palpable   Spleen not palpable
Other systems normal

Analysis

Pallor and ecchymosis suggest that it is a primary hematological disease. Anemia without hepatosplenomegaly is either a deficiency anemia or marrow failure. Vitamin **B$_{12}$ deficiency anemia** may present with thrombocytopenia, but fever is not a presenting feature and the child does not appear "sick". Besides, there may be pigmentation of knuckles suggestive of B12 deficiency. Thus, **marrow failure** is more likely. Absence of hepatosplenomegaly and lymphadenopathy may be against an **acute lymphatic leukemia,** and favors an **aplastic anemia**. However, gum hypertrophy in the absence of dental caries and a poor oral hygiene may suggest **acute myeloid leukemia** of M4 type. In severely malnourished children (this child is malnourished), gum hypertrophy may be due to a deficiency of vitamin C, i.e., **scurvy**. However, hypertrophied gums in scurvy bleed with pressure. Besides, patients with scurvy do not usually present with a severe anemia. Other causes of gum hypertrophy include drugs such as **phenytoin** or **cyclosporine**. However, the details of the drugs consumed are not available in this child.

■ INVESTIGATIONS

Hb 4.8 gm   TLC 5,300/c.mm   N 03 L 92 E 05
Platelets 70,000/c.mm ESR 103 mm at end of 1 hour
PS – normocytic, normochromic anemia, few microcytes seen
Retic 1% (corrected retic 0.3%)
MCV 78 fL   MCH 27 pg   MCHC 31 g/dL   RDW 14%
Bone marrow aspiration: Hypocellular marrow

Analysis

Though the total leukocyte count is within the normal range, marked neutropenia in association with anemia and thrombocytopenia obviously indicates a pancytopenia. The corrected reticulocyte count is quite low and is consistent with a poor marrow response. The indices also suggest a normocytic anemia, though a few microcytes are reported on peripheral smear examination. Hypocellularity of the marrow aspirate needs to be confirmed with a trephine biopsy because a dilute aspirate can simulate hypocellularity. In addition, one can miss a diagnosis of aplasia on aspirate alone, because one may hit the pockets of normo or even hypercellularity that exist even in an aplastic marrow.

■ FURTHER INVESTIGATION

Diagnosis was confirmed by bone marrow biopsy. The gum hypertrophy in this child was because the patient was being treated with cyclosporine.

FINAL DIAGNOSIS

Bone marrow aplasia.

KEY MESSAGES

- While the normal reticulocyte count is around 1%, one needs to look at the corrected reticulocyte count (or reticulocyte index) to accurately judge the response of the marrow to any severe anemia.
- Marrow aspiration needs to be supplemented with a trephine biopsy to confirm the diagnosis of aplasia.

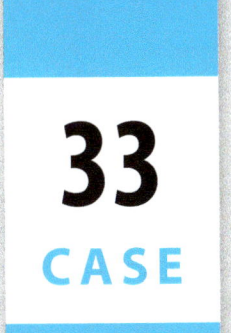

CASE 33: Ecchymosis with Joint Swellings

■ HISTORY

A 4-year-old male child presented with a painful swelling of the right knee without any apparent injury, since the last 4 days. There was no history of fever or any other associated symptoms. On direct questioning, though there was no history of any petechiae, an isolated ecchymotic spot was noticed at about the same time on the elbow.

- No history of sore throat or diarrhea in the recent past
- No history of any ocular symptoms
- No history of any other joint swellings, now or in the past
- No history of excessive bleeding from the umbilical cord at birth
- No history of epistaxis
- No family history of similar disorder (including siblings)

Analysis

An acute painful swelling of a single large joint suggests **arthritis**. In the absence of any fever whatsoever, an acute **infective** pathology is unlikely. While it could be a non-infective inflammatory disorder (in evolution) like a **rheumatic** arthritis or any other **rheumatological** disorder, the ecchymotic spot on the elbow remains unexplained. In children, trauma may not be reported, particularly if the toddler is alone at the time of sustaining the injury. In that case, an injury could explain both the ecchymosis and the joint swelling (**traumatic** arthritis). However, if there is definitely no injury, then in this afebrile child one may even consider a **coagulation disorder** resulting in both hemarthrosis and ecchymosis.

■ PHYSICAL EXAMINATION

Fairly built and nourished
Weight 17 kg
Temp/pulse/respiration normal
Tense tender swelling of the right knee
A single ecchymotic patch on the right elbow
Liver just palpable, soft
Other systems normal

Comfortable, not sick looking
Height 98 cm
No pallor

Spleen not palpable

Analysis

The only positive findings are a tense tender knee joint swelling with an ecchymotic spot on the elbow. In view of the history of a *spontaneous* swelling and in the absence of any other findings, one may consider this to be a **hemarthrosis**. Therefore, it may suggest a bleeding disorder due to a **coagulation factor deficiency**. It may be congenital or acquired. Usually, spontaneous hemarthrosis is not a feature of **acquired** disorders.

Amongst the inherited coagulation disorders, hemophilia is the commonest. **Prothrombin complex factor deficiency** such as deficiencies of Factors II, V, VII and X are usually acquired and rarely inherited. Specifically, Factor VII deficiency has a high prevalence of spontaneous CNS bleeds in addition to other manifestations. **Factor XII deficiency** does not present clinically as a bleeding disorder. **Factor XIII deficiency** commonly has its onset in infancy, with bleeding after separation of the umbilical cord stump (though a severe deficiency of other factors can also result in the same manifestation.) **Factor XI deficiency** (often called hemophilia C) can occur in both sexes as it has an autosomal recessive inheritance. However, spontaneous hemorrhage is rare. Similarly in von Willebrand's disease, spontaneous hemarthrosis is very rare. So this child must be suffering from either **factor VIII** or **IX deficiency** (hemophilia A and hemophilia B respectively). Clinically they are *indistinguishable* from one another.

■ INVESTIGATIONS

Hb 8 gm%
Platelet count normal
PTT prolonged
Factor IX activity - less than 1%
Factor VIII normal activity

WBC normal
Platelet clumps seen on peripheral smear
PT normal

■ FINAL DIAGNOSIS

Factor IX deficiency.

■ KEY MESSAGES

- Deep bleeds induced by relatively minor trauma are classically due to coagulation disorders. However, the history of trauma may not always be forthcoming.
- Deficiency of specific coagulation factors can often be diagnosed clinically, without factor assays.

Ecchymosis with Joint Swellings

RELEVANT INFORMATION

Interpretation of tests

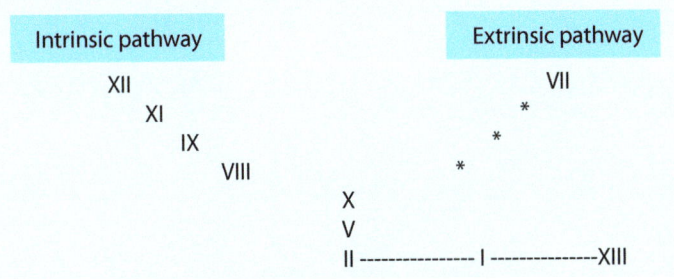

Prolonged PTT is seen in - L limb of the "Y" and the stem
Prolonged PT is seen in - R limb of the "Y" and the stem
Therefore BOTH abn means - X, V, or II def (or, in DIC)
- Inherited abn of these are rare, individual differentiation by factor assays

Only PTT abnormality   - XII (never presents clinically), XI, IX, & VIII

Abn PTT corrected by: Plasma   Adsorbed Serum
              VIII   yes   no
              IX   no   yes

These correction tests are not routinely done in pvt labs, but if asked for, give a valuable guide and save the cost of doing all the individual assays instead of one.

Factor I (fibrinogen) def. is rare - Thrombin Time (TT) abn in addition to abn PT & PTT
Factor XIII - urea stability test
Correct group of tests to be asked for in bleeding disorders; Plt count, BT, PT, PTT, TT, UST
Factor IX is present either in fresh frozen plasma or factor concentrates, BUT NOT in cryoprecipitate
- 1 mL of plasma increases factor IX activity by 1%
- It is sometimes difficult to control buccal mucosal bleeds in spite of adequate factor concentrations in plasma because of fibrinolytic factors in saliva, which lyse the clot formed, so drugs like EACA are necessary, to counter this effect.

It is very important to achieve a peak concentration of any factor during treatment of active bleeding episode and therefore adequate quantity of replacement fluid must be transfused.
Bleeding time and clotting time are very crude tests and are unreliable, except prolonged BT as a indicator of platelet functional defect.

34 CASE

Anemia in a 15-month-old

■ HISTORY

A 15-month-old female child presented with severe pallor noticed by the parents over the last 1 month. She was apparently well prior to this observation by the parents. There was no history of any acute illness, fever, bleeding from any site, jaundice or breathlessness.

Hailing from the Maratha community, this child was born of a non-consanguineous marriage, after a full-term normal delivery. She maintained average growth and normal development through infancy. She was breastfed for a year; supplementary semisolid food was introduced after 5 months of age.

No history of high colored urine.

No relevant past or family history.

She was found to have a hemoglobin of 4 gm% and hence, was transfused with blood at a primary care facility without any detailed hemogram. She remained well for another 4 months. Thereafter, she was noticed to be pale again. However, she remained otherwise well without any other symptoms. At this time, she was referred to a tertiary center for further management.

Analysis

As this child did not present with symptoms suggestive of cardiac decompensation in spite of severe anemia, it is a *chronic anemia*. A common cause of such a chronic anemia is a deficiency anemia. At this age, this would classically be an **iron deficiency anemia**, which is seen in a setting of prolonged milk feeds and delayed weaning; however, this child has been weaned at 5 months of age. Further, though iron deficiency anemia may recur if there is a continued occult blood loss, it will rarely do so within 4 months of a blood transfusion; in fact, it would rarely need a blood transfusion in the first place. Since this anemia is also *recurrent*, in an apparently healthy child it may suggest a **hemolytic anemia** or **bone marrow aplasia**. As this anemia manifested for the first time at 15 months of age, amongst congenital hemolytic anemias, it is likely to be **thalassemia major**, hereditary spherocytosis, **combined hemoglobinopathy** or an enzyme deficiency. While a family history of a similar disorder, or a history of consanguinity would have favored the diagnosis of congenital hemolytic anemia, its absence cannot rule it out. Though one expects a history of jaundice in **hereditary spherocytosis**, the parents may not have noticed it. **Pyruvate kinase deficiency**, while possible, is rare. **G6PD deficiency** is rare in girls. **Acquired hemolytic anemia** is usually acute, manifests with jaundice and is rare at this age. While **leukemia** can almost be ruled out as this child is otherwise asymptomatic and has remained so in between two episodes of presentation, bone marrow aplasia is possible, especially in view of the recurrence of anemia within 4 months of a transfusion. Therefore, this child is likely to have a congenital hemolytic anemia or a bone marrow aplasia.

■ PHYSICAL EXAMINATION

Average built and nourished	Irritable	Not sick looking
Weight 9.5 kg	Length 77 cm	Head ⊙ 46 cm
Temp normal	Pulse 125/min	RR 35/min
Severe pallor	Pigmentation of knuckles	
Glossitis and oral ulcers present	No koilonychia or platynychia	
Purpuric spots on the skin	No ecchymosis or bleeding from any other site	
No bony tenderness	No lymphadenopathy	

Liver 6 cm + firm, mildly tender	Liver span 9 cm	Spleen not palpable
Jugular venous pressure raised	Hepatojugular reflux positive	

Soft systolic murmur present - functional
Other systems normal

Analysis

Severe anemia with clinical evidence of thrombocytopenia in the form of purpura indicates involvement of two cell lines. *Clinically, two-cell line involvement should be viewed as a three-cell line affection till proved otherwise,* as the white cell abnormality is often not apparent on history or physical examination. Therefore, we need to consider bone marrow aplasia, leukemia or hypersplenism as a possibility. Since there is no splenomegaly and no background cause to suspect **hypersplenism**, it is ruled out. Similarly, it is unlikely to be **leukemia** because though the illness has been going on for the last 4 months (without any specific treatment), she has not developed any splenomegaly or lymphadenopathy. Also, she does not look "sick". On the other hand, a **bone marrow aplasia** may manifest gradually and may be considered in this child.

The enlarged liver in this child may represent cardiac failure or may also be a part of the primary hematological disease. There are definite signs of cardiac failure in the form of a tender hepatomegaly and an increased jugular venous pressure with a hepatojugular reflux. Further, the absence of splenomegaly suggests that the hepatomegaly may not be due to the primary hematological disease, as generally both the organs enlarge together in primary hematological disorders. Hence, we may consider the anemia in this child to be *without hepatosplenomegaly*. Thus, hemolytic anemia is ruled out. Anemia without hepatosplenomegaly is either deficiency anemia or bone marrow aplasia. As discussed in the analysis of history, iron deficiency is unlikely. While we consider a bone marrow aplasia, the presence of pigmentation of knuckles suggests a **vitamin B$_{12}$ deficiency** as the cause of aplasia. Glossitis and oral ulcers further support the diagnosis. Thus, the clinical diagnosis in this child is a megaloblastic anemia. Recurrence of anemia suggests that replacement therapy was never prescribed in this child.

■ INVESTIGATIONS

Hb 5 gm%
WBC 15,000/c.mm
Retic count 1%
Serum vitamin B_{12} level was low

Macrocytic hypochromic anemia
P 65 L 30 E 2 M 3
ESR 45 mm

Hypersegmented neutrophils seen
Platelet count 60,000/c.mm
Serum iron and folic acid normal

■ FINAL DIAGNOSIS

Vitamin B_{12} deficiency anemia.

■ KEY MESSAGES

- A common cause of anemia in an apparently healthy child without hepatosplenomegaly is a deficiency anemia.
- Koilonychia or platynychia when present, indicate iron deficiency but their absence does not rule it out. Pigmentation of knuckles favors vitamin B_{12} deficiency.
- Thrombocytosis is a feature of iron deficiency anemia, while thrombocytopenia that of B_{12} deficiency.
- Vitamin B_{12} deficiency can be considered to be an acquired cause of bone marrow aplasia.

CASE 35

Severe Anemia Noticed Incidentally

■ HISTORY

A 9-year-old female child presented with fever for the last 8 days. The fever was moderately high without any other significant accompanying symptoms.

When the patient was taken to a medical practitioner for treatment of fever, she was noticed to have severe pallor and hence was referred to the hospital.

No history of bleeding from any site.
No history of worm infestations.
No history of breathlessness.
No past history of any significant illness.
No family history of anemia.

Analysis

Severe pallor noticed during an acute febrile illness may suggest an anemia that has **developed acutely** or a **pre-existing chronic anemia** unrelated to the present febrile illness. Severe anemia with fever may suggest **acute leukemia**, **bone marrow aplasia or malaria**. (Pallor may also denote shock state without anemia, but the child would be very sick in such a situation). However, as the pallor was severe and yet, had not led to any cardiac decompensation (it was noticed incidentally) it is likely to be a chronic anemia and hence unrelated to the present febrile illness. An asymptomatic chronic anemia may be a **deficiency anemia**, **congenital hemolytic anemia** (compatible without a blood transfusion) or **malaria**. Bone marrow disease is unlikely, as it would have presented with other symptoms over time.

■ PHYSICAL EXAMINATION

Fairly built and poorly nourished
Weight 23 kg
Height 130 cm
Temp. normal   HR 95/min
RR 24/min   BP 95/55 mm of Hg
Severe pallor
Hemolytic facies   No icterus
Circumoral pigmentation
Glossitis
Koilonychia +

Liver 2 cm +, soft, not tender
Spleen 2 cm + firm
Soft systolic murmur
No signs of cardiac failure
Other systems normal

Analysis

Severe pallor, hemolytic facies and a firm splenomegaly suggest a **chronic hemolytic anemia**. However, there are some *odd points*. While any chronic, severe anemia would lead to growth failure, it is an essential feature of a congenital hemolytic anemia presenting at this age. Since this child's height is near normal, congenital hemolytic anemia is unlikely. Chronic hemolytic anemias presenting at 9 years of age (without any blood transfusion in the past) may be hereditary spherocytosis or thalassemia intermedia (which is a phenotypic variant of thalassemia major with decreased transfusion requirements and therefore presents late). Considering the severity of this child's anemia, in spherocytosis the splenomegaly should have been larger and jaundice should also have been present, while in thalassemia there should have been features of marked extramedullary hematopoiesis, i.e., *significant hepatosplenomegaly* and a florid hemolytic facies. This child does have a mild hemolytic facies thereby suggesting some extramedullary hematopoiesis; however the other features mentioned earlier are absent. Thus, it is unlikely to be chronic hemolytic anemia. Circumoral pigmentation and glossitis suggest deficiency anemia and koilonychia favors an **iron deficiency** state. Occasionally a *long standing, severe* iron deficiency may lead to a small degree of extramedullary hematopoiesis, thereby explaining the mild hemolytic facies. Though significant organomegaly is characteristically not associated with deficiency anemia, a mild splenomegaly is compatible with iron deficiency anemia in 10-15% of the cases. Splenomegaly may also indicate **malaria**. Thus, it may denote old malaria and may be unrelated to the present illness and anemia may be deficiency anemia.

■ INVESTIGATIONS

Hb 2.6 gm%
MCV 66 fL
Serum iron 35 pg/dL
Peripheral smear - dimorphic anemia
RDW 27%
TIBC 353 pg/dL
Retic count 1%
Hematocrit 9%

Analysis

Low MCV with high RDW may be seen in iron deficiency anemia or thalassemia major.

However, a low reticulocyte count is against thalassemia major and may favor iron deficiency anemia. Since it can rise within 2-3 days of iron administration, and at times even due to food rich in iron, a high reticulocyte count also would not have ruled out iron deficiency anemia.

Low serum iron and high TIBC prove iron deficiency anemia. Dimorphic cytology on peripheral smear may suggest a mixed deficiency.

■ FINAL DIAGNOSIS

Deficiency anemia, predominantly iron deficiency.

KEY MESSAGES

- Hemolytic facies may also be seen occasionally in iron deficiency anemia. Absence of hepatosplenomegaly differentiates it from chronic hemolytic anemia.
- Growth failure is a significant feature of hereditary chronic hemolytic anemias.
- Malaria being endemic in our country, a small firm splenomegaly may represent old malarial infection and may be unrelated to the presenting illness.

RELEVANT INFORMATION

Iron deficiency is extremely common in clinical practice. While the usual clinical features are well known, it is important to note subtle clinical manifestations like a poor school performance, which may often be brushed aside as a minor complaint. Obviously, there are no "tonics" to enhance school performance, but administration of iron in a child who has iron deficiency, can help. Similarly, if ever there is a need to satisfy the parental demand for a "tonic", an iron containing preparation should be prescribed.

Treatment of iron deficiency can always be accomplished with oral iron preparations; parenteral iron is almost never required. Even in severe iron deficiency anemia, parenteral iron does not lead to a quicker response; in fact, the absorption of oral iron is naturally enhanced. The iron preparation being used should be a "complete" hematinic, i.e., it should contain iron, folic acid, and vitamin B_{12} in therapeutic concentrations. The "newer" iron salts offer no advantage over the traditional salts, and are not cost-effective in comparison to the older salts.

CASE 36

Generalized Weakness for a Few Months and Recent Facial Asymmetry

■ HISTORY

A 4-year-old child presented with a history of (H/o) generalized weakness over the last 6 months and facial asymmetry noticed over the last 2 weeks. He was well prior to the onset of this problem.

Analysis

Non-neurological "generalized weakness" suggests muscle tiredness. This could be a symptom of slowly progressive **hypoxia** (interstitial lung disease), **hypoperfusion** (cardiac failure), or **chronic anemia**. Hypokalemia and hypomagnesemia mostly present as an acute onset of neurological weakness (paresis); rarely, chronic hypokalemia may occur in renal tubular disorders and present as tiredness. **Diabetes mellitus** may also present as generalized weakness, but usually over a shorter period of a few days or weeks and hence unlikely in this child. Thus, one should ask for mild breathlessness on exertion (interstitial lung or cardiac disease) and pallor. On direct questioning, the mother confirmed that she had noticed pallor over the last 2 months. Since the symptoms started 6 months ago, it means that the onset of anemia was >6 months ago. Then, as the anemia slowly progressed it reached a point when the mother noticed the pallor. Thus, this child has slowly progressive anemia. It is unlikely to be **congenital hemolytic anemia** as it would have started much earlier; nor an **acquired hemolytic anemia** which mostly presents as acute anemia. **Bone marrow infiltrative disorders** or bone marrow aplasia may present as chronic progressive anemia but usually, the child looks unwell or sick. Chronic **deficiency anemia** has to be considered as it is the most common cause of chronic anemia in our population. To differentiate the probable cause of anemia, one could ask for abdominal distension if noticed by parents. It would help differentiate between deficiency anemia (without hepatosplenomegaly) and marrow infiltration.

■ PHYSICAL EXAMINATION

Comfortable
Wt 17 kg   Ht 100 cm
HR 110/m   RR 23/m   BP 100/50 mm Hg   Pallor ++
Liver 4F+, not tender, span 9 cm   Spleen 2F+
JVP normal, soft systolic murmur grade 2 (functional), Left LMN facial nerve palsy
Other systems normal

Analysis

This healthy child has severe anemia with a functional murmur and hepatosplenomegaly. It suggests bone marrow infiltration that has not disturbed the general health of the child. Thus, it rules out malignancy (leukemia) and myelodysplastic or myelofibrotic marrow disorders. Storage disorders such as Gaucher's disease present with similar findings but the sequence (organomegaly first and then anemia), and duration (often much longer) of presentation and are different; besides, there is no suggestion of affection of another system (neurological), and so, unlikely. Further, left facial LMN palsy in this situation of marrow infiltration suggests that enlargement of skull bones may be pinching the outgoing structures from the cranium. This leads us to the diagnosis of osteopetrosis as a possibility.

■ INVESTIGATIONS

CBC showed pancytopenia without any abnormal cells

Bone marrow aspiration failed suggesting thickened marrow

X-ray of skull showed thickening and dense bones, especially at the base (appearance of bone within bone)

Genetic study confirmed the diagnosis of osteopetrosis.

■ FINAL DIAGNOSIS

Osteopetrosis.

■ KEY MESSAGES

> Chronic anemia with or without hepatosplenomegaly differentiates deficiency anemia/marrow aplasia from marrow hypercellularity (hemolytic anemia and marrow infiltration). Patients suffering from marrow diseases are sick but there are exceptions. Osteopetrosis is a noninflammatory localized disease restricted only to bones though structures leaving the cranium may be pinched by thickened skull bones.

■ RELEVANT INFORMATION

In osteopetrosis, there is a defective osteoclast function which includes—osteoclasts being unable to resorb the bone effectively due to the relevant enzyme deficiency which leads to disruption of normal bone homeostasis. There are two different types of the disease that are (1) a malignant variety presents in infancy and the other may present anytime later in life. It is a genetically determined disease and (2) a genetic study offers a complete diagnosis. Bone marrow transplantation is the only available therapy.

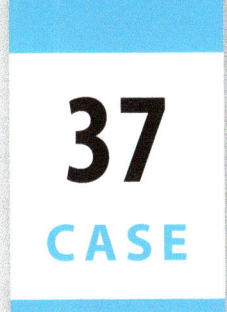

37 CASE

Fever for 2 Weeks with Constitutional Symptoms

■ HISTORY

A 10-year-old child was presented with a fever and loss of appetite and weight for 2 weeks. There were no other symptoms. The fever was moderate to high, temporarily responding to paracetamol with a normal interfebrile period. He was prescribed two sets of antibiotics without any diagnosis; his complete blood count (CBC), urinalysis, and chest X-ray were normal. He had suffered from a viral infection a few days prior to the onset of this fever which had settled by itself without any treatment; otherwise, he had been a healthy child.

Analysis

History suggests an acute onset of probably a **noninfective disease** as evidenced by a normal interfebrile period, absence of localizing symptoms, and failed antibiotic therapy. **Partially treated infections** can be kept in mind, especially acute bacterial infections that present without any localizing symptoms like subacute endocarditis. In case it is a noninfective illness, one should look out for any clinical features that suggest **rheumatological** diseases (arthritis, mouth ulcers, and skin rash) or **hematological** diseases (pallor, petechiae, and lymph node swellings). The history of (H/o) having suffered a recent viral infection may be relevant in the sense that immune complications of such infections are known to appear after an interval of a few days. However, there is no clue to any specific organ involvement yet.

■ PHYSICAL EXAMINATION

Sick look
Temp. 102°F   HR 112/m   RR 28/m   BP 115/75 mm Hg
Moderate pallor   No purpura   No skin rash
No lymphadenopathy or joint swelling or tenderness
Liver 2 cm, soft, not tender, span 9 cm   Spleen 2 cm
Other systems normal

Analysis

A sick look with moderate anemia suggests a progressive disorder of inflammatory origin. Splenomegaly without any significant hepatomegaly favors a hematological disorder either a hemolytic disorder or an infiltrative disorder of the marrow. The absence of jaundice almost rules out a hemolytic process; and therefore, bone marrow infiltration is the likely possibility (leukemia or other similar disorders). Malaria is unlikely as the fever has gone on for 2 weeks, the child looks sick, and yet there don't seem to be further complications.

■ INVESTIGATIONS

Hb 7 g% WBC 12,000/cmm P 52 L 43, M 3 E 2 PC 50,000/cmm
S ferritin 2,500 ng/mL   S triglycerides 500 mg/dL S fibrinogen 80 mg/dL
PS no abnormal cells
Bone marrow: Hemophagocytosis

Analysis

Bicytopenia with marrow showing hemophagocytosis, raised ferritin and triglycerides and reduced fibrinogen favor the diagnosis of hemophagocytic lymphohistiocytosis (HLH) which is further proved by high CD-25 and low NK cells.

Final Diagnosis

Hemophagocytic LymphoHistiocytosis (HLH) (probably secondary to the viral infection that this child suffered in the recent past).

■ KEY MESSAGES

Prolonged fever without localizing symptoms is mostly, not due to acute bacterial infection; subacute infections such as tuberculosis, brucellosis, Epstein–Barr virus (EBV) or *Cytomegalovirus* (CMV) viral infections, toxoplasmosis, and kala azar may be considered. Besides, noninfective inflammatory disorders (rheumatological or hematological) also have to be considered. Anemia and splenomegaly favor hematological diseases.

■ RELEVANT INFORMATION

Hemophagocytic lymphohistiocytosis is an immune-mediated disorder secondary to many triggers; such as infections of all types, autoimmune disorders, malignancy; and drugs such as anticonvulsants and antibiotics (cotrimoxazole and vancomycin). Rarely HLH may be due to a primary immune defect—perforin deficiency, that is genetically determined. It may be present very early in life and is often fatal. Diagnosis is suspected when there is a persistent fever without any clue to infections, in the presence of bicytopenia or pancytopenia, and splenomegaly with or without hepatomegaly. Occasionally, it may also be present as specific organ affection. Macrophage activation syndrome is similar to HLH though it presents as a complication of a rheumatological disorder and not as a primary hematological disease. Clinically, a high index of suspicion is necessary; once suspected, it has to be followed by further confirmatory tests which may pick up typical laboratory findings as in this child. The treatment consists of etoposide, steroids, cyclosporine, and if necessary other chemotherapeutic drugs. A bone marrow transplant can also be considered.

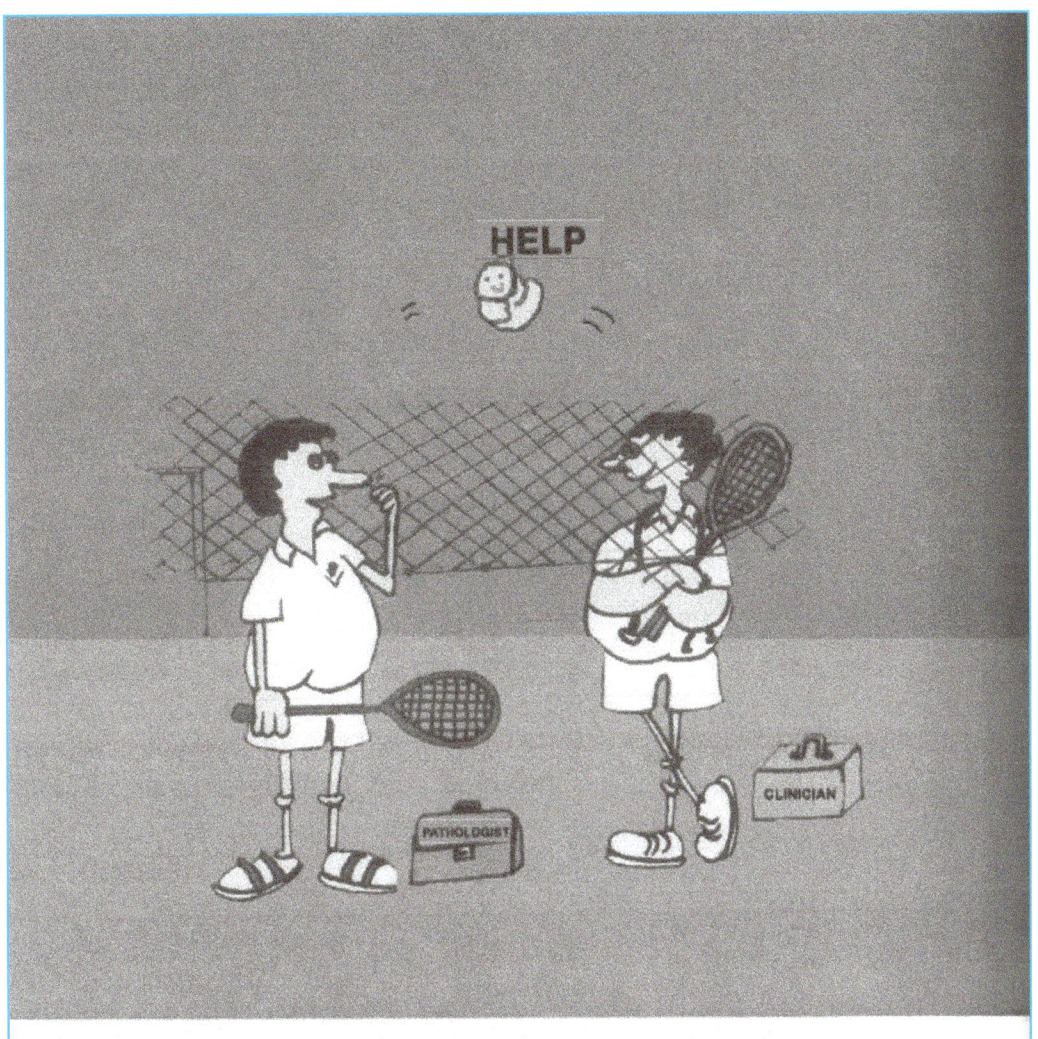

Pyrexia

BACK TO BASICS

Fever is a pyrogenic response to a variety of stimuli. The most common cause of fever is infection. However, non-infective inflammation and malignancy also result in fever. Occasionally, diseases affecting the temperature-regulating mechanism may also cause fever, such as central fever or an autonomic disturbance. Other rarer causes include heat fever, dehydration fever, drug fever, poisoning and hyperthyroidism.

The initial physical examination in a child presenting acutely with high fever, is primarily aimed at ruling out serious infections such as meningitis/pneumonia/sepsis/diphtheria/surgical inflammatory conditions such as acute appendicitis. The physical examination on subsequent days should carefully search for a focus of infection.

The etiology of the infection must be clinically evaluated. *Acute bacterial and viral infections* present with fever. (Chronic bacterial or viral infections may present without fever). A v*iral infection* often presents with high fever at the onset, which usually subsides by day 3-4. The child appears nearly normal during the interfebrile period. The infection is mostly *generalized* and affects the entire system (upper and lower respiratory tract) or multiple systems (respiratory and gastrointestinal). History of contact with a similar infection almost clinches the diagnosis of a viral infection. As against this, an acute *bacterial* infection often starts with moderate fever, which peaks early in infections which localize quickly (tonsillitis, UTI, pneumonia, meningitis), but may peak after a couple of days in cases where early localization is absent (typhoid fever). During the interfebrile state, the child continues to be sick. A bacterial infection does get *localized* sooner or later. The site of infection needs to be evaluated on the basis of localizing symptoms. Therefore, bacterial infections usually manifest with symptoms related to specific organ involvement within the first few days. However, there are a few exceptions. Symptoms of urinary tract infection may remain elusive especially in an infant. Typhoid fever, bacterial endocarditis and bacteremia/septicemia due to any cause may manifest with fever alone without any initial localizing symptoms.

Recurrent infections need a proper evaluation. Recurrent viral infections are common in early childhood, with increasing contact with other children in the community. It does not call for further investigations. Unlike recurrent viral infections, recurrent bacterial infections are always secondary to some underlying structural, functional or an immunological defect and should be thoroughly investigated. It should be a rule to investigate any child who presents with recurrent bacterial infections, especially within a short period. Thus, prescribing an antibiotic for the second time within a short period for a recurrent bacterial infection, is not rational without further relevant investigations.

Recurrent fever may be mistaken easily for persistent fever, unless a detailed history is sought from the parents with leading questions. The causes of persistent fever are quite different from those of recurrent fever and naturally, the management also differs a lot.

Mycobacterial, fungal and parasitic infections may present with a subacute onset of fever, without localization. In non-infective inflammatory diseases, fever may be the only symptom for the first few weeks, until subtle manifestations arise such as a skin rash, vague arthralgia or myalgia, mouth ulcers, nail abnormalities, alopecia, etc. It is important to realize that many of these symptoms or signs come up *sequentially* and not necessarily simultaneously, and hence a detailed enquiry about such symptoms in the past is mandatory. Malignancy presents with a wide spectrum of manifestations but occasionally, fever may be the only symptom at the onset of the disease. Non-localizing malignant disorders include leukemia, lymphoma and neuroblastoma.

Once these diseases are ruled out, rarer conditions may be considered. Some of them such as drug fever may not have any laboratory proof and at times, it may be prudent to withdraw all the drugs as a trial.

In the absence of clinical clues, it is ideal to investigate for the cause of fever before employing empiric antibiotic therapy.

A complete hemogram must be obtained from a reliable source, preferably performed on an automated counter. It needs to be interpreted with caution. The total leukocyte count has a limited role, especially if it is borderline abnormal. Marked neutrophilic leukocytosis is also seen in non-infective systemic inflammatory disorders besides an acute severe bacterial infection. However, leukopenia is a feature of typhoid fever, also a severe bacterial infection. Mild to moderate neutrophilic leukocytosis can be seen in acute viral and many common bacterial infections. Thus, the total number of leukocytes and neutrophils/lymphocytes are often of no great help in differentiating viral from bacterial infections or non-infective disorders. Eosinopenia is an important feature of an *acute* bacterial or viral infection while in other infections (tuberculosis/malaria) and inflammatory disorders, the eosinophil count may be normal or even mildly elevated. Thrombocytosis is a feature of both acute bacterial infections and systemic inflammatory diseases. Thrombocytopenia is seen in malaria, dengue and typhoid fever. Repeat counts may be ordered to follow the progress of serious diseases, but mild changes in either direction should not be considered significant.

ESR is a good screening test to consider in cases of pyrexia of unknown origin. It is of no help in a fever of a short duration. A high ESR (close to 100) suggests a systemic inflammatory disease or malignancy and may also be seen in tuberculosis. Mild to moderate elevation of ESR is seen in many diseases and is non-specific.

Routine imaging modalities such as a chest X-ray or an abdominal ultrasound, may fail to depict any abnormality and even then, CT or MR scans may demonstrate a lesion.

Additional tests may be necessary, such as CSF (in infants) and bone marrow examination (older children) to diagnose the cause of fever that is elusive with clinical and other laboratory parameters.

Interpretation of CBC

Reliable with automated counter results

Hb	TC	P	L	E	Platelets	Disease
N	+++			0	N or +	Acute bacterial infection
N	Low	++	++	0	N or Low	Typhoid fever
N	++	++		0	N	Acute viral infection
N	+		++	+	N	Chronic infection/TB
N	+++	+++		+	High	Systemic inflammatory disease
Low	+/−			+	Low	Malaria
Low	+++		+++		Low	Acute lymphatic leukemia

CASE 38

Fever for 2 Months

■ HISTORY

A 10-month-old infant presented with fever for the last 2 months. The fever had been high and continuous, temporarily responding to antipyretics for a few hours. He had been very irritable and difficult to manage at times. He had lost his appetite and weight over the last 2 months.

There were no significant symptoms other than fever.

The bowel pattern and urination had been normal.

He had undergone many laboratory tests without any clue to the diagnosis. These tests included a hemogram, urinalysis, chest X-ray, blood culture, urine culture, Widal's test, Paul-Bunnell test, tests for brucellosis, leptospirosis, dengue fever, and a Mantoux test.

He had been treated empirically with different antibiotics and antimalarials without benefit.

No relevant past or family history.

No history of contact with any specific infection.

Birth history normal.

His growth and development had been normal until the onset of this illness.

Analysis

It is most *unlikely* that this infant has an **acute bacterial infection**, as the fever has lasted too long without any localizing symptoms or any complications and there has also been no response to multiple antibiotics. A chronic infection such as **tuberculosis** may present with continuous high fever as seen in disseminated/miliary disease. However, *at this age* the disease would have lead to many other manifestations by now. Other chronic infections without localizing symptoms include **CMV, toxoplasmosis, malaria, EB virus, brucellosis**. High persistent fever may be the only initial manifestation of **systemic inflammatory disorders** also, and therefore should be considered in this child though such diseases are not common at this age. Similarly, infiltrative disorders (**malignancy/histiocytosis/sarcoidosis**) are also a possibility, though there is no definite clue on the history. Thus, the history alone does not offer any specific clue to the diagnosis in this child and a chronic infection or an infiltrative disorder is equally possible. Physical examination may help to localize the disease.

■ PHYSICAL EXAMINATION

Fairly built, poorly nourished	Sick looking	Irritable
Weight 6 kg	Length 70 cm	Head ⊙ 44 cm
Temp. 102°F	Pulse 130/min	RR 35/min
No respiratory distress	Moderate pallor	No lymphadenopathy

Two nodular swellings on the scalp, firm to hard, not mobile, fixed to the underlying bone, not tender

Other bones normal	Joints normal	No skin rash
Liver just palpable, soft	Spleen not palpable	Other systems normal

Analysis

The only positive findings on physical examination in this infant are *nodular swellings on the skull* and *moderate pallor*. Obviously, the cause of fever is related to the bony swellings. Etiologically, such a nodular swelling may be due to **tubercular osteomyelitis, histiocytosis** or **malignancy**. Tuberculosis at this age, manifests either as a primary lesion in the lung or disseminates to other organs, as in miliary tuberculosis or TBM. Isolated tuberculosis of bone is rare at this age. Therefore, this is likely to be either histiocytosis or a malignancy. A **primary bone malignancy** involving the skull is rare at this age and hence it is likely to be secondary spread from a distant malignancy such as a **neuroblastoma**. Most other malignant diseases do not present with secondaries but are localized to an organ (Wilm's tumor/hepatoblastoma/retinoblastoma/brain tumor) or present as hematological disorders. Acute leukemia may involve the periosteum and cause bony pain but not a nodular bony swelling. A soft tissue swelling is known with leukemia (chloroma in a myeloid leukemia).

Anemia without hepatosplenomegaly (a just palpable, soft liver is normal) may be a deficiency anemia, marrow aplasia or anemia of chronic disease. In relevance to bony swellings in this child, it may either be deficiency anemia or related to a chronic disease. Chronic infections that were considered on history are unlikely, considering the physical findings in this child. Class I histiocytoses usually presents only with bony lesions and only when the disease is extensive, the child may have systemic manifestations like fever or a multisystem involvement and therefore less likely in this child. While class II histiocytoses can present as a generalized disease with fever, irritability and weight loss (as in this child), they are usually associated with hepatosplenomegaly and symptoms of CNS involvement (aseptic meningitis).

Between histiocytosis and neuroblastoma, it is the latter that is more subtle and occult in presentation. Thus, it may favor a diagnosis of neuroblastoma.

■ INVESTIGATIONS

Hb 8 gm% Microcytic hypochromic anemia
WBC 20,000/c.mm P 75 L 20 E 3 M 2 ESR 120 mm
Biopsy from the nodule over the skull confirmed the diagnosis of neuroblastoma.

■ FINAL DIAGNOSIS

Neuroblastoma.

KEY MESSAGES

- Thorough examination of bones and joints is vital in every undiagnosed persistent fever.
- ESR is a good screening test in prolonged fevers.
- Neutrophilic leukocytosis does not always indicate acute bacterial infection.
- If two sets of antibiotics have failed to produce a desirable response, change of diagnosis is mandatory rather than change of antibiotics.

RELEVANT INFORMATION

The differences in the outcome of patients with a neuroblastoma are striking. Infants younger than 1 year have a good prognosis, even in the presence of metastatic disease, whereas older patients with metastatic disease fare poorly, even when treated with aggressive therapy. Unfortunately, approximately 70–80% of patients older than 1 year present with metastatic disease (usually to lymph nodes, liver, bone and bone marrow). Fewer than half of these patients are cured, even with the use of high dose therapy followed by autologous bone marrow or stem cell rescue. More than 90% of patients have elevated homovanillic acid (HVA) and/or vanillylmandelic acid (VMA) detectable in urine. Mass screening studies using catecholamines in neonates and infants in Japan and Europe have demonstrated the ability to detect neuroblastoma before it clinically manifests.

CASE 39

Low Fever, Cough and Failure to Thrive

■ HISTORY

A 2-month-old infant presented with a history of low-grade fever and episodic cough for the last 1 month. He was apparently normal till 1 month of age. The symptoms were not progressing in severity, though the parents reported a poor weight gain. He was seen by a doctor, but the details of treatment were not available.

- No history of feeding difficulty or breathlessness
- No history of vomiting
- No history of choking while feeding
- Antenatal and perinatal period normal
- Average birth weight
- Exclusively breastfed
- No history of contact with TB

■ ANALYSIS

Significant cough at this age always denotes definite underlying disease necessitating investigations. Episodic cough for a month primarily suggests an airway disease. In the absence of symptoms referable to the nose, it is likely to be a lower airway involvement. **Aspiration syndrome** presents either with an acute pneumonia or a chronic cough without fever, and is hence unlikely in this infant. Also, there is no history of choking or vomiting. Fever denotes a probable **infection** or an **infiltrative disease**. *Low-grade fever* for a month with poor weight gain suggests a **chronic disease,** and when it denotes an infection, it almost always denotes a *persistent infection*. As against this, though **recurrent bacterial infections** may mimic a persistent disease, they present with recurrent *acute* manifestations, i.e. recurrent *high fever*. Though a malnourished infant may fail to respond with high fever even in acute bacterial infections, this child was normal (not malnourished) when his illness started. In other words, *this illness started with a low fever in a normally nourished infant,* thereby suggesting a chronic persistent infection, which may be **congenital** or **acquired**. A congenital infection is not localized to the respiratory system alone; so this is most likely to be an acquired infection. It may be a chronic infection such as **tuberculosis**, fungal infection or whooping cough. In early infancy, tuberculosis and **fungal infections** usually occur in immunocompromised hosts, though they may also occur in infants with a normal immune status. Specifically, prolonged antibiotic therapy may lead to fungal infections. A history of contact with tuberculosis in the family is a strong indicator of the disease in infancy, but its absence does not rule out such a possibility, as the neonate may have been exposed to tubercular infection at the time of birth, in the maternity home. Whooping cough (**pertussis**) can present with severe cough and poor weight gain and therefore, is another possibility in this child. Amongst other chronic diseases, infants with **cystic fibrosis** or **congenital immune deficiency** may present with either persistent or recurrent severe bacterial infections, but the infant usually runs high fever. **Acquired immune deficiency** does not present so early in infancy. Chronic infiltrative diseases such as **histiocytosis** may present with fever and poor weight gain, though cough is not a prominent feature.

■ PHYSICAL EXAMINATION

Poorly nourished
Weight 2.8 kg (birth weight 2.5 kg)
Temp. 99°F   Pulse 118/min
No lymphadenopathy

Sick looking
Length 53 cm
RR 32/min
No cyanosis

Head Θ 38 cm
No respiratory distress
No clubbing

Resp. system – Chest movements bilaterally symmetrical
Resonant all over
Liver 7 cm +, firm, not tender
Other systems normal

TVF/VR normal
Normal breath sounds   Bilateral crepitations
Liver span 9 cm   Spleen 2 cm +, firm

Analysis

Physical examination reveals bilateral crepitations without any localizing signs. This suggests bilateral airway disease or a disseminated alveolar disease. Absence of respiratory distress denotes a slowly progressive disease without respiratory dysfunction. The liver and spleen are not only enlarged but also firm, thereby indicating a pathological organomegaly and not merely pushed down organs. This hepatosplenomegaly denotes dissemination of the disease beyond the respiratory system. This favors a disseminated infection such as tuberculosis/fungal disease or histiocytosis. Miliary tuberculosis presents with minimal or no cough, unlike this infant who presented with significant cough. Hence, this must be a **tubercular bronchopneumonia** with dissemination through the bloodstream to the liver and the spleen. However, a **fungal infection** or **histiocytosis** cannot be ruled out completely and further investigations may help.

■ INVESTIGATIONS

Hb 8 gm%   WBC 9,500/c.mm   P 42 L 53 E 3 M 2   ESR 75 mm
Tuberculin test negative
Chest X-ray – bilateral bronchopneumonia
CT scan of chest - multiple nodular lesions on both sides
Bronchoalveolar lavage showed *Mycobacterium tuberculosis*

Analysis

Bilateral shadows on the chest X-ray may suggest bronchopneumonia, however nodular lesions seen on the CT scan of the chest denote tuberculosis or histiocytosis. Lesions secondary to malignant disease are rare in children.

Bronchoalveolar lavage proved the diagnosis of tuberculosis.

Tuberculin test is expected to be negative in a malnourished infant with disseminated disease. It may revert to a positive reaction after 2-3 months of successful treatment.

FINAL DIAGNOSIS

Disseminated tuberculosis with bronchopneumonia.

KEY MESSAGES

- Respiratory disease with hepatosplenomegaly in early infancy is usually a manifestation of a disseminated infection such as tuberculosis or an infiltrative disease like histiocytosis.
- Significant cough denotes an airway disease and such a symptom is rare in tuberculosis except in the case of endobronchial disease or bronchopneumonia.

CASE 40

High Fever, Cough and Failure to Thrive

■ HISTORY

A 3-month-old infant presented with high fever and cough, off and on for the last 6 weeks, and failure to thrive. Born after a full-term normal delivery, he was all right for the first 3 weeks of life. Thereafter he developed an episode of fever, which was treated with antibiotics without a definite diagnosis, and got better. The fever returned within a few days again and this time, he was diagnosed to have a pneumonia. He was hospitalized and treated accordingly. He improved partially but was never normal. He was irritable and did not feed well.

He was exclusively breastfed.
No history of diarrhea, vomiting or any other significant symptoms.
Family history of asthma in the father.
He was immunized with BCG, OPV and hepatitis B vaccines at birth and had no untoward reaction.

Analysis

Recurrent *high* fever usually signifies a *recurrent* infection; it may signify a persistent infection only of a kind whose inherent symptomatology is one of intermittent fever, e.g., malaria. On the other hand, a low grade fever almost always denotes a persistent infection. *Recurrent* fever and cough suggests **recurrent respiratory infection**. It may be due to an **aspiration syndrome** as a result of upper GI anomalies such as **GER**, a cardiac defect in the form of a **left to right shunt**, congenital immune deficiency or cystic fibrosis. Fever is not a prominent symptom of aspiration syndromes; instead they present with severe cough. Fever is also not a predominant feature of cardiac defects, while breathlessness is (which is absent here). Hence in this infant, an aspiration syndrome and a cardiac defect are unlikely. **Congenital immune deficiency** and cystic fibrosis are both possible. Immune deficiency presenting so early in infancy is mostly severe combined immune deficiency, which manifests with disseminated infections at multiple sites and the BCG vaccine may lead to a non-healing ulcer with possible spread of BCG infection (BCGitis). As this infant did not present with infection at multiple sites, nor had any abnormal response at the BCG vaccination site, congenital combined immune deficiency is unlikely. B-cell immune deficiency presents usually after 3–6 months of life as maternally transmitted antibodies protect the infant for the first few months of life. **Acquired immune deficiency (HIV)** does not present so early in infancy. **Cystic fibrosis** is also a multisystem disorder affecting primarily the respiratory and the gastrointestinal tract. However, clinical manifestations in early infancy are often restricted to the respiratory tract, and the infant may not present with diarrhea though investigations may reveal intestinal malabsorption. A chronic infection such as **tuberculosis** or a **fungal infection** is also a possibility as it may simulate recurrent respiratory infections. However, the presence of high fever is against such a possibility.

■ PHYSICAL EXAMINATION

Sick looking malnourished infant
Weight 2.8 kg (Birth weight 2.6 kg)   Length 55 cm   Head ⊖ 38 cm
Temp. 101°F   HR 140/min   RR 50/min   Chest retractions present
No clubbing   No cyanosis   BCG scar seen
Resp. system – Bilateral crepitations Vesicular breath sounds
Liver 3 cm +, soft, not tender   Liver span 5 cm   Spleen just palpable
Other systems normal

Analysis

The physical signs in this infant suggest a generalized airway disease or a disseminated alveolar disease. The disease is progressive as is evident by the failure to thrive. Tachypnea denotes respiratory dysfunction, and therefore a widespread respiratory involvement. The history of recurrent high fever suggests recurrent infection as discussed earlier. Such a widespread recurrent lower respiratory tract infection is likely to be bacterial, and due to either **immune deficiency** or **cystic fibrosis**. Though **tuberculosis** may also present with similar physical findings, such a widespread lung involvement is expected to be accompanied with signs of a disseminated disease in the form of a hepatosplenomegaly. Though the liver is palpable, it is soft and the liver span is normal; therefore it is unlikely to be pathological. The spleen is also just palpable, and therefore the "apparent" hepatosplenomegaly in this child may be due to a pushed down effect as a result of a progressive airway disease with tachypnea. In that case, clinically, this is not a disseminated disease with multisystem involvement, and therefore unlikely to be tuberculosis. However, if this hepatosplenomegaly is considered significant, then TB needs to be ruled out. The presence of a normal BCG scar denotes an intact T cell immune function. As mentioned earlier, a B-cell immune deficiency does not present so early, as maternally transmitted antibodies protect the infant for the first 3–4 months. Hence, immune deficiency disorders also seem to be less likely. Therefore, it is likely to be cystic fibrosis.

■ INVESTIGATIONS

Hb 8 gm%   WBC 12,000/c.mm   P 60 L 38 E 0 M 2
Chest X-ray – bilateral streaking, no pneumonia or pleural disease.
CT scan of chest – bilateral multiple small cavities
ABG – metabolic alkalosis.

Analysis

Metabolic alkalosis is a surprise, as one would have expected respiratory acidosis in this infant with progressive respiratory failure. This is typical of cystic fibrosis due to loss of chlorides (and sodium) in the sweat, resulting in metabolic alkalosis.

CT scan of the chest showing multiple cavities also favors the diagnosis of cystic fibrosis.

Other causes of multiple cavities on a CT scan of the chest are bronchiectasis or congenital cystic disease. Both conditions are localized to a few segments and present only if infected. Progressive deterioration in early infancy is not a feature of such diseases.

■ FURTHER CONFIRMATIVE TESTS

Sweat chlorides and sodium were high.

Molecular diagnosis confirmed the diagnosis of cystic fibrosis with delta 508 antigen.

Knowing that cystic fibrosis is a genetically determined defect, it was decided to investigate the father who claimed to be suffering from asthma. He was also positive for the cystic fibrosis gene, though he had a milder form of clinical presentation.

■ FINAL DIAGNOSIS

Cystic fibrosis.

■ KEY MESSAGES

- Severe bacterial infections in an exclusively breastfed infant suggest a serious underlying functional or anatomical defect.
- High fever in an infant needs to be considered as a serious bacterial infection and demands urgent investigations to diagnose correctly. Antibiotic therapy without relevant prior investigations is irrational and dangerous.
- A plain chest X-ray may not demonstrate airway and interstitial disease; a CT scan of the chest is useful in such cases to demonstrate the lesions clearly.
- Metabolic alkalosis in a child with respiratory distress strongly suggests cystic fibrosis.

■ RELEVANT INFORMATION

It is an autosomal recessive disorder. Most of the carriers are asymptomatic. Infants present with progressive pulmonary infection (typically with pseudomonas) with or without diarrhea.

Even those who do not have diarrhea do have laboratory evidence of pancreatic insufficiency. In older children and adults, the disease manifests with chronic cough simulating asthma, without pancreatic insufficiency. Sweat chloride test is difficult to carry out and not diagnostic, as it may be abnormal in many other conditions. Elevated sweat chlorides are seen in malnutrition, hypothyroidism, panhypopituitarism, hypoparathyroidism, cholestasis, atopic dermatitis, ectodermal dysplasia, adrenal insufficiency, MPS and glycogen storage disease. The list seems to be ever increasing. Thus, molecular diagnosis should be attempted. Though there are 900 mutations known, the most common mutation is delta 508. However, other mutations are getting reported now from India. A negative result may not rule out the disease.

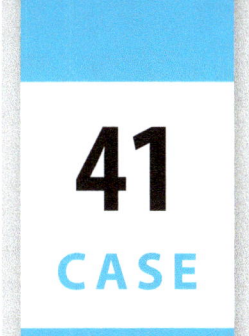

Fever for 2 Months: Case 1

■ HISTORY

An 8-year-old child presented with fever for the last 2 months. He was apparently well 2 months ago when he developed fever. The fever had been high grade, coming in two spikes per day with a normal intervening period. There were no other symptoms at that time. After initial symptomatic therapy, he was prescribed amoxicillin for 5 days without any response. At that stage he was investigated. His laboratory test results were as follows:

    Hb 11 gm%   WBC 23,000/c.mm   P 72 L 24 E 4   ESR 80 mm
    Platelets 4.5 Lacs/c.mm Routine urine normal   Widal test negative

Considering it to be an acute bacterial infection, based on the neutrophilic leukocytosis, he was prescribed IV Cefotaxime and Amikacin for the next 7 days. He was partially better and hence, the same drugs were continued.

However in spite of continuation of antibiotics, the high fever appeared again and he started complaining about a vague pain in the joints without any swelling. This was ascribed to the high fever. He was reinvestigated at this juncture, and the results were as follows:

    Hb 9 gm%   WBC 35,000/c.mm   P 82 L 14 E 3 M 1   ESR 105 mm
    Platelets 5.4 Lacs/c.mm Chest X-ray normal   Blood and urine culture normal
    Widal test negative   Abdominal USG normal

He was advised a CSF examination and CT scans of the chest, abdomen and brain.

The parents decided not to investigate further, and preferred hospitalization at a referral center.

Analysis

Any fever of a long duration, with increasing neutrophilic leukocytosis but without any localization should arouse the suspicion of a non-infective fever, especially if two sets of antibiotics have failed. In this setting, a **bacterial infection** is possible only in the form of a **hidden abscess,** such as a **subdiaphragmatic, perirenal** or **intraspinal** abscess or **deep-seated muscle abscesses** or **osteomyelitis.** Even then, it is expected to manifest with local symptoms over a period of 2 months. In such cases, antibiotic therapy can fail, and the fever would abate only after drainage of the abscess. If this is not a bacterial infection, neutrophilic leukocytosis is a feature of a severe ongoing inflammation. A falling hemoglobin and an increasing platelet count, without any other positive laboratory tests, support the diagnosis of a **systemic inflammatory disorder**. In the absence of a definite history of swelling, the vague pain in the joints does not have any interpretive value. Since there are no other specific symptoms, it may evolve into any of the systemic inflammatory disorders. However, **systemic lupus erythematosus (SLE)** seems less likely since the leukocyte counts are usually normal or low (as against this case), and it is more common in females. Considering the pattern of fever, **systemic onset juvenile idiopathic arthritis** (formerly known as systemic onset JRA) can be a possibility.

■ PHYSICAL EXAMINATION

Fairly built and nourished	Weight 24 kg	Height 120 cm
Temp. 102°F	Pulse 118/min	RR 26/min
Looks sick	No lymphadenopathy	Mild pallor

Joint examination – Minimal fullness of few interphalangeal joints
Mild restriction of movements of left wrist and right ankle joint

No bony tenderness	No skin rash	No mouth ulcers
Liver not palpable	Spleen not palpable	

Other systems normal

Analysis

There is definite evidence of involvement of two major joints and a few small joints in the form of either restriction of movements or fullness. Hence, the diagnosis is probably evolving into a systemic onset juvenile idiopathic arthritis. The clinical findings of joint involvement may have appeared recently, and thereby facilitated the diagnosis. However, even prior to the development of such signs, a diagnosis of systemic inflammatory disorder could have been definitely considered (as analyzed after the history).

■ INVESTIGATIONS

Hb 8 gm%	Normocytic normochromic anemia		
WBC 38,000/c. mm	P 85 L 10 E 5	ESR 120 mm	Platelet count 7.5 Lacs
ANA weakly positive	Anti-dsDNA negative	RA factor negative	

Analysis

High neutrophilic leukocytosis, high platelet count and a high ESR suggest an active systemic inflammatory disease. A weakly positive ANA is non-specific and is seen in a variety of inflammatory and other disorders. Anti-dsDNA is also negative (this test is specific for systemic lupus and should be ordered only when ANA is strongly positive). A negative RA factor is no surprise, as it is present only in 5% of cases of juvenile chronic arthritis (the polyarticular variety) and not in systemic onset disease. The diagnosis of systemic onset juvenile idiopathic arthritis is clinical; there is no specific test. Moderate anemia with a normocytic, normochromic morphology indicates an anemia of chronic inflammation.

FINAL DIAGNOSIS

Systemic onset juvenile idiopathic arthritis.

KEY MESSAGES

- The diagnosis of systemic inflammatory diseases is clinical and is based on an evolving pattern over a few months.
- A definite label cannot be applied to a disease till a specific pattern develops.
- No single test can be considered to be sensitive and specific of a particular disease; it may at best, be supported by laboratory tests. However, the tests may help rule out other conditions in clinically doubtful situations.
- Until a specific diagnosis is possible, therapy is restricted to anti-inflammatory drugs only.

RELEVANT INFORMATION

	Polyarthritis	Monoarthritis	Systemic onset
RA factor	5% (older girls)	Rare	Rare
ANA	40–50%	75–80%	10%

CASE 42

Fever for 2 Months: Case 2

■ HISTORY

An 8-year-old female child presented with fever for the last 2 months. She was apparently well prior to the onset of this illness. The fever had been high grade, coming in two spikes per day with a normal intervening period, without any other localizing symptoms. She had undergone many laboratory tests and on two occasions her WBC counts were reported to be high. It led to therapy with multiple antibiotics without any relief.

On direct questioning, the parents reported an evanescent skin rash at the peak of fever. It appeared anywhere on the body without any specific predilection to any particular area and disappeared by itself as the fever reduced. It was macular and not itchy.

History of mouth ulcers in recent past
No other relevant past or family history.

Analysis

This female child has persistent fever *without localization*. Most of the bacterial infections would have localized within a few days of the onset, and either got better with antibiotic treatment or developed complications. **Tuberculosis** may present with a persistent fever without localization, but *persistent, high grade* fever is relatively less common, and a skin rash is an unusual feature. Viral infections would have been self-limiting, and those that persist with fever for such a long period would have localizing signs (**EB virus**). These signs would, of course, be apparent only on physical examination. WBC counts have been reported to be high at times, and with bacterial infections ruled out, it could suggest a **systemic inflammatory disease**. A skin rash at the peak of fever is in favor of systemic vasculitis. Past history of mouth ulcers also supports such a diagnosis. Malignancy may present with high persistent fever, and a skin rash may also be a feature (as in **Hodgkin's lymphoma**). A high WBC count may also be compatible with a **leukemia,** but persistent fever for 2 months without any deterioration, is less likely.

■ PHYSICAL EXAMINATION

Fairly built and nourished		Weight 24 kg	Height 120 cm
Looks "sick" at the peak of fever, but looks well when fever is temporarily controlled			
Temp. 102°F	Pulse 110/min	RR 28/min	BP 100/65 mm
No skin rash	No mouth ulcers	Patches of alopecia	No edema
Whitish lines on nails	No lymphadenopathy		
Moderate pallor	Bones and joints normal		
Liver just palpable, soft	Spleen not palpable		
Other systems normal			

Analysis

The only positive physical findings in this child are alopecia, nail changes and moderate pallor. Pallor without hepatosplenomegaly is likely to be due to nutritional deficiency, bone marrow hypoplasia or anemia of chronic diseases. Fever as a presenting symptom may suggest that the anemia is that of a chronic disease. Absence of lymphadenopathy, hepatosplenomegaly and any other abnormal findings (suggestive of mediastinal or abdominal lymphadenopathy) rule out Hodgkin or non-Hodgkin lymphoma. A leukemia can neither be confirmed nor completely ruled out with these physical findings; relevant investigations will be needed. Alopecia and nail changes, though not specific, may suggest a diagnosis of **systemic lupus**. Though there are no other classical features of SLE like a facial rash etc., they may evolve over time. However, the high leukocyte counts reported in the past, are unusual in SLE. **Bone marrow hypoplasia** may also present with fever (and pallor); the mere absence of purpura may not rule out such a possibility.

■ INVESTIGATIONS

Hb 8 gm%
WBC 9,500/c.mm
Platelet count 5.5 Lacs
Urinalysis normal
ANA strongly positive
Other antibody tests were negative
Serum creatinine/blood urea normal
Liver function tests normal

Normocytic normochromic anemia
P 82 L 12 E 4 M 2
ESR 110 mm
Chest X-ray normal
Anti-dsDNA positive

Analysis

The hematological parameters rule out a leukemia and bone marrow hypoplasia. While a strongly positive ANA may favor a diagnosis of lupus especially in a female child, it is also seen in other conditions, though usually in low titers. However, a positive anti-dsDNA is specific for the diagnosis of lupus. The disease is likely to evolve further over time. However, at present there is no evidence of any kidney or other organ involvement.

■ FINAL DIAGNOSIS

Systemic lupus erythematosus (SLE).

■ COMMENT

The high leukocyte counts reported in this case earlier in the history are unusual. SLE is typically characterized by normal leukocyte counts or leukopenia. In established SLE, such counts almost always indicate some occult infection. However, it may be possible to explain such counts *early* in the course of the disease before hematological involvement sets in, or they remain unexplained.

KEY MESSAGES

- A detailed history, including the relevant recent past events, are important to arrive at a diagnosis in patients without obvious localizing symptoms or signs.
- Majority of the collagen vascular disorders clinically evolve over a few months and till then, the diagnosis remains uncertain. Naturally, up to this point, the drug treatment is also restricted to symptomatic therapy only.
- Once a systemic inflammatory disorder is suspected, every organ must be evaluated for possible involvement, as the therapy and the prognosis would change.
- Majority of the inflammatory diseases are syndromic in nature, and the diagnosis is based on clinical patterns more than laboratory tests.

RELEVANT INFORMATION

The ANA test should always be done by immunofluorescence and not by the Elisa method. It is a screening test; it does not determine which of various known and unknown nuclear antigens the antinuclear antibody is specific for. Nonspecific elevated ANAs may be detected in healthy children (in low titer) and in various rheumatic and nonrheumatic diseases like ITP, Crohn disease, autoimmune hepatitis, Graves' disease, malaria, rarely leukemia/lymphoma and due to various drugs.

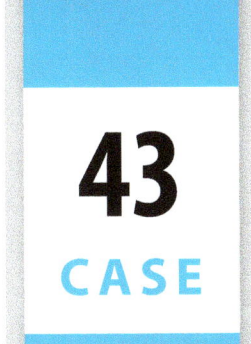

CASE 43

Fever for 3 Months

■ HISTORY

A 6-year-old child presented with fever for the last 3 months. She was apparently well prior to the onset of this illness. The fever had been mild to moderate in intensity, and initially did not disturb the child's routine activities. However, after 3 weeks of persistence of fever, she started feeling weak and stopped attending school and also stopped playing. She had become irritable, and was vomiting off and on since the last 2 months. There was also a loss of appetite, and she was constipated in general for the last 2 months. There were no urinary complaints and no history of cough.

She was treated for these complaints but the details of treatment are not available.

No relevant past or family history.

No contact with any specific infections.

Analysis

This child has been getting *progressively sick*. Vomiting off and on in a child at this age is significant unlike in infancy. Infants vomit for many stray triggers such as crying, physical activity and feeding besides an illness. However, *vomiting in an older child is significant* though it may or may not specifically localize the disease to any particular organ. Thus, a detailed enquiry should be made about subtle symptoms, which may offer clues to a particular organ involvement. *Constipation* may be a nonspecific symptom arising simply out of a poor intake and hence may not be very useful, so also symptoms such as loss of appetite and loss of weight. However, *irritability* in this child (at this age) represents a behavior change and must be given due importance, especially if there is no complaint of pain or any other specific disturbance to account for the same. Such a behavior change in the presence of significant vomiting may be a symptom of **encephalopathy**. While a history of headache would have substantiated this inference, its absence does not rule it out. Encephalopathy may be caused by an infection, systemic inflammatory disease, malignancy or a metabolic disease. In view of fever for 3 months, the encephalopathy in this child is likely to be infective in origin, the infection being a **chronic CNS infection**. Such infections include **partially treated bacterial meningitis**, **brain abscess** secondary to acute bacterial meningitis, **tubercular meningitis** or **fungal meningitis**. **Viral infections** are short lasting and present with an acute onset of a change in sensorium and convulsions. Acute bacterial meningitis and a brain abscess would have had a stormy course and would have significantly deteriorated if not treated adequately, and hence rather unlikely. A brain abscess would also have led to focal convulsions. Thus, the encephalopathy in this child is probably due to a tubercular or a fungal meningitis.

■ PHYSICAL EXAMINATION

Fairly built, poorly nourished child looks "sick"
Weight 15 kg Height 105 cm
Temp. 100°F Pulse 95/min RR 26/min BP 100/60 mm
Mild pallor No skin rash No significant lymphadenopathy
Bones and joints normal

CNS - irritable child No meningeal signs
MacEwen's sign negative Fundus normal
No motor deficit No other abnormality
Other systems normal

Analysis

Malnutrition at this age is always due to a chronic underlying disease. Absence of any localizing abnormality on physical examination makes it impossible to define the anatomy and the pathology of the disease. However, considering that the history was suggestive of an encephalopathy, this may be a chronic CNS disease.

■ INVESTIGATIONS

Hb 10 gm% WBC 8,000/c.mm P 42 L 48 E 4 M 6
ESR 35 mm Mantoux test negative Chest X-ray normal

CSF - clear fluid Normal pressure Proteins 150 mgm%
Cells 60/HPF Mostly lymphocytes Sugar 40 mgm%
Smear negative Culture negative
(Blood sugar 105 mgm% done simultaneously)

CT scan of brain – basal exudates with mild hydrocephalus
CT scan of chest – showed necrotic right hilar lymph nodes

Analysis

A mild increase in the proteins and cells in the CSF and a borderline low sugar confirms the diagnosis of a low-grade meningitis. Basal exudates and mild hydrocephalus as seen on the CT scan of the brain, suggests a basal meningitis with obstructive hydrocephalus. Though such findings are typical of tubercular meningitis, they may be mimicked by fungal meningitis as well. However, the necrotic hilar lymph nodes found on the CT scan of the chest strongly suggest tuberculosis in our epidemiology. Nevertheless, fungal meningitis cannot be ruled out totally.

■ FURTHER TESTS

ZN stain for tuberculosis and India ink preparation to rule out fungal infection were negative. CSF BACTEC culture was also negative. PCR for tuberculosis was positive.

FINAL DIAGNOSIS

TB meningitis.

COMMENT

This case exemplifies the fact that in the absence of any positive findings on physical examination, the diagnosis totally rests on the history.

KEY MESSAGES

- Subtle symptoms such as vomiting may assume significance, especially in an older child.
- Unexplained irritability and behavior change localizes the disease to the nervous system.
- Diagnosis of tuberculosis is often difficult to prove, but circumstantial evidence should be strong enough to consider anti-TB treatment.
- A slow increase in intracranial pressure may present as irritability more than a headache (just as a slowly progressive cardiac or respiratory failure presents as easy fatiguability rather than breathlessness).

CASE 44

Fever for 6 Months

■ HISTORY

A 5-year-old child presented with fever for the last 6 months. He was apparently well, prior to the onset of this illness. The fever had been erratic; it was present on most of the days though varying in intensity. It responded to antipyretics, though temporarily. There had been no other symptoms. The appetite had been near normal. There was no significant loss of weight.

No relevant past or family history.

He had been investigated extensively and treated with multiple antibiotics without relief.

Analysis

As there are no localizing symptoms, the anatomy and the pathology of the disease is not obvious. In terms of etiology, **bacterial infections** seem unlikely, as most of them would have either localized over a short-time, and then improved on treatment or deteriorated. On the other hand, in **tuberculosis,** localization may sometimes be delayed, but not for as long as 6 months. However, as the localizing symptoms may be so vague that the parents easily overlook them, it may still be a possibility. Chronic parasitic infections like **kala-azar** may present with a prolonged fever without any other symptoms; however, most of them would have an associated weight loss. Recurrent **malaria** may simulate a persistent fever for 6 months, though on close scrutiny there are will be afebrile periods in between. **Systemic inflammatory disorders** can also be almost ruled out, as they would have developed either a joint or any other organ involvement, or a skin rash, over time. **Malignancy** is not considered for similar reasons. Infiltrative disorders like **histiocytosis** and **sarcoidosis** may go on for a long-time and need to be considered. **Heat fever** will not go on for so long; since no continuous drug is being used, **drug fever** is also unlikely. **Hyperthyroidism** is also unlikely as there is no significant weight loss. As this fever is reported to respond to antipyretics, **central fever** or autonomic dysfunction seems to be less likely. Hence at this stage, there is no clue to the probable diagnosis, on analysis of the symptoms. That would justify considering rare causes of fever. Whenever one meets this situation of a dead end at the end of analysis of the history, either the informant has offered inadequate details or it may be a **rare infection**. It is possible that physical examination may provide some additional help.

■ PHYSICAL EXAMINATION

Fairly built and nourished	Weight 18 kg	Height 103 cm
Does not look sick	Fairly comfortable	
No pallor	No lymphadenopathy	No icterus
Bones and joints normal		

Liver 7 cm +, firm, not tender Liver span 11 cm Spleen 5 cm +, firm
No engorged veins over abdominal wall   No ascites
Other systems normal

Analysis

This child has a prolonged pyrexia with hepatosplenomegaly. Presence of prolonged fever, in the absence of liver dysfunction (no loss of appetite or loss of weight) rules out a primary hepatocyte disease. Since there is no history of hematemesis or engorged abdominal veins or ascites on physical examination, the splenomegaly may not be a feature of portal hypertension in this child. Also, venous obstruction as the cause of hepatomegaly is ruled out. Therefore, this hepatosplenomegaly may be due to reticuloendothelial hyperplasia or a storage disorder. Persistent fever suggests **reticuloendothelial cell hyperplasia due to infection** and in fact, is against a **storage** disorder. Such infections include **tuberculosis**, Ebstein-Barr virus infection, **leptospirosis, kala-azar**, and **malaria**. However, EB viral infection would have improved over a few weeks, and leptospirosis/tuberculosis would have either improved on treatment or deteriorated. Absence of significant pallor/pigmentation rules out kala-azar and malaria. This infection has been such that neither has it led to any complications nor has it been controlled by the antibiotics used so far. Therefore it is an unusual infection, which is very slowly progressive, and not responsive to commonly used antibiotics. The exact etiology cannot be guessed and needs to be proved by appropriate tests. It is certainly not a **malignancy** as the fever has been going on too long with a reasonably normal health.

■ INVESTIGATIONS

Hb 10 gm%	WBC 8,000/c.mm	P 65 L 30 E 3 M 2
Platelets normal	ESR 105 mm	

Chest X-ray normal
Abdominal USG showed enlarged liver and spleen   No other abnormalities
CT abdomen showed microabscesses scattered all over the liver parenchyma and also in the spleen
There were few similar microabscesses in both kidneys.
CT chest normal.

Analysis

Evidence of *microabscesses* in various organs is a feature common to **brucellosis** and **plague**. Septicemic plague is characterized by microabscesses, but is an acute illness and therefore ruled out in this case. Since the antibiotic of choice for brucellosis is either streptomycin or tetracycline, and since these antibiotics are rarely used in routine clinical practice, such infections remain uncontrolled.

Granulomas may simulate microabscesses and are seen in tuberculosis and sarcoidosis. Since the CT scan of the chest is normal, tuberculosis is unlikely. Sarcoidosis is uncommon, but cannot be ruled out.

Subsequently, brucellosis was confirmed by serological tests.

■ FINAL DIAGNOSIS
Brucellosis.

■ KEY MESSAGES

- Unusual infections must be kept in mind to evaluate PUO presenting with hepatosplenomegaly.
- Routine imaging techniques such as X-ray or USG may fail to delineate finer abnormalities in an organ and CT or MR scans may be necessary.
- Unusual infections may go on for long-time without serious complications, as much as some malignant disorders which may remain undiagnosed for a long-time and still be compatible with life.
- Hepatosplenomegaly alone is a fairly nonspecific sign to evaluate any infection.

CASE 45

Fever for 12 Months

■ HISTORY

A 10-year-old child presented with a history of fever for the last 1 year. The fever has been erratic, and was present on most of the days. It fluctuated from a mild to often a high fever, and was not responsive to antipyretics. It used to return to normal by itself, at times with sweating. There were absolutely no other symptoms, nor any significant past or family history. The child had been eating well and remained active whenever there was no fever. He had been thoroughly investigated without any clue to the diagnosis.

Several empirical treatment modalities had failed.

Analysis

Whenever a child presents with fever for such a prolonged period, it is important to rule out fictitious fever. Hence, the temperature must be recorded by a proper thermometer and only after confirming the persistence of fever, further action should be planned. As this child has remained so well in spite of the long duration of fever, it is *quite unlikely* that this fever is due to an **infection, malignancy** or a **systemic inflammatory disorder**. These conditions do not remain stable for such a long-time. Either there would have been some improvement with treatment or a deterioration. **Heat fever** and **drug fever** can be ruled out merely by the persistence of fever for so long. A **hyperthyroid** state may lead to fever, but there would have been a loss of weight and diarrhea. The important clue to the diagnosis in this child is a *poor response to antipyretics*, which is suggestive of either a **central fever** or **autonomic dysfunction**.

In view of the fact that this child does sweat, it is unlikely to be an autonomic disturbance. However, it would be important to note any evidence of autonomic dysfunction on physical examination.

■ PHYSICAL EXAMINATION

Well-built and nourished child   Does not look sick
No positive findings on general and systemic examination
No evidence of autonomic dysfunction.

Analysis

As expected, there are no abnormal findings on physical examination. It favors a diagnosis of central fever. Common causes of a central fever are **acute encephalopathy with a hypothalamic dysfunction.** An acute severe **pontine lesion** may also result in high fever. However, all such conditions are *too acute* and they would not last for so long without other manifestations. As this child has fever for a year, the pathology is *chronic persistent* rather than acute. Considering a **hypothalamic tumor** as one possibility, the fundus was examined for the presence of papilledema. However, it did not reveal any abnormality. Knowing that hypothalamic/pituitary tumors may not present clinically with an increased intracranial tension, he was subsequently subjected to a CT scan of the brain. It showed a hypothalamic tumor, as the cause of the prolonged fever.

◾ FINAL DIAGNOSIS

Hypothalamic tumor.

◾ KEY MESSAGES

- Fever not responding to antipyretics is likely to be due to a central cause, especially if it is prolonged.
- In spite of a prolonged fever if the child remains healthy, it could be a clue to a central fever.
- Fictitious fever and drug fever must be ruled out in such cases.

◾ RELEVANT INFORMATION

Unlike other brain tumors, hypothalamic tumors may remain silent for a long-time or present with atypical manifestations, often apparently unrelated to the central nervous system. Endocrine manifestations include short stature or diabetes insipidus as the presenting features. Adrenal and thyroid functions may also be affected and should be assessed by relevant laboratory tests. Central fever may be the only presenting feature of a hypothalamic tumor. Papilledema and visual field defects (for bilateral hemianopsia) must be closely looked for. Even with evidence of increased intracranial pressure, the tumor may be difficult to localize clinically and at times may simulate pseudotumor cerebri.

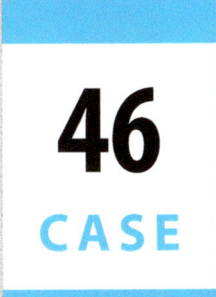

CASE 46

Fever and Cough for a Few Days

■ HISTORY

A 10-year-old child presented with moderate fever and a mild cough for 4 weeks. When he was seen on the 4th day of the illness by his doctor, there were apparently no positive findings on physical examination. Nevertheless, he was empirically treated with amoxicillin for a week, without response. At that stage, investigations revealed a total leukocyte count of 16,000/c.mm; P 68%, L 28%, E 2%, M 2%, and the chest X-ray was normal. The antibiotic was now changed to a macrolide.

There was still no response in the fever and cough after another 5 days. Clinically, the child was not tachypneic or toxic, and there were still no positive findings on physical examination. At this point, the tests were repeated: WBC count 14,500/c.mm; P 58%, L 34%, E 4%, M 4%, and the ESR was 60 mm at the end of 1 hour. The chest X-ray was also repeated, and it now showed a right upper zone consolidation with an air bronchogram.

Considering drug resistance, IV cefotaxime and amikacin were started. When there was no response after a few days, a chest X-ray was repeated yet again, and it showed a persistence of the pneumonia. At this stage, lung puncture was attempted for a bacteriological diagnosis. It revealed *Staphylococcus epidermis* sensitive to all antibiotics. Finally, the child was put on Vancomycin and Imipenem. However, since the fever continued in spite of these antibiotics, he was referred to a tertiary center.

Analysis

If we analyze the history from the onset of the illness, fever and cough for 4 days *without* any positive findings suggests a **respiratory infection**, which has not yet localized to any specific part of the respiratory system. It could possibly be a **disease in evolution** (infective or even non-infective). Ideally, at this stage it may be irrational to start an antibiotic; either one should carefully wait for further localization, or investigate. Further, when this child's leukocyte counts were nonspecific and the chest X-ray was normal, atypical community acquired acute bacterial infection seemed unlikely. However, treatment for **atypical bacterial infections** in the form of macrolides may have been justified, since their clinical features (as well as the counts and the X-ray) may not be specific. Subsequently, this child was diagnosed and treated as an acute bacterial pneumonia on the basis of radiology (with still no clinical signs). However, an **acute bacterial pneumonia** presents with *clinical and* radiological signs, within the *first few days* of onset of the illness. Further, a neutrophilic leukocytosis with eosinopenia would have been expected, and if an acute bacterial pneumonia fails to respond to antibiotics, it is likely to develop complications such as empyema, lung abscess or sepsis. Since this child had none of these features, it is unlikely that this was an acute bacterial pneumonia. Development of pneumonia after 2 weeks of onset of the illness, itself suggests a **subacute infection** such as tuberculosis or a **non-infective inflammatory pathology**. Therefore, the fact that there was no response to further antibiotics is not surprising. Systemic inflammatory disorders like **Wegener's granulomatosis** may be a possibility; other features may evolve over time. **Tuberculosis** also needs to be considered, because in tuberculous consolidation the disease often starts in a segment of a lobe and then progresses slowly. Thus in the initial stages, there may be minimal or no clinical signs. Further, an obstructed bronchus due to a lymph node may lead to a collapse consolidation, and since the air entry is compromised, it may lead to a paucity of clinical signs. Other subacute infections like **fungal infections** are unlikely in this immunocompetent host (previously healthy child). *Staph. epidermis* was obviously picked up from the skin and should have been ignored.

■ PROGRESS

This child was subjected to a CT scan of the chest, which showed caseating mediastinal lymph nodes with a collapse consolidation. The tuberculin test was negative. However, with a clinical setting of tuberculosis, this child was put on anti-TB therapy. He responded within 2 weeks, and progressed satisfactorily thereafter on a compliant treatment. The tuberculin test was repeated after 6 weeks and was positive then. Bronchoalveolar lavage may have been tried in this child, which may have proved the diagnosis of tuberculosis.

■ FINAL DIAGNOSIS

Tuberculous collapse consolidation.

■ KEY MESSAGES

- A subacute onset of pneumonia without toxicity or dyspnea, is unlikely to be due to acute bacterial infection.
- A persistent clinical and radiological pneumonia may be due to a wrong diagnosis, provided other possibilities like complications (empyema/lung abscess) or a drug resistant infection have been ruled out.
- If two antibiotics have failed, the diagnosis must be revised.
- Reversal of a negative tuberculin test to positive, is a retrospective indication of a correct diagnosis and successful treatment.

■ RELEVANT INFORMATION

It is well-known that the tuberculin test may be negative in active tuberculosis due to immune suppression caused by the bacterial load. On successful treatment, the immune status returns to normal and the tuberculin test becomes positive.

In a recovering pneumonia, the clinical symptoms and signs disappear much before radiological clearance, which may even take a few weeks. In other words, persistence of a radiological shadow after clinical recovery does not need continuation of treatment. However, its eventual clearance must be documented. Persistence of the radiological shadow beyond a few weeks (without clinical symptoms), may suggest a congenital malformation of the lung such as a cyst or a sequestration.

Bronchoscopy with bronchoalveolar lavage (BAL) is an ideal procedure in the evaluation of a persistent pneumonia. It offers a direct visualization of the bronchial tree, besides allowing drainage of secretions, and also helps to obtain material for bacteriology and histopathology.

47 CASE

Fever and Cough with Large Expectoration

■ HISTORY

A 15-year-old male child presented with a high-grade continuous fever, cough with large amount of expectoration and breathlessness on exertion for the last 3 weeks. There was a past h/o similar episodes off and on for the last 7–8 years, and he was also hospitalized several times for the same, in the past. He had never suffered from an episode of acute breathlessness in the past, but over the last 2 years, he complains of breathlessness on exertion with each episode of fever and cough, which has been gradually worsening. He has been treated with antibiotics and anti-TB drugs without lasting benefit. There has been no history of frequent upper respiratory symptoms (nasal discharge) or headache associated with the fevers. There has also been no history of frequent episodes of diarrhea in the past.

Analysis

A prolonged history of repeated cough and breathlessness on exertion may have suggested a **cardiac disease**. However, predominant cough with a large amount of expectoration, a relatively minor degree of breathlessness without any acute exacerbations, fever as a predominant symptom and a history spanning over several years without cardiac decompensation, rules out a cardiac disease. Cough with a large amount of expectoration suggests either **bronchiectasis** or a **lung abscess**. As this child has had similar episodes in the past, it is unlikely to be a lung abscess; hence, it must be bronchiectasis. However, breathlessness is a rare feature in bronchiectasis as the disease is usually limited to some bronchial segments. Even though the lung parenchyma may be involved secondarily, its extent is usually small. Hence, lung function is usually well maintained in spite of severe bronchial involvement and repeated infections. It may so happen that such a child may get breathless acutely, due to an acute exacerbation of infection leading to a pneumonia. But this child seems to have never presented with acute onset breathlessness. Gradually progressive breathlessness in a respiratory disease is often seen in an **interstitial lung disease**. However, the history of predominant cough with large expectoration rules it out. Therefore, this is likely to be an extension of the bronchiectasis into the lung parenchyma (**spreading bronchoalveolar disease**) involving *large areas* of the lung. Such a progressive, destructive bronchopulmonary disease has therefore lead to a slow decompensation of lung function. **Recurrent lower respiratory infections** are always secondary to some underlying disorder, either structural or functional. When seen in the same anatomical site, they suggest a **congenital malformation** but when seen in different areas as seen in this case, they suggest **immune deficiency, ciliary dyskinesia**, or **cystic fibrosis**. **Multidrug resistant tuberculosis** could also present with similar complaints; however this kind of a prolonged history over several years makes it unlikely. Considering the above possibilities, a detailed family history was again sought, at which time the history of death in an elder sibling at 18 years of age was reported. This child had also suffered similar symptoms over several years.

(Often such a history is deliberately hidden by the patients, possibly in an attempt to escape from the same diagnosis in another sib). This positive family history may favor the inherited disorders like immune deficiency or cystic fibrosis.

■ PHYSICAL EXAMINATION

Poorly nourished child   Wt 28 kg   Ht 140 cm
Temp. 100°F   HR 105/min   RR 28/min, no respiratory distress
clubbing of nails   No cyanosis
RS examination
Chest symmetrical, no flattening in any area
Trachea central, apex beat normal, TVF markedly decreased posteriorly at the left base
Impaired note posteriorly at the left base with absent breath sounds (VR absent)
Scattered crepitations all over on both sides, bronchial breath sounds at multiple areas
Liver 2 firm, spleen not palpable
Other systems normal.

Analysis

Scattered coarse crepitations all over the chest, with clubbing suggests **extensive bronchiectasis**. Bronchial breathing suggests consolidation or a cavity; multiple areas suggest cavities (markedly dilated bronchial segments simulate cavities). The signs at the left base suggest either an **atelectasis** or a **cavity** (both, with an obstructed bronchus), or a **pleural disease**. Since, there is other evidence of multiple cavities, this is also likely to be a cavity with an obstructed bronchus (due to thick viscid secretions). It may be a pleural disease resulting from an extension of the chronic bronchopulmonary infection (such as thickened pleura). Atelectasis is unlikely with dilated bronchial segments.

Similarly, fibrocaseous cavitatory disease due to **tuberculosis** is also less likely, because clinical signs such as flattening of the chest and a pulled mediastinum are lacking. Also, in fibrocaseous TB, unilateral disease is more common. If it is bilateral, it again suggests an underlying **immune deficiency** (including **HIV**) or multidrug resistant TB. Immotile cilia syndrome may be characterized by dextrocardia (its absence does not rule it out); however, absence of symptoms of sinusitis makes it less likely. HIV infection is also unlikely as the disease is spanning over several years and is restricted to repeated respiratory infections responding temporarily to antibiotics. Since, there is no history of frequent diarrhea, cystic fibrosis is unlikely. **IgA deficiency** may also be a strong consideration in this situation.

■ INVESTIGATIONS

Hb 8 gm% WBC 12,000/c.mm P 65 L 30 E 2 M 3
ESR 65 mm at the end of an hour
Chest X-ray – honey comb appearance, with multiple bilateral cavities.
Sputum culture – *Klebsiella* and *Candida albicans*
Sweat chloride – normal Serum IgA - zero

Analysis

Klebsiella and *Candida* in sputum culture favors a diagnosis of immune deficiency which has been proved.

■ FINAL DIAGNOSIS

Severe IgA deficiency.

■ KEY MESSAGES

- Recurrent bacterial lower respiratory infections are always due to some underlying cause and such a child should be investigated early in the course of the disease.
- Recurrent infections restricted to the respiratory tract alone are likely to be due to local structural or functional defects in the lungs or airways. Those due to structural defects present with localized lesions, and are not progressive, though they are recurrent. On the other hand, functional defects are progressive and generalized.

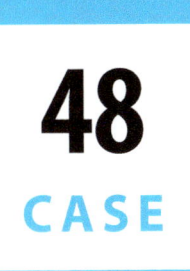

CASE 48

Fever with "Changing Pneumonia"

■ HISTORY

An 8-year-old child presented with a continuous high fever and mild cough for the last 4 days. He was diagnosed as a case of pneumonia, on the basis of a chest X-ray showing left middle zone haziness, and a WBC count of 25,000/c.mm P 78 L 15 E 5 M 2. He was treated with IV Augmentin and symptomatic therapy. There was no response and the fever continued to be high even after 6 days of treatment. The WBC count was repeated; it was now 40,000/c.mm P 82 L 14 E 4. The chest X-ray was also repeated, which showed a regression of the left sided haziness, but appearance of haziness in the right lower zone. The antibiotics were changed to Cefotaxime and Amikacin. However, there was still no response after another 5 days.

On day 16 of the illness, he developed a seizure. The CSF was normal.

No past history of any significance.

Analysis

The initial history is apparently suggestive of an **acute bacterial pneumonia**; however the progress and the investigations are unusual. Though this child has a high neutrophilic leukocytosis, an eosinophil count of 5% is not expected in an acute infection. Further, though the fever has persisted and the counts have worsened in spite of antibiotic therapy, the X-ray has shown a regression of the initial lesion on the left side. Meanwhile, a new lesion seems to have developed on the right side. An **inhaled foreign body** can present like this as *'changing pneumonias'*, but in a younger child; it is unlikely at this age. Further, severe cough is an important feature of an inhaled foreign body and the secondary infection is usually amenable to antibiotic treatment, at least temporarily. Therefore, a foreign body inhalation is unlikely. The fact that the first lesion has regressed, suggests that the antibiotic therapy was successful. However, the appearance of a new lesion on an apparently successful antibiotic therapy is very unusual, raising the possibility that it may not be an infection at all. Fever of non-infective origin may be due to **inflammatory diseases** or a **malignancy**. A malignant lesion will not disappear so soon, hence it is likely to be a systemic inflammatory disease.

A seizure on *day sixteen* of the illness is unlikely to be a **primary intracranial infection**; it would have manifested initially with symptoms like headache and vomiting, *followed by* a change in sensorium and a seizure. It is also unlikely to be an infective **complication of** an **extracranial** disease (e.g., brain abscess in a cyanotic heart disease or an extension from mastoiditis); they would also have presented with intracranial symptoms and a focal seizure. Therefore, it is likely to be a **non-infective** complication (either **vascular** or **immune mediated**) of this febrile disease.

Therefore, if this is a systemic inflammatory disease as discussed above, the appearance of a seizure in such a disease suggests a neurological involvement in a systemic inflammatory disease.

Investigations were planned accordingly:

■ INVESTIGATIONS

Hb 9 gm% Normocytic normochromic anemia
WBC count 45,000/c. mm P 84 L 10 E 6 Platelet count 8.5 Lacs
ESR 120 mm at the end of hour CRP strongly + ve
ANA + ve p-ANCA + ve c-ANCA + ve
CT scan of brain showed infarct in the territory of anterior cerebral artery
CT scan of chest showed pneumonia on the right and the left side

Analysis

Increasing neutrophilic leukocytosis without eosinopenia, thrombocytosis, and a high ESR and CRP favor a systemic inflammatory disease. Presence of multiple antibodies and specifically p-anca and c-anca support such a diagnosis. The cerebral infarct suggests a vasculitic process.

Subsequently, the child was diagnosed as Wegener granulomatosis.

■ FINAL DIAGNOSIS

Wegener granulomatosis.

■ KEY MESSAGES

- Eosinophil count is important to take note of. Acute bacterial or viral infection presents with eosinopenia, while absence of eosinopenia in a setting of an "acute infection" may suggest either a parasitic infection or a non-infective disorder.
- Continuation of fever in spite of sudden disappearance of a radiological lesion is unusual; appearance of a new lesion while on compliant treatment is against an acute bacterial infection. It is, in fact, suggestive of an immunological disease.

■ RELEVANT INFORMATION

Wegener granulomatosis is characterized by histologic evidence of granulomatous inflammation, presence of pulmonary nodules, cavitatory pulmonary lesions, or invasive bony disease. It is a type of small vessel vasculitis, a differential diagnosis being Churg-Strauss syndrome. Rheumatoid factor is positive in a low titer in two-thirds of the patients, whereas antinuclear antibody is present in 10–20% of the patients. Complement levels are normal.

Despite some limitations, when used appropriately, the ANCA (antibody to nuclear cytoplasmic antigens) test provides a tool that can aid greatly in the diagnosis of small vessel vasculitis. Patients with clinical evidence of ANCA positive small vessel vasculitis, who lack granulomatous inflammation, are classified as having microscopic polyangiitis (MPA).

All are forms of small vessel vasculitis with multiorgan involvement, and all are associated with ANCA. In contrast to WG, the indirect immunofluorescence staining pattern in MPA and Churg-Strauss syndrome is often perinuclear (pANCA). In WG, it is cANCA +ve.

pANCA positivity alone can be observed in a number of other diseases that would not qualify as small vessel vasculitis. These include inflammatory bowel disease, Kawasaki disease, polyarteritis nodosa, Felty's syndrome, and infections, such as HIV and endocarditis.

CASE 49

Fever with Irritability in an Infant

■ HISTORY

A 1-year-old child presented with fever and irritability for 5 days. He started with high fever that would respond to paracetamol only to recur again after 6–8 hours. Irritability started soon after fever and continued even when fever subsided temporarily with paracetamol. It was difficult for mother to keep the child quiet. It was only in small periods of sleep that child would be quiet. There was no vomiting or any other symptoms. He was treated with antibiotic on day 3 of fever because of neutrophilic leukocytosis.

Analysis

Infection is the most common cause of fever. Had it been a viral infection, usually there would have been associated cold and cough and there would have been a natural recovery over 5 days. Similarly by day 5, bacterial infection would have localized and is therefore unlikely. Malaria is characterized by an erratic pattern of fever and is therefore less likely. So, this seems to be a **non-infective fever** due to systemic inflammation as suggested by neutrophilic leukocytosis. Extreme irritability suggests pain. **Intracranial infection** can present as fever with irritability, but there should be additional features such as vomiting, seizures and drowsiness with progressive deterioration. **Earache** is a common cause of pain and often follows upper respiratory infection, but this child has no such symptoms. Further, over 5 days, the ear would have started discharging and the pain and irritability would have been relieved by now. **Abdominal pain** would have been colicky and if continuous, would not have lasted for so long without other symptoms or further worsening. Hence, this extreme irritability could suggest generalized pain as in myalgia or bony pain. Considering the age of this child, **Kawasaki disease** or **systemic onset of Juvenile idiopathic arthritis** is likely though **leukemia** must be ruled out.

■ PHYSICAL EXAMINATION

Conscious, Extremely irritable
Temp. 102°F
Weight 9.5 kg
Conjunctiva pink, no discharge
No lymphadenopathy
Systemic examination normal

Pulse 145/min
Length 75 cm
Mouth normal
Development normal

RR 40/min
Head C. 45 cm
No skin rash

Analysis

This febrile irritable child has no localization except conjunctival infection without discharge. It may suggest non-infective inflammation. At this stage, no definite diagnosis can be made after physical examination, but if we correlate with the history, this child seems to be in a stage of evolution of an inflammatory disease. We need to watch carefully for further development of clinical clues/signs, but it may be worth investigating for specific vasculitides like Kawasaki disease because early diagnosis can prevent permanent disability in terms of coronary artery aneurysm.

■ INVESTIGATIONS

Results were compared with previous reports done on day 3.

	Earlier	*Day 3*
Hb	9 gm%	8 gm%
WBC count	17,000/c.mm	22,000/c.mm
Polymorphs	73	85
Platelet count	3.4 L/c.mm	4.5 L/c.mm
ESR	60 mm	85 mm

Urinalysis normal   Chest X-ray normal   Blood culture no growth
2D Echo normal

Analysis

Increasing neutrophilic leukocytosis, thrombocytosis and ESR indicate systemic inflammatory disorder in an evolving stage. Normal echocardiogram does not rule out coronary artery disease as it may take time to appear. Diagnosis of Kawasaki disease is largely clinical; further, at this age of 1 year, one has to be extra cautious because atypical or incomplete Kawasaki disease is more common at this age and should not be missed. Thus, in this infant the present manifestations are highly likely to represent Kawasaki disease and hence one may not wait for further manifestations such as skin rash, red strawberry tongue, cervical large lymph node, etc. It is best to administer IVIG in this case presuming it to be Kawasaki disease. Anyway there is no specific test for this disease and it is the constellation of findings in a typical setting that makes a diagnosis of Kawasaki disease.

■ FINAL DIAGNOSIS

Kawasaki disease.

KEY MESSAGE

Fever beyond 5 days that has not yet localized should alert the clinician to rule out Kawasaki disease. Typical manifestations develop over time; at the same time, waiting for a "definite" diagnosis may be a bit late especially in infants who run a higher risk of coronary heart disease. So one has to strike the right balance between an early suspicion that may run a risk of overdiagnosis and waiting for all typical manifestations which might delay the diagnosis. The only other systemic inflammatory disease known to present at this early age is systemic onset Juvenile Idiopathic Arthritis, but Kawasaki disease is probably much more common at this age than systemic-onset juvenile idiopathic arthritis (SOJIA).

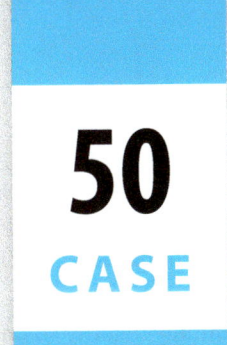

CASE 50

Fever with Irritability

■ HISTORY

An 8-year-old healthy male child presented with a history of a fall on his back, while playing on the school ground. Immediately after the fall, he could not get up, though he was fully conscious and was able to move all his limbs. He was rushed to a medical facility, where the X-ray showed a minor vertebral fracture involving D10. He was put in a plaster jacket and allowed to go home. After 3 days, he started running fever. Initially, it was mild but after a few days it became more severe. There was neither any pain at the site of the injury, nor any other accompanying symptoms. He was treated with paracetamol initially and later with oral ampicillin without any relief. After 10 days of persistent fever, he started getting irritable and had lost his appetite. The plaster was removed for inspection, expecting local infection. But there was no evidence of infection. At this stage, routine investigations were ordered.

    Hb 10 gm%   normocytic normochromic anemia
    WBC 8,000/c.mm   P 22 L 70 M 5 E 3   Platelets adequate
    X-ray spine revealed findings similar to the previous X-ray.
    At this stage of the illness, he was referred for evaluation of the cause of fever.
    The child has been in perfect health prior to this illness with no history of any minor or major illnesses whatsoever.

Analysis

In this child, a trivial fall has resulted in a fracture. Hence, it is likely to be a pathological fracture. Such a fracture may result from either a generalized bony disorder like osteoporosis, or a local bony abnormality. Since the child has been in perfect health prior to this event, the former seems unlikely. A local abnormality could be in the form of a congenital bony cyst, which would obviously remain undetected prior to this event, being asymptomatic. However, the fever remains unexplained on the basis of such an abnormality. Therefore, unless we dissociate the two complaints and take the fever as unrelated, we need to consider a localized bony pathology which can be associated with fever. This is possible with an inflammatory bony pathology, e.g., a TB spine. However, if such a pathology is arising out of an infection, it should have initially presented with fever and pain at the local site. On the other hand, such a pathology could be a part of a systemic inflammatory disorder. However, isolated vertebral involvement without any other manifestations, as the presenting complaint is quite unusual. These disorders would either present with isolated involvement of other organs (joints, kidney, skin, etc.) more commonly, or a few weeks or months of systemic/constitutional symptoms before specific organ involvement. Therefore, one needs to consider a condition that is neither infective nor a systemic inflammatory disorder, and yet, can cause a localized destruction of the vertebral body and can cause fever. Thus, this may be a malignant disease; either a local malignancy in the form of a bone tumor or a generalized malignancy which also affects the bone, such as a leukemia.

In this setting, a hemoglobin of 10 gm% in a child who has been absolutely healthy so far, may also be viewed with suspicion. Though iron deficiency anemia is not uncommon in any socioeconomic group of children due to faulty eating habits, a normocytic, normochromic anemia suggests a different cause for the same.

■ PHYSICAL EXAMINATION

Child in plaster jacket Well built and nourished Weight 30 kg   Height 128 cm
Temp. 102°F   Pulse 120/min   RR 30/min
Severe pallor   No purpuric spots or skin rash   Bony tenderness present
No lymphadenopathy

Liver 3F +, firm, not tender   Spleen 1F +, firm
No ascites   No engorged veins over abdomen
CVS - soft systolic murmur   No signs of cardiac failure
Other systems normal

Analysis

Physical examination reveals severe pallor in this child, within a few days of the hemoglobin being reported as 10 gm%. This suggests a rapidly progressive primary hematological disease. An acute onset febrile illness with severe anemia, hepatosplenomegaly and bony tenderness in a child who has been absolutely healthy so far, leaves no other diagnosis other than acute leukemia. A serious illness could have been suspected in this child before he started running fever, only if one analyzed it to be a pathological fracture and evaluated accordingly.

■ INVESTIGATIONS

Hb 6 gm%   TLC 5,400/c.mm   P 08 L 97, occasional blasts seen
Platelet count 90,000/c.mm.
Bone marrow aspiration proved the diagnosis of acute lymphoblastic leukemia.

■ FINAL DIAGNOSIS

Acute lymphoblastic leukemia.

■ KEY MESSAGES

- One must evaluate the probability of occurrence of a presenting symptom in a given setting, which may provide clues to the etiology, as illustrated in this case.
- Significant lymphocytosis could be due to a disease primarily leading to lymphocytosis, or it could represent neutropenia and hence relative lymphocytosis.

RELEVANT INFORMATION

Approximately 10% of patients with ALL have disseminated intravascular coagulation (DIC) at the time of diagnosis, usually as a result of sepsis. Consequently, some patients may present with hemorrhagic or thrombotic complications. A large number of ecchymoses is usually an indicator of a coexistent coagulation disorder such as DIC.

Although patients may present with symptoms of leukostasis (e.g., respiratory distress, altered mental status) because of the presence of large numbers of lymphoblasts in the peripheral circulation, leukostasis is much less common in patients with ALL than in patients with AML, and occurs only in patients with very high WBC counts, i.e., several hundred thousand/mL.

Immunochemistry, cytochemistry, and cytogenetic markers aid in categorizing the malignant lymphoid clone.

In more than 90% of ALL cases, specific genetic alterations can be found in the leukemic blasts. These alterations include changes in chromosome number (ploidy) and structure; about half of all childhood ALL cases have recurrent translocations. Standard cytogenetic analysis is an essential tool in the workup of all patients with leukemia, because the karyotype of the leukemic cells has important diagnostic and therapeutic implications. In addition, molecular techniques, including reverse-transcriptase polymerase chain reaction (RT-PCR), Southern blot analysis, and fluorescence in situ hybridization (FISH), have helped improve diagnostic accuracy. Molecular analysis can identify translocations that are not detected by routine analysis of karyotype and can distinguish lesions that appear identical cytogenetically but differ at the molecular level.

Historically, the prognosis of patients with T-cell ALL has been worse than that of patients with B-lineage ALL. With the use of intensive chemotherapy, however, the outlook for patients with T-cell leukemia appears improved.

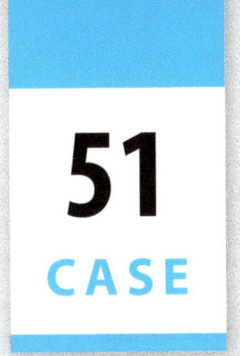

CASE 51

Fever Followed by Generalized Convulsion

■ HISTORY

An 8-month-old infant presented with fever for the last 15 days and convulsions on the day of admission to the local hospital. He was apparently well 2 weeks ago, when he started getting a mild to moderate degree of fever without any other obvious symptoms. He was treated for the first 4 days with paracetamol, and then prescribed an oral antibiotic for 5 days after which he seemed to be partially better. However, he was never afebrile for more than 24 hours at any time. He did not feed well during this period and was irritable. On day 15 of the illness, he developed a generalized convulsion lasting for 15 minutes followed by drowsiness. He was hospitalized for the same and the doctor noted the following positive findings:

Drowsy, but arousable
Anterior fontanelle boggy, not pulsatile
No meningeal signs
Left hemiparesis (upper motor neuron)
CSF - clear fluid   cells 200/c.mm   P 60 L 40   Sugar 25 mgm%   Proteins 300 mgm%

A diagnosis of partially treated bacterial meningitis was made and he was treated with IV Ceftriaxone and Ampicillin for the next 15 days. He improved clinically and a repeat CSF examination showed:

Cells 80/c.mm   P 50 L 50   Sugar 30 mgm%   Proteins 100 mgm%
Blood sugar was not assessed simultaneously any time.

He was discharged. He remained well for another 2 weeks and then started getting fever again and had a recurrence of convulsions for which he was referred to a tertiary center.

Analysis

This child had mild to moderate fever for 2 weeks before he had his first convulsion. He was never afebrile even though he appeared to get better partially after oral antibiotics. While poor feeding could be a feature of many childhood diseases, significant irritability in the absence of symptoms referable to any particular organ/system (in presence of fever) suggests an **infective encephalopathy** (generalized cortical dysfunction) and/or **raised intracranial pressure**. Subsequent development of a convulsion favors such a possibility. Acute bacterial meningitis generally presents with high fever followed by a convulsion within the first few days. As this child was not treated with any antibiotic for the first few days, if he had bacterial meningitis he would have deteriorated rapidly. Thus, this must have been a slowly developing **subacute meningitis**. On the day of admission to the local hospital, he had signs suggestive of an encephalopathy (drowsiness) with raised intracranial pressure (non-pulsatile boggy fontanelle) and also focal signs in terms of a hemiparesis. Classically, chronic meningitis such as tuberculous meningitis or a fungal infection is characterized by focal signs in a global disease. In the light of these findings, the CSF picture suggests a chronic meningitis such as a TBM. The CSF abnormalities are quite disproportionate as the sugar is very low but the proteins and cells are not very high. Further, though this child did improve clinically, the CSF did not return to normal as would have been expected in a bacterial meningitis. Thus, there was a disparity between the clinical course of the illness and the CSF picture. Such a disparity again favors **TBM** or **fungal meningitis**.

He remained well thereafter for 2 weeks and then threw up another convulsion. If it was a partially treated bacterial meningitis (at the time of discharge), such a recurrence of the convulsion after being well for 2 weeks was unusual, and would have meant development of a brain abscess, which would have presented with a focal convulsion and localizing signs.

■ PHYSICAL SIGNS

Poorly built and nourished

Weight 5.5 kg	Length 65 cm	Head ⊙ 45 cm	Chest ⊙ 40 cm
Temp normal	Pulse 120/min	RR 35/min	BP 80/50 mm of Hg
Moderate pallor	No lymphadenopathy	Bones and joints normal	
Palmar erythema	Tachycerebral response		

CNS – drowsy, but responding to stimuli   Anterior fontanelle boggy
Sutures separate   No neck stiffness
Left hemiparesis with upper motor neuron facial palsy
Liver 3 cm +, firm, not tender   Liver span 7 cm   Spleen 2 cm, + firm
Other systems normal

Analysis

This child has classical signs of intracranial infection with *hydrocephalus* as suggested by the increased head circumference, boggy fontanelle and sutural separation, *encephalopathy* as depicted by drowsiness and *vasculitis* as noted by the dense left sided hemiplegia due to affection of the middle cerebral artery.

A combination of a subacute infective encephalopathy with focal signs and hydrocephalus makes the typical triad of **TBM**. In addition, this child is malnourished and has hepatospleno-megaly suggestive of disseminated disease.

Intracranial space occupying lesion may also lead to increased intracranial pressure with encephalopathy, but a dense hemiplegia is unlikely. A supratentorial space occupying lesion is ruled out as it would have resulted in a focal seizure as the *initial* manifestation. An infratentorial lesion may be considered on physical examination, though there would have been localizing signs relevant to the site of space occupation, such as cranial nerve palsies or cerebellar signs. The original history of fever for 2 weeks followed by a convulsion and an abnormal CSF is against a space occupying lesion.

INVESTIGATIONS

Hb 8 gm% WBC 8,000/c.mm P 50 L 42 E 3 M 5 ESR 65 mm
Mantoux test negative Blood sugar 90 mgm%
CSF – proteins 500 mgm% sugar 30 mgm% cells 350/cmm P 20 L 80
CSF smear and culture negative CSF PCR +ve for *Mycobacterium tuberculosis*
Chest X-ray normal
CT scan showed marked hydrocephalus with basal exudates and infarct in the territory of left MCA.

Analysis

A moderate increase in proteins and the cell count (with lymphocytic predominance) and a low sugar in the CSF, suggests active subacute meningitis. The hydrocephalus with an infarct favors a tuberculous meningitis. Though PCR results are known to be false positive and when interpreted in isolation, may not be dependable, in this case the positive PCR confirms the diagnosis (in this clinical situation). Though the CSF smear and culture is negative for tuberculosis, it does not rule out a TBM, as the sensitivity of these tests is not very high. Even a negative Mantoux test can be compatible with a diagnosis of TBM, depending on the host immune response. A normal chest X-ray may not rule out a pulmonary lesion; a CT scan of the chest may pick it up.

FINAL DIAGNOSIS

Tuberculous meningitis.

KEY MESSAGES

- Detailed history of origin, duration and progress of symptoms coupled with the nutritional, immunization and contact status helps in differentiating a partially treated bacterial meningitis from TBM.
- Global encephalopathy with focality and hydrocephalus is typical of TBM. Evidence of dissemination to other organs is common in infants.
- The immunological response in tuberculosis is extremely variable. As a result, a temporary improvement in the clinical status does not necessarily suggest a favorable therapeutic response to antibiotics and is often misleading, by indicating a non-tuberculous disease.

RELEVANT INFORMATION

Though tuberculous meningitis may occur at any age, it commonly presents between the ages of 6 months and 3 years, but generally not <3 months. The classical presentation includes a subacute infective encephalopathy with hydrocephalus, raised intracranial pressure, vasculitis involving different sites and multiple cranial nerve affection. However, as most of the manifestations are immune mediated, the presenting features depend upon the host response. Thus TBM may present with a wide spectrum of manifestations, at one end of the spectrum being meningitis without encephalon involvement (as in acute bacterial meningitis) and at the other end, an encephalopathy without meningitis (as in viral encephalitis). In miliary TB, nervous system involvement may not be clinically apparent but may be evident only by CSF examination. Rarely, TBM may present as an isolated clinical abnormality such as an acute hemiplegia or a movement disorder. Confirmation of the diagnosis is difficult in such cases and is possible only with evidence of tuberculosis elsewhere in the body. Hepatosplenomegaly in infants is a strong pointer to disseminated tuberculosis. A pulmonary lesion on the chest X-ray is seen in only one-third of the patients of TBM, though a CT scan of the chest may pick up more abnormalities.

CASE 52

Frequent Fever with Inability to Walk

■ HISTORY

A 2-year-old male child presented with a progressive inability to walk and stand for the last 1 year. On direct questioning, the parents informed that he suffered from repeated episodes of fever during infancy. For each episode, he got some treatment from the local doctor. There was a temporary relief from the fever, but the parents were sure that he was never well, and in fact, was getting progressively weaker. They also gave a history of irritability and pain if made to stand and walk.

He was born after a full-term gestation and a normal vaginal delivery with an average birth weight. He was normal for the first-6 months and had attained normal milestones. Thereafter, with recurrent fever episodes his motor development was delayed, but his social and adaptive development was normally maintained. He has barely started walking at 18 months of age, but thereafter had a progressive difficulty in walking and standing.

He was mainly breastfed for the first 1 year without much semisolid food. Thereafter, he was weaned off breastfeeding, but did not eat well as he was always sick.

- No history of upper limb involvement
- No history of edema or breathlessness
- No history of consanguinity
- No history of joint pain or swelling
- Bladder and bowel functions normal
- No relevant family history

Analysis

This child has a *painful* inability to stand and walk, due to a progressive pathology starting sometime in infancy and gradually worsening over time. It is unlikely to be a neurological disease as most of the neurological diseases present with *weakness without pain*. (Pain may be seen in early preparalytic stage of poliomyelitis or may be localized pain as seen in involvement of the nerve roots. In both the conditions, weakness is a predominant symptom and pain is not a presenting complaint). Generalized weakness reported by the parents, and delayed motor development after 6 months of age with normal mental milestones, suggests severe malnutrition and is also corroborated by the dietary history (late weaning and poor intake of food). Generalized pain without swelling in a malnourished child denotes bony pain as in **scurvy** or **osteopenia**. If it is osteopenia, it must be due to non-nutritional rickets (**renal tubular acidosis**), as vitamin D deficiency is seen in a well-nourished, fast growing child and not in a malnourished child.

Recurrent episodes of fever may represent either **malaria** or **urinary tract infection**. A child suffering from recurrent malaria would have presented with significant anemia more than severe malnutrition and would have been normal in between the febrile episodes. On the other hand, a painful inability to walk and stand may be related to poorly treated recurrent urinary tract infections resulting in metabolic rickets. A child with renal tubular acidosis does not present with recurrent fever and is hence ruled out.

■ PHYSICAL EXAMINATION

Poorly built and nourished
Looks "sick", irritable
Pulse 118/min
Signs of rickets and bony deformities present
Eyes – no cataract or any other abnormality

Weight 5.4 kg
Severe pallor
Resp. 40/min

Length 68 cm
No respiratory distress
BP 110/84 mm
Joints normal
No edema

CNS – generalized hypotonia
Liver 1 cm +, soft
Kidneys and bladder not palpable
CVS – soft systolic murmur, functional
RS – harsh breath sounds, no foreign sounds

Delayed motor milestones
Spleen not palpable

Normal mentation

Analysis

This is a severely malnourished and pale child with active rickets, who has tachypnea without distress, suggesting metabolic acidosis. It may suggest renal tubular acidosis or chronic renal failure, but the presence of hypertension in this child rules out renal tubular acidosis. Therefore, it is likely to be chronic renal failure due to chronic nephritis. In the absence of edema or a history of oliguria or hematuria, it is not a glomerulonephritis. In view of recurrent fever, it may be pyelonephritis. This child must have developed chronic renal failure as a result of poorly managed recurrent urinary tract infections.

The delayed motor milestones are most probably due to the severe malnutrition. The soft systolic murmur denotes severe anemia, which is due to chronic renal failure in addition to the nutritional deficiency. There is no evidence of an obstructive uropathy in the form of palpable kidneys or bladder, though clinically, it cannot be definitely ruled out. However, recurrent urinary tract infection may have resulted from a vesicoureteral reflux.

■ INVESTIGATIONS

Hb 5 gm% normocytic normochromic
Urinalysis – pus cells ++
Antibiogram – resistant to most of the drugs
Serum creatinine 5.2 mgm%
Serum Na 128 mgm%
Serum Ca 7.5 mgm%
Abdominal USG normal
DMSA scan – scarring of both kidneys

WBC 9,000/c.mm   P 67 L 30 E 2 M 1
Urine culture – heavy growth of *Klebsiella*

Blood urea 120 mgm%
Serum K 7.2 mgm%   Serum bicarb 8 mEq/L
Serum P 6.2 mgm%   Serum alk. phos 450 KA
MCU grade V reflux

Analysis

Urinary tract infection is proved by the bacteriological results. Presence of drug resistant *Klebsiella* suggests chronic infection. A VUR of grade V has resulted in damage to the kidneys as depicted by scarring on the DMSA scan. There is also evidence of chronic renal failure in terms of high serum creatinine and potassium, low bicarb level, rickets and severe normocytic normochromic anemia.

■ FINAL DIAGNOSIS

Chronic pyelonephritis due to grade V vesicoureteral reflux, leading to chronic renal failure and rickets.

■ KEY MESSAGES

- Urinary tract infection must be properly diagnosed prior to administration of antibiotics, and investigated to rule out structural or functional abnormality.
- Abdominal USG and MCU are minimal investigations necessary after the first attack of urinary tract infection is treated and controlled, especially in young children.
- In case of detection of an abnormality, a DMSA scan is indicated to consider long-term antibiotic prophylaxis to prevent subsequent renal damage.

CASE 53

Fever, Lethargy and Refusal to Feed

■ HISTORY

A 4-month-old infant presented with fever off and on for the last 4 weeks. During the first 3 weeks of fever, there were no other accompanying symptoms and no specific diagnosis was attempted. During this period, he was treated twice with amoxycillin for 5 days each, with temporary improvement.

Presently, the parents complained of fever for the last 7 days and lethargy and refusal to feed since the last 4 days. The fever was moderate to high grade, responding temporarily to antipyretics. The mother had noticed lip smacking and abnormal movements of the limbs, along with increasing drowsiness, since the last 2 days. She also reported two episodes of excessive inconsolable crying, lasting for a few minutes, which resolved on their own. He developed decreased movements of the left lower limb a day prior to hospitalization.

The birth history was normal and the neonatal period was uneventful. The developmental history prior to the illness was normal.

Analysis

This infant has presented with a **recurrent/persistent infection** without localization for the first 3 weeks. However, by the 4th week the disease has localized to the **intracranial** compartment. It is unlikely that the **previous illnesses** were **unrelated** and this is a separate infection. Recurrent infections due to **immunodeficiency** are characterized by unusual infections and/or a poor response to treatment. Hence, it is more likely that this is a persistent pathology, denoting a gradually progressive **subacute intracranial infection**. Lip smacking and abnormal movements of the limbs denote convulsions. Along with drowsiness and the episodes of excessive crying, it suggests an **encephalopathy** with **increased intracranial pressure**. There is also an evidence of **localization** in the form of decreased movements of the left lower extremity. Thus, this child has a subacute infective encephalopathy with increased intracranial pressure and focal signs. This favors **tuberculous meningitis** or a **partially treated bacterial** meningitis. At this age, tuberculous meningitis is rare. **Fungal infections** may occur in nursery graduates after having received excessive antibiotics and can be indolent; however there is no such history in this child. If it is a partially treated bacterial meningitis, focal signs may suggest complications like a **brain abscess** or a **subdural empyema**.

■ PHYSICAL EXAMINATION

Fairly built and poorly nourished

Weight 4.5 kg	Length 62 cm	Head ⊙ 45 cm	Chest ⊙ 38 cm
Temp. 101°F	Pulse 135/min	RR 45/min	BP 100/65 mm of Hg

Mild pallor Anterior fontanelle bulging and non-pulsatile
No prominent veins over the scalp No meningeal signs

CNS - drowsy, responding to painful stimuli   Pupils constricted left >right
Left 6th nerve palsy   Other cranial nerves normal
Fundii shows venous congestion
Mild weakness of left lower limb   Hypotonia in all the limbs
DTR exaggerated   No clonus

Liver just palpable   Spleen not palpable
Other systems normal

Analysis

The fact that this infant's length is normal but he is underweight, suggests that this is not a very longstanding illness. The milestones being normal also corroborate that he was well up to 3 months of age.

The large head circumference, along with a boggy fontanelle and systemic hypertension, indicates raised intracranial pressure. It may be due to either **hydrocephalus**, or some **space occupying lesion** such as a brain abscess or a subdural empyema, as suggested by the localizing signs (weakness of the left lower limb and the pupillary inequality). Pupillary inequality may also suggest impending **herniation**. The sixth cranial nerve palsy could be a **false localizing** sign denoting raised ICP. However, it could also be "truly" localizing in meningitis (sixth nerve compromised by exudates in the subarachnoid space). Thus, this infant is mostly suffering from a subacute meningitis with hydrocephalus and localizing lesions. Hence, this is likely to be a partially treated bacterial meningitis with a **brain abscess** or a **subdural empyema**. In the rare event of it being tuberculous meningitis, one would have expected it to be a part of a disseminated disease. Absence of hepatosplenomegaly rules out disseminated/miliary TB.

■ INVESTIGATIONS

Hb 7 gm%   normocytic, normochromic anemia
WBC 9,000/c.mm   P 64 L 32 E 1 M 3

In view of the raised intracranial pressure, lumbar puncture was deferred on admission.

CT scan of the brain showed multiple brain abscesses of varying sizes, the largest being 4 × 3 cm, with perilesional edema and shift of the midline, with mild hydrocephalus.

The brain abscesses were evacuated by burr holes in the skull. CSF collected from the ventricles showed evidence of ventriculitis.

Analysis

Normocytic normochromic anemia suggests anemia of chronic infection. In view of a partially treated bacterial infection, there is no neutrophilic leukocytosis. The CT scan of the brain proved the diagnosis of brain abscesses.

∎ FINAL DIAGNOSIS

Multiple brain abscesses.

∎ COMMENT

Usually, a partially treated meningitis would give rise to complications like a subdural effusion/empyema; brain abscesses occur more often in association with certain predisposing conditions like bacterial endocarditis, cyanotic heart disease, etc. However, abscesses are also known to occur as a complication of a persistent neonatal infection/inadequately treated neonatal meningitis/ventriculitis; and in young infants as a complication of bacterial meningitis. In fact, brain abscesses may be the result of antibiotic therapy administered to a neonate for mere prophylaxis of infection, without realizing the actual presence of infection. Brain abscesses arising out of a partially treated bacterial meningitis may remain asymptomatic for a long time and lead to permanent developmental delay.

∎ KEY MESSAGES

- Recurrent symptoms with a short intervening period of normalcy may be a manifestation of a persistent disease.
- Antibiotics should not be prescribed in the absence of localizing symptoms or signs, especially in infants. Prior to starting antibiotics, the physician must be sure of it not being an intracranial or a urinary infection; CSF examination is mandatory.

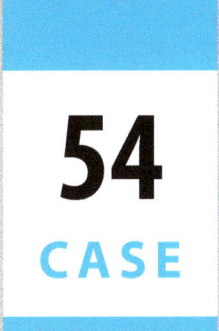

CASE 54

Fever with Neck Swelling

■ HISTORY

A 10-year-old child presented with a mild to moderate fever for 4 days, without any other symptoms. He was diagnosed to have acute tonsillitis and was treated with antibiotics. After 3 days of antibiotic therapy, the parents noticed a swelling on both sides of the neck, which was followed by difficulty in swallowing and breathing, a day later. The neck swelling was mildly painful only when touched. On the next day, his voice had gone down in intensity and subsequently he could not vocalize. Moderate fever continued.

No history of cough.
No history of drooling of saliva.
No relevant past or family history.

Analysis

This child seems to have developed a *rapidly progressive* neck swelling after a few days of fever, which has impinged upon the oropharynx as is evident by the difficulty in swallowing. It has also involved the trachea and/or larynx, as suggested by the difficulty in breathing and loss of voice. An **acute infection** in or around the oropharynx may lead to **severe cellulitis** (bull's neck) and result in a bilateral neck swelling; however, difficulty in breathing or a loss of voice is unlikely in most such infections, except **diphtheria**, which needs to be considered. A **retropharyngeal abscess** may lead to a difficulty in swallowing and breathing, but it is very painful and is not likely to cause a swelling in the neck. It could also be **lymph node swellings** on both sides of the neck. Since, this neck swelling was painful only when touched, it is unlikely to be due to an acute inflammation. Any lymph node swelling that develops acutely can be mildly painful (even if non-inflammatory). If lymph nodes in the retropharyngeal area and the upper mediastinum are enlarged, they may result in difficulty in swallowing and breathing. Laryngeal involvement, either due to direct extrinsic pressure or due to involvement of the nerves, may lead to loss of voice. If the neck swelling is presumed to be due to a **non-inflammatory** enlargement of the lymph nodes, it is likely to be a **malignant** disease in view of its fast progress. In retrospect, the tonsillar enlargement that was diagnosed as acute tonsillitis, must not have been inflammatory; instead, it represented a lymphoreticular disorder.

■ PHYSICAL EXAMINATION

Well built and nourished
Mouth kept open for breathing
Weight 32 kg
Temp. 99°F Pulse 120/min
Respiratory distress

Looks "sick" and in agony
No drooling of saliva
Height 136 cm
RR 45/min
Inspiratory stridor present

Bilateral large, firm to hard, mildly tender lymph nodes in the neck without signs of inflammation - both anterior and posterior cervical groups.
Submandibular, submental, suprasternal and supraclavicular lymph nodes also enlarged.
No other group of lymph nodes palpable
Tonsils large in size but not inflamed
Liver not palpable Spleen not palpable
Other systems normal

Analysis

Massive lymphadenopathy of an acute onset, extending into the mediastinum as evident by the laryngeal involvement, in a previously healthy child, suggests a rapidly progressive pathology. Absence of signs of inflammation rule out an acute infective process. Firm to hard lymph nodes suggest a malignant process like a leukemia or a lymphoma. **Hodgkin's lymphoma** is unlikely because it does not present so acutely. Similarly, a **leukemia** is also unlikely because one would have expected at least some hepatosplenomegaly along with such a massive lymphadenopathy. Besides, at least clinically, there is no significant pallor or any evidence of thrombocytopenia. Therefore, a **non-Hodgkin's lymphoma** is more likely. Other conditions that can cause such a lymphadenopathy could be **tuberculosis/histiocytosis**; however, they are chronic illnesses and therefore not considered here.

■ INVESTIGATIONS

Hb 8 gm% WBC count 12,000/c.mm P 35 L 61 E 4
ESR 120 mm at the end of 1 hour
Chest X-ray normal
Abdominal USG - no evidence of enlarged lymph nodes No ascites
Blood gas - showed hypoxia with hypercapnia
Excision biopsy – non-Hodgkin's lymphoma

Analysis

The high ESR suggests a malignancy. Though the chest X-ray is normal, mediastinal lymphadenopathy may be seen on a CT scan. The blood gas picture is a result of acute respiratory obstruction. Excision biopsy confirms the diagnosis.

■ FINAL DIAGNOSIS

Non-Hodgkin's lymphoma.

KEY MESSAGES

- Tonsils are large in size between 8 and 12 years of age, as this is the age of a rapid growth of the lymphoreticular system. To diagnose tonsillitis, the tonsils must be "inflamed", with an exudate, not just enlarged.
- Malignant disorders in children often present as an acute illness unlike in adults and hence, nutritional status is preserved in children.
- Malignancy may present as a medical emergency, in which case, relevant investigations must be carried out urgently before using any specific therapy.

RELEVANT INFORMATION

Childhood NHL (non-Hodgkin's lymphoma) generally presents as bulky extramedullary (usually extranodal) disease with or without demonstrable dissemination. The distinction between NHL and acute leukemia is arbitrary. NHL may present with a variable spectrum of manifestations from a clinically localized disease to overt leukemia. Most treatment protocols now define acute leukemia on the basis of marrow involvement greater than some threshold (typically, a blast count >25%), irrespective of the presence of bulky extramedullary disease. In contrast, a tumor accompanied by marrow involvement less than this threshold constitutes stage 4 lymphoma. Localized disease presents as firm, non-tender lymphadenopathy, tonsillar hypertrophy or a mass in virtually any location. However, NHL is primarily an extranodal disease in children.

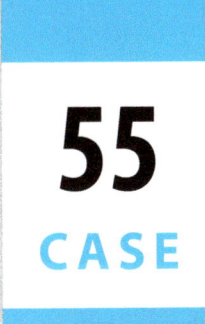

55 CASE

Fever with Severe Abdominal Pain

■ HISTORY

A 5-year-old child presented with a high-grade continuous fever for the last 8 days. He developed significant vomiting and severe abdominal pain 4 days prior to admission to the hospital. The pain was localized to the upper abdomen and was continuous. The vomitus was not bile stained. The parents also noticed that the child appeared pale over the last 2 days.

There was no history of any change in the bowel pattern. The color of the urine was reported to be normal. The appetite was poor and he had lost 2 kg of weight.

There was no significant past or family history.

Analysis

High fever of an acute onset suggests an **infection**. Initial high-grade fever followed by severe upper abdominal pain a few days later, either suggests a localization of the infectious process to an organ situated in the upper abdomen, or a complication of the infective disease or its treatment (e.g., drug induced gastritis). Upper abdominal pain may arise from the stomach, pancreas, liver or the gallbladder. Persistent fever for 8 days is unlikely to be due to gastritis. Rarely, a **basal pneumonia** may present with upper abdominal pain (in a child with fever) due to affection of the diaphragmatic pleura and thereby mimic an intra-abdominal pathology. However, such a pain is localized to the side of the pneumonia and not all over the upper abdomen. An **acute pyopericarditis** may present similarly, but the pain is more retrosternal with the child leaning forwards, in an attempt to relieve discomfort. Primary **cholecystitis** is rare in children. High-grade continuous fever may suggest enteric fever followed by a complication like cholecystitis; however such a cholecystitis rarely *presents* clinically as severe abdominal pain. In acute **pancreatitis**, pain is a presenting feature but would not take 4 days to manifest. Therefore, this is likely to be an acute infection of the liver—viral, pyogenic, or amebic. Acute **viral hepatitis** is ruled out since there is no history of a high colored urine and jaundice. Therefore, this may be a pyogenic or amebic infection of the liver, in the form of a **liver abscess**. **Amebic hepatitis** is a generalized affection of the liver and may also present with fever and acute abdominal pain, though the pain may not be so severe. Also, it is rare in children. Pallor when complained of by the parents, almost always signifies a low hemoglobin. However, this being their recent observation, in the absence of a history of blood loss, it is difficult to correlate it with the other presenting complaints. Amongst primary hematological disorders, **sickle cell disease** can present as a sickling crisis with abdominal pain and pallor, triggered by an infection (which can explain the fever). Sometimes an acute infective pathology can lead to a state of shock; such patients may occasionally report sudden pallor.

■ PHYSICAL EXAMINATION

Fairly built and nourished child Weight 16 kg Height 106 cm
Appears sick and in agonizing pain
Temp. 103°F Pulse 130/min RR 36/min BP 80/50 mm of Hg
Moderate pallor No icterus Delayed capillary refill

Abdomen - distended more in upper part severe tenderness mainly in the upper part
guarding and rigidity of right hypochondrium and epigastrium.
Liver 6 cm +, firm, Liver span 13 cm Marked *superficial tenderness* over liver
Spleen not palpable No ascites Other systems normal

Analysis

Physical examination localizes the disease to the liver. Severe tenderness to an extent that the patient does not allow easy palpation, suggests a severe inflammatory pathology of an acute onset such as a **liver abscess** or a **severe viral hepatitis**. Severe hepatitis usually presents with jaundice and rarely with high persistent fever. Thus, it is most likely to be a liver abscess. This child seems to be in compensated shock as suggested by the delayed capillary refill and a normal blood pressure. A pale appearance could be explained on this basis. However, he may be actually anemic also. Often, anemia due to pre-existing nutritional deficiency, which is quite common, may confuse the clinical picture of the primary illness. In this case, such an anemia may have been complicated by the acute severe destructive inflammatory pathology.

■ INVESTIGATIONS

Hb 7 gm% Microcytic hypochromic anemia with high RDW
WBC 25,000/c.mm P 88 L 12 E 0 Platelets 4.5 Lacs/c.mm
Serum bilirubin normal SGPT mildly raised Alk. phos. normal
Abdominal USG—Markedly enlarged liver with a single large liver abscess

Analysis

A normal serum bilirubin favors a localized liver pathology. Marked neutrophilic leukocytosis and thrombocytosis favors an acute infection. The diagnosis of a liver abscess is confirmed by the abdominal USG. While differentiation between a **pyogenic** and an **amebic liver abscess** may be difficult, amebic liver abscesses are rare in children and hence this patient should be treated with antibiotics. This child also has a deficiency anemia, which may have been aggravated by the acute severe infection.

■ FINAL DIAGNOSIS

Pyogenic liver abscess.

KEY MESSAGES

- Severe tenderness of the liver represents an acute severe inflammation (acute hepatitis) or acute severe congestion (CCF).
- Absence of jaundice is a feature of a localized liver disease.
- Pallor may or may not mean anemia in a setting of an acute severe infection and may sometimes represent a shock state.

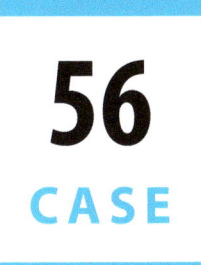

CASE 56

Prolonged Fever with Jaundice Later in the Illness

■ HISTORY

A 2-year-old child presented with fever for the last 2 weeks. The fever was high at onset, would respond to paracetamol for a few hours before rising again, the child's behavior in the interfebrile period was normal and the fever continued to be rhythmic every 6 hours. There was mild cold and cough that subsided in 3 days, but the fever continued. By the end of 1 week, he was more sick, and developed abdominal distension that gradually increased over the next week. In the last 2 days he was also noticed to have jaundice. He had lost appetite and weight and was getting sicker. He was treated with antibiotics without any improvement.

Analysis

High fever at onset that was rhythmic and partially responding to paracetamol, with the behavior of the child being normal in the interfebrile period, with mild cold and cough, suggests **probable viral infection**. However, most viral infections settle over a few days; so this child may have started as a viral fever but has developed some complications. He seems to have a progressive disease as is evident by the worsening health status. Gradually increasing abdominal distension denotes organomegaly—mostly an enlarged liver with or without splenomegaly. Jaundice that was noticed 2 days ago indicates hepatocyte involvement. So, what started as an extra-hepatic infection seems to have caused **hepatitis** as a complication. This may happen in typhoid fever or malaria wherein child manifests with jaundice, but abdominal distension is not a presenting complaint (though, in typhoid, there may be mild distension in the form of "fullness" that may be noticed by the physician). Moreover, the pattern of fever does not suggest either of these infections. In this child, abdominal distension was noticed much before jaundice came up, suggesting the involvement of reticuloendothelial system in the liver to begin with, which has subsequently led to hepatocyte disease. So, this seems to be an **immunological complication** to the initial infection, which is now manifesting as continuous fever. **Leptospirosis** is one such infection which may present as a biphasic fever with the second immune phase resulting in dysfunction of the affected organs such as jaundice due to liver involvement or renal failure due to kidney disease. However, the initial illness in leptospirosis is often characterized by severe myalgia; further cough and cold is not a feature. So, this is likely to be some other infection to begin with, which has now lead to immunologic complications.

■ PHYSICAL EXAMINATION

Sick looking child　　　　　　Irritable not in distress　　　　　Temp. 102°F
HR 120/min　　　　　　　　　RR 35/min　　　　　　　　　　BP normal
Weight 10 kg　　　　　　　　　Length 86 cm　　　　　　　　　Head Cir 48 cm
Severe pallor　　　　　　　　　Icterus +　　　　　　　　　　　No lymphadenopathy
Bones and joints normal　　　　　　　　　　　　　　　　　　　Spleen 3 F+, no ascites
Abdomen distended, liver 4 F+, firm, span 9 cm, not tender
Other systems normal

Analysis

Severe pallor indicates a hematological disease; in the light of our earlier discussion, it indicates a hematological complication. Since the child does not show any signs of hypovolemia or shock, this pallor is not due to hemorrhage. Anemia with hepatosplenomegaly indicates either hemolytic anemia or bone marrow infiltration. Jaundice may suggest hemolytic anemia but sickness and marked hepatomegaly are out of proportion to what is expected in any hemolytic anemia. Hence, it may be bone marrow infiltration. As hematological manifestations were not primary to start with, it is secondary involvement of bone marrow and not primary bone marrow disease. Such an infiltration in bone marrow may be due to histiocytosis. It may be either Langerhans's histiocytosis or hemophagocytic lymphohistiocytosis. Between the two types of histiocytosis, HLH is more likely as it presents with severe pallor and much more sickness.

■ INVESTIGATIONS

Hb 5 gm%　　　　　　　　　　WBC 1,300/c.mm　　　　　　　P 60 L 37 M 2 E 1
Platelets 0.4 Lakh/c.mm　　　　　S. bil. 4 mg% (D 2.3 mg%)　　　ALT 200 IU
AST 350 IU　　　　　　　　　　Alk phos 45 IU　　　　　　　　INR 1.6
Serum proteins 6.5 gm%　　　　　Albumin 3.5 gm%　　　　　　　Globulin 3 gm%
Serum triglycerides 400 mg%　　　Serum ferritin 1,650 mg%
Bone marrow showed hemophagocytosis

Analysis

This child has pancytopenia with hepatocyte involvement due to HLH as evident by bone marrow showing hemophagocytes, with high ferritin and triglycerides. This must have followed some infection that may have been viral. It is secondary HLH and not primary.

■ FINAL DIAGNOSIS

HLH secondary to probable viral infection.

KEY MESSAGE

Acute bacterial infection localizes within first few days while acute viral infection recovers within few days. If fever continues beyond a week, one may have to consider either non-localizing bacterial infection such as tuberculosis or more often non-infective immune-mediated disorder. Often diagnosis evolves over time in immune disorders. Such disorders may be either immune complications secondary to infection or at times autoimmune disorders. Both types of disorders are difficult to diagnose in initial stages of the disease and it is only when some organ gets involved that the diagnosis is thought of. However in such cases, misuse of antibiotics must be avoided as it is not difficult to exclude acute bacterial infections—if the continuing fever is due to an acute bacterial infection, there would be other symptoms either of localization or of complications.

CASE 57

Fever with Weakness of the Right Side

■ HISTORY

A 14-month-old male child born of a 3rd degree consanguineous marriage, presented with fever and weakness of the right side of the body since the last 15 days. He was apparently well 3 weeks ago when he started getting loose stools, 5-6 per day, watery, foul smelling without mucus or blood. The motions lasted for 3 days and got better without treatment. A day later, he developed a moderate degree of fever and on day 2 of the fever, the parents noticed that he had developed weakness of the right half of the body. He became irritable around the same time and on direct questioning, the parents informed that he was probably not able to see or hear, as he did not respond to their calling him, but kept quiet when picked up. The fever continued; he was admitted on day 15 of the fever.

Over these last few days, no new symptoms have developed and weakness has remained static.
No history of refusal of feeds
No history of convulsions
No other relevant past or family history
Birth history normal
Immunized up to date.

Analysis

This child had an **acute diarrhea** followed by neurological manifestations after a brief period. **Neurological complications** of diarrhea include toxic encephalopathy, metabolic disturbances and thrombosis due to dehydration. This acute infection, which could be **bacterial** or **viral**, could also extend to the central nervous system. If it was viral, it could have lead to viral encephalitis. If it was bacterial, the fact that the fever continued even after the stools stopped, suggests that either the diarrhea was a manifestation of some systemic bacterial infection, or the development of a complication. However, it is unlikely to be a bacterial infection because *this child never had high fever to begin with*. Since the diarrheal episode was self-limiting, it may have been a viral infection. The subsequent neurological events could well be **unrelated** to the diarrheal episode. However, since some viral infections may have a biphasic course and immune-mediated complications may occur in the second phase of the disease, this also remains a small possibility.

An acute onset, static weakness of the right half of the body suggests a **vascular episode**. Irritability for 15 days on the background of a neurological event, suggests either a **raised intracranial pressure** or a diffuse encephalopathy. Almost concurrent with the neurodeficit, the parents also noticed that the child was not responding to visual and auditory stimuli. Irritability may also be related to visual and/or auditory impairment. Children who suddenly develop visual or auditory impairment after having a normal vision and hearing, become irritable as they get confused due to the acute handicap (since they cannot relate to the surroundings). This visual/auditory defect could be due to visual and auditory *impairment* or visual and auditory *inattention*. It is unlikely that multiple scattered lesions have developed at the same time, giving rise to hemiplegia as well as affection of the visual and auditory pathways. Thus in this child, the reported failure to respond to visual and auditory stimuli may signify "inattention", and along with irritability, denotes an altered sensorium due to a **diffuse encephalopathy**. In view of fever for 2 weeks, this is likely to be a **subacute infective encephalopathy**.

■ PHYSICAL EXAMINATION

Fairly built and nourished
Weight 9 kg   Length 75 cm   Head Ⓞ 46 cm   Chest Ⓞ 44 cm
Drowsy, responds to external stimuli   Irritable on disturbance
Temp. 100°F   Pulse 120/min   RR 35/min   BP 80/50 mm of Hg
Severe pallor   No lymphadenopathy   No meningeal signs
Bones and joints normal
Anterior fontanelle dimple   Sutures not separate

CNS –
Vision - does not focus on objects   Pupils normal in size but not reacting to light
No roving eye movements or nystagmus   Bilateral optic atrophy
Hearing could not be assessed
Bilateral 6th nerve palsy   Other cranial nerves normal
Right upper motor neuron hemiparesis with (UMN type) facial palsy
DTR -knee and ankle jerks brisk on both sides, other reflexes normal
No ankle clonus   Plantar extensor on both sides
Cerebellar signs could not be tested   Sensory system apparently normal

Liver just palpable   Spleen not palpable
Other systems normal

Analysis

Drowsiness when associated with irritability on arousal suggests an **encephalopathy** (as against this, a drowsy child who is not irritable on arousal may be physiological, i.e., sleepy or drug induced). Bilateral 6th nerve palsy is a false localizing sign, indicating **raised intracranial pressure**. If it was a true localizing sign, it would have been unilateral and often associated with a lower motor neuron type of 7th nerve palsy on the same side. Pupils bilaterally not reacting to light, suggest affection of the afferent visual pathway in the form of optic nerve involvement, before the level of optic chiasma. In the setting of a raised intracranial pressure, bilateral optic atrophy indicates the occurrence of papilledema in the recent past (this bilateral optic atrophy also denotes that this child has a **visual impairment** rather than inattention, as was thought earlier in the analysis of the history). Bilateral extensor plantars in presence of a unilateral upper motor neuron lesion suggests **hydrocephalus**. An abnormal increase in the head circumference may be a sign of hydrocephalus, but in the absence of a previous record, it is difficult to correlate the present parameters. Apparently, the head circumference in this child is appropriate for the age and length of the child. However, normally in a well nourished child, the head and chest circumference equal by 1 year of age, whereas in this child, the head circumference is larger than the chest by 2 cm. This may be interpreted as a large skull size in favor of hydrocephalus. An acute static upper motor neuron hemiparesis indicates a **vascular lesion**. Therefore, this is a subacute infective encephalopathy with raised ICP with hydrocephalus, with a focal neurodeficit due to a vascular lesion. In our epidemiology, a subacute infection is almost always **tuberculosis**; however, a **partially treated bacterial** meningitis can also be a possibility. It is worth noting that absence of hepatosplenomegaly indicates a localized tuberculous disease, without dissemination to multiple organs, which is expected for this nutritional status. **Viral** infections may also result in widespread neurological lesions but without hydrocephalus. Similarly, vascular lesions may also be seen in **sickle cell disease** and **collagen vascular diseases**. However, the presence of hydrocephalus and raised intracranial pressure rule them out. Rarely, multiple vascular lesions may occur in **Moyamoya disease**, diagnosis of which is proved on angiography.

■ INVESTIGATIONS

Hb 5 gm% microcytic hypochromic
WBC 20,200/c.mm P 30 L 62 E 4 M 4
Hb electrophoresis normal Mantoux test -ve
CSF - clear fluid, proteins 150 mgm%, sugar 40 mgm%, cells 50/c.mm mostly lymphocytes
CT scan showed basal exudates, hydrocephalus with dilated lateral, 3rd and 4th ventricles, periventricular edema, and hypodense lesions in the left motor cortex.

Analysis

The CSF abnormalities confirm meningitis; the nature of the abnormalities favor the possibility of TBM. The CT scan findings support the diagnosis. However, it could not be confirmed bacteriologically. MT was expected to be positive; a negative Mantoux may be due to immune suppression caused by the bacterial load and will revert on successful treatment. Microcytic hypochromic anemia indicates iron deficiency.

■ FINAL DIAGNOSIS

Tuberculous meningitis.

■ KEY MESSAGES

- A good nutritional status is not against the diagnosis of tuberculosis, especially in well breastfed infants.
- Every effort should be made to confirm the diagnosis bacteriologically, though the results may often be negative.

■ RELEVANT INFORMATION

It is important to distinguish impairment from inattention. In visual inattention, the child "sees" but does not "register" or "interpret". This can happen when the visual association areas are affected or when the sensorium is altered. In visual impairment there is a lesion along the visual pathways. Presence of roving eye movements or nystagmus definitely indicates visual impairment due to a lesion in the anterior segment of the visual pathways, e.g., refractory error, retinal problems, etc. Similarly, auditory impairment occurs due to damage to the auditory pathway up to the cochlear nerve only. Lesions beyond the cochlear nerve rarely give rise to total deafness. Auditory inattention is classically seen in autism, but is also seen in Landau-Kleffner syndrome and adrenoleukodystrophy.

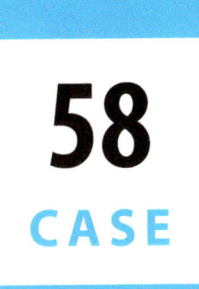

CASE 58
"Osteomyelitis" that would not Get Better or Worse!

■ HISTORY

An 8-year-old child presented with a history of (H/o) fever for 2 days; he was treated with paracetamol, and he was completely alright by the second day. The fever recurred after 36 hours followed by pain and swelling in the left thigh—he was diagnosed with acute osteomyelitis based on neutrophilic leukocytosis and computed tomography (CT) scan suggestive of (s/o) osteomyelitis. The blood culture was sterile. Two antibiotics failed to produce a response; meanwhile, the neutrophilic leukocytosis and radiology remained the same. It was decided to drain the affected site—histopathology confirmed osteomyelitis, but the culture was negative. Considering this to be an antibiotic-resistant infection, a third set of antibiotics was started, and this time continued for 2 weeks without benefit. Simultaneously, immunodeficiency was ruled out by relevant tests. At this stage, the parents sought a second opinion. On direct questioning, though fever and pain continued over the last month, there was no deterioration of health, and he would eat whenever the fever was partly controlled.

Analysis

When seen superficially, the history seems typical of acute osteomyelitis. When antibiotics are changed within a few days or a week, even an infection that is sensitive to the antibiotic used may fail to show a definite improvement when it comes to bone infections. However, since antibiotics were used all the time, even if they were different sets of antibiotics, a community-acquired infection should have shown at least some partial improvement. If the infection was resistant to the antibiotics used, the child should have worsened with local or systemic complications. It is important to note that the initial fever settled down by the second day without specific therapy and the child remained well before the long story started. So, the initial fever should not be interpreted to be the onset of acute osteomyelitis as it would not have abated by itself. Considering it to be a different illness altogether followed within 2 days by unrelated acute osteomyelitis is also far-fetched. Besides, the child has maintained near-normal health status despite three sets of failed antibiotics over a month. In other words, this is **not a bacterial infection** at all. This osteomyelitis could be an immune-mediated phenomenon— either an immune reaction to the first trivial infection or more likely, a primary immune disorder itself—an **autoimmune disease**.

■ PHYSICAL EXAMINATION

Not sick looking
Wt 26 kg Ht 122 cm
Temp. 100°F HR 85/m RR 20/m
Left mid-thigh swelling, mildly warm and tender, small swelling on the lower part of the left tibia
Other systems N

Analysis

There is clinical evidence of an inflammatory lesion in the midthigh and also, in the lower part of the left leg. Since this child is not looking sick, it is likely to be a noninfective inflammatory disease. As discussed above, investigations were interpreted to be in favor of osteomyelitis, though the etiology was elusive. But infection seemed to be ruled out based on the clinical arguments put forth above. So, a diagnosis of immune-mediated osteomyelitis was considered. Antibiotics were withdrawn and the child was treated with naproxen to which he responded well.

■ FINAL DIAGNOSIS

Chronic Recurrent Multifocal Osteomyelitis.

■ KEY MESSAGES

> Acute bacterial infection and acute noninfective inflammation present in a similar way but there are subtle differences. The patient suffering from acute bacterial infection is usually sick, while this is not so in the case of an immune disorder. Even the laboratory test results are also similar except that bacteriological proof can be obtained in acute bacterial infection. But we also know that for various well-known reasons, one may not get such proof even in a genuine infection. At such times, the differentiation between infection and noninfective inflammation needs a careful clinical analysis of the whole story as exemplified by this case.

■ RELEVANT INFORMATION

Autoinflammatory diseases are not uncommon. There is a wide spectrum of presentations ranging from poorly localizing illnesses such as periodic fever syndromes to specific organ affection as in this case. Diagnosis is suspected clinically and may be proved only when a specific organ is affected by ordering specific relevant immunological tests. A therapeutic trial is rational in such a situation and most children improve with the use of nonsteroidal anti-inflammatory drugs (NSAIDs). Use of steroids/intravenous immunoglobulin (IVIG)/other biologicals is reserved for specific purposes.

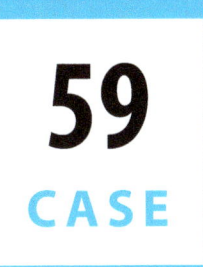

CASE 59

Fever Off and On, but the Child Remains Healthy!

■ HISTORY

A 12-year-old child presented with moderate to high fever off and on for 2 months. Each episode would last for a few days and recur after a few days. No other symptoms. Several tests were inconclusive, and two sets of antibiotics had failed. On direct questioning, he was well during the interfebrile period as well as during the inter-episode period; there was no deterioration in his health status.

Analysis

As this child's health is not affected, it may suggest recurrent self-limiting viral infections or theoretically, a partially treated bacterial infection. However, it is rare to suffer from multiple **recurrent viral infections**, and certainly not at this age. Similarly, a **partially treated bacterial infection** would present with some localization and hence is unlikely in this child. No localization over a period of 2 months, poor response to management and yet, maintaining normal health, suggests a **noninfective disorder**. Such disorders could be either rheumatological or malignant diseases. **Malignancy** in children who present with fever may be either leukemia or lymphoma. Neuroblastoma is not common at this age and would have presented with continuous high fever and the child would not have remained well in between fever episodes. **Rheumatological disorders** presenting with a high fever such as systemic-onset juvenile idiopathic arthritis (SOJIA) would have had other manifestations such as arthritis or skin rash by now. Hence diseases of both these groups are less likely. Since it seems to be a noninfective disease, it may be an autoimmune disorder without any specific organ affection.

■ PHYSICAL EXAMINATION

Not sick looking	Wt 35 kg	Ht 152 cm
TPR and BP normal	No pallor	Significant lymph node enlargement
Skin rash	Joint pain or swelling	Mouth ulcers
Systemic examination normal.		

Analysis

This is a healthy child without any abnormality on physical examination. Since he has a fever that is documented (and is hence not a fictitious fever), the disease process seems to be still evolving. Based on our analysis of the history, we can consider the diagnosis of an autoimmune disorder without localization at present. One should watch for further progress but try not to do more (random) tests or use antibiotics at this stage. The family will need proper counseling to allay anxiety.

■ INVESTIGATIONS

As many tests done earlier have been negative, one may at best consider repeating complete blood count (CBC) and erythrocyte sedimentation rate (ESR)/C-reactive protein (CRP) which would help to decide the need for further tests, if any, such as bone marrow examination, imaging, and other immunological tests; such as antibody tests. If CBC and ESR/CRP are normal, it is best to wait and watch without any intervention.

■ FINAL DIAGNOSIS

Periodic Fever syndrome.

■ KEY MESSAGES

> It is possible to consider a group diagnosis (infective or noninfective disorders) during the initial few days of fever in any child, by carefully analyzing a detailed history, thorough physical examination, and relevant tests if required. If we remain clueless at this point, and "seriousness" has been ruled out, it is rational to wait and watch for further progress with repeat clinical examination. In case of suspected seriousness, one should hospitalize the child and start an antibiotic covering common infections as per local epidemiology, but only after sending out relevant tests.

■ RELEVANT INFORMATION

Periodic fever syndrome is now referred to as recurrent fever syndrome without any evidence of infection or other causes. It is an autoinflammatory disease caused by dysregulation of the innate immune system. It is *not* an autoimmune disorder due to acquired (adaptive) immune malfunction. This disorder results from genetic mutations. There are many types of clinical presentations and subsequent progress, depending upon the type of mutations. Familial Mediterranean fever presents with severe pain in the abdomen, chest, or joints and resolves over a few years. PFAFA presents with recurrent fever, aphthous stomatitis, pharyngitis, and adenitis. The disease starts around 2–5 years and resolves mostly by 10 years. Tumor necrosis factor receptor-associated periodic syndrome (TRAPS) presents around adolescence or early adulthood with abdominal pain, diarrhea, skin rash, and severe myalgia. Hyperimmunoglobulin D disorder and neonatal-onset multisystem inflammatory disease are other types of recurrent fever syndromes. Prognosis is variable—some of them may last life-long while others resolve over time. They are treated mostly with NSAIDs but other drugs including biologicals are tried in severe cases.

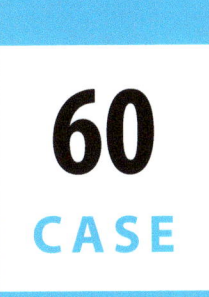

CASE 60

Frequent Wheezing in an Infant

■ HISTORY

An 8-month-old infant presented with an acute onset of cough and breathlessness of 2 days duration. The cough has been severe and the breathlessness started a day after the cough began. There was mild fever at the onset but it subsided without any treatment within 12 hours.

There was a past history of wheezing episodes since the age of 3 months; he had to be nebulized on a few occasions and was hospitalized for the same at 6 months of age.

There was a family history of asthma and atopy (in his father, uncle and grandfather).

He was prescribed prophylactic inhaled steroids for the last 3 months but did not have a significant beneficial effect, in spite of compliant treatment.

Analysis

This infant has been getting frequent wheezing episodes since the age of 3 months and some of the attacks have been severe. Since he has failed to respond satisfactorily to inhaled therapy in spite of compliant treatment, a **review** of the **diagnosis** may be called for. The poor response could be due to a **wrong technique** of inhalation, uncontrolled **trigger factors**, or a wrong diagnosis. Even in the presence of a strong family history of asthma, it is worth noting that asthma rarely starts so early in infancy. In other words, everything that wheezes may not be asthma. Conditions simulating asthma at that age are **aspiration syndromes** due to a variety of causes, **viral infection induced hyper-reactive airway disease** and rarely cystic fibrosis or **alpha-1-antitrypsin deficiency**. Since repeated infections is a hallmark of **cystic fibrosis** and there is no such history in this case, it is unlikely.

■ PHYSICAL EXAMINATION

Fairly built and nourished   Weight 7.5 kg   Length 69 cm
Temp. normal   Pulse 110/min   Resp. 45/min   Mild respiratory distress
Rest of the general examination – normal
Resp. system – Harsh breath sounds, bilateral wheezing, occasional crepitations scattered all over the chest
Other systems normal

Analysis

A fairly nourished child with generalized signs of airway disease, without fever, suggests a **non-infective condition**. The past history of episodic breathlessness requiring hospitalization denotes acute exacerbations of airway obstruction. This condition is **simulating asthma**. The strong family history would support such a diagnosis. However, as it has manifested so early in infancy, other possibilities need to be considered, as discussed in the analysis of the history. Since there is no clinical evidence of any failure to thrive, or any other organ/system affection, cystic fibrosis is quite unlikely. Therefore, aspiration syndromes and wheeze associated lower respiratory infections (viral) need to be considered. Since there is no history of fever at all, repeated viral infections are also less likely, **aspiration syndrome** being the likely possibility.

■ INVESTIGATIONS

Routine hemogram- normal
Chest X-ray showed prominent bronchovascular markings.
Barium swallow - showed esophageal stricture
Esophageal pH monitoring suggested a gastroesophageal reflux

Analysis

The stricture visualized on the barium swallow must have resulted from the gastroesophageal reflux (peptic stricture). Congenital esophageal strictures are extremely rare. In this case, subsequent repeated esophageal dilatation improved the cough and wheezing episodes.

■ FINAL DIAGNOSIS

Gastroesophageal reflux disease with an esophageal stricture.

■ KEY MESSAGES

- Everything that wheezes is not asthma, though it is also true that every child with asthma does not wheeze.
- "Asthma" starting early in infancy must be investigated for other causes such as an upper GI anomaly, a congenital heart defect with left to right shunt, hyper-reactive airway disease induced by viral infections or prematurity or neonatal lung damage, cystic fibrosis, alpha-1-antitrypsin deficiency, etc.
- While GERD (gastroesophageal reflux disease) is usually known to be associated with a history of frequent vomiting leading to failure to thrive, lack of any of these features does not rule out GERD.

RELEVANT INFORMATION

Gastroesophageal reflux (GER) in infants is "physiological" and when it results in pathological symptoms, it is referred to as gastroesophageal reflux disease (GERD). It presents with a wide range of symptoms. Contrary to expectations, vomiting is often not present. Classical manifestations are mainly related to the respiratory tract. Recurrent or chronic cough due to microaspiration is easily mistaken as a primary respiratory disease (e.g., asthma or pneumonia). Chronic pharyngitis may be the only feature of undiagnosed GERD. Aspiration into the airways may present as an acute life-threatening episode of apnea and cyanosis or sudden infant death syndrome (SIDS). Failure to thrive, excessive inconsolable crying and unresponsive anemia may be other subtle manifestations of GERD in infants and are usually overlooked. Untreated GERD may result in esophageal stricture and accompanying respiratory complications. Neurologically handicapped children are especially prone to GERD.

However, the diagnosis is not easy; a reflux may only be picked up if the radiological tests are done with meticulous care and dedication, with adequate time spent for the procedure.

The commonly asked for barium study needs to be planned properly. Amount of barium used for the study should be nearly equal to the average single milk feed for that age and should be of the consistency of milk. It should be administered in the same way in which the infant usually takes a feed or through a spoon. The study should span over half an hour to detect reflux occurring at any given time and the infant must not be kept in any slanting position. 24 hours esophageal pH monitoring may be the most ideal, but may neither be practical nor necessary. Esophagoscopy helps in detecting any other lesion that may accompany or complicate GER. A radionuclide milk scan can only demonstrate pulmonary aspiration, but fails to detect the cause.

Principles of medical treatment consist of lowering the acidity of gastric secretions and stimulating gastric emptying. The success of treatment is judged by weight gain, improvement in hemoglobin and absence of any symptoms referable to GERD. Failure of compliant medical therapy or the occurrence of a life-threatening episode anytime would deserve surgery.

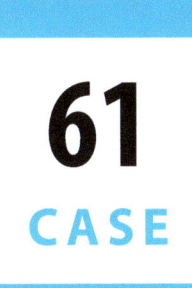

CASE 61

Recurrent Hematuria in a 4-year-old

■ HISTORY

A 4-year-old male child presented with recurrent episodes of gross hematuria over the last 2 years. He has had three such episodes so far. Each time he had a painless passage of red colored urine throughout micturition, without any clots, lasting for 4–5 days, remitting on its own, without any treatment. He remained well in between these episodes and had a normal growth and activity.

On direct questioning

History of mild puffiness of face during the last episode.
No history of oliguria, dysuria or fever.
No history of joint pain or swelling, skin rash, abdominal pain or hematochezia.
No history of any drug intake.
No relevant family history.

Analysis

Every red colored urine may be complained of by the patient as hematuria, but the urine may also be "red" due to other causes which need to be differentiated. (On the other hand, sometimes a microscopic hematuria may be complained of only as a high colored urine, and may be missed on the history unless a detailed enquiry is made.) A red urine that is not due to hematuria may be due to hemoglobinuria, myoglobinuria, consumption of pigments in **food** or **drugs**. Associated symptoms help to differentiate these conditions. Children with **hemoglobinuria** or **myoglobinuria** are usually quite sick and present as an acute illness. Besides, recurrence of hemoglobinuria is rare, and is therefore unlikely in this child. Since there is no history of consumption of any relevant foods or drugs, this child is likely to have hematuria.

It is important to decide whether the hematuria is glomerular or extraglomerular. The history of mild puffiness of face obtained on direct questioning in this child, may suggest a **glomerular** pathology. However, the urine in such cases is often cola colored and not bright red as reported in this child. Besides, other symptoms of glomerular involvement such as oliguria and edema are absent in this child. It is important to realize that symptoms such as *mild edema or oliguria* are difficult to recognize for the parents, and may be missed when not reported on their own, unless specifically asked for. Therefore, while a definite history of such symptoms is diagnostic of a glomerular disease, absence of such a history does not rule it out. On the other hand, the same symptoms when brought out only after direct questioning, may at times, be an erroneous perception of the parents. Therefore, in this case if we do consider the history of puffiness of face, it suggests a glomerular disease. Amongst these, recurrent gross hematuria may be seen in **IgA nephropathy**, **Alport's syndrome** or **thin glomerular basement membrane disease.** Absence of family history and a history of deafness may not rule out Alport's syndrome. Though Alport's syndrome is known to be more progressive as compared to IgA nephropathy, a 2 years period is too small to comment or make a distinction between them. While **acute (post streptococcal) glomerulonephritis** does not recur, chronic glomerulonephritis like **membranous** or **membranoproliferative** glomerulonephritis usually present as a nephrotic/acute nephritic syndrome in older children, and not as recurrent gross hematuria with periods of normalcy in between. Chronic **glomerulonephritis associated with systemic diseases** like SLE may be slowly progressive; however, it is usually seen in older girls.

On the other hand, if we ignore the mild puffiness of face reported only once, and that too on direct questioning, this may be **extraglomerular hematuria**. Urinary tract **infection** is unlikely in the absence of a history of fever and dysuria. Absence of colicky abdominal pain and painful hematuria suggest that **urolithiasis** is unlikely. Renal **tuberculosis** may present with painless hematuria but would disseminate over time. **Wilm's tumor** should have presented with an abdominal mass by now (if the parents have not noticed, it will be revealed on physical examination). **Idiopathic hypercalciuria** is a possibility since it is a common cause of such hematuria.

■ PHYSICAL EXAMINATION

Fairly built and nourished   Weight 16 kg   Height 100 cm
TPR normal   BP 80/60 mm of Hg
No puffiness of face or edema feet
Other systems normal

Analysis

Since there is no abdominal mass felt, Wilm's tumor is unlikely. While the other conditions leading to extraglomerular hematuria discussed above may not have any positive clinical findings, the same may be true for the glomerular diseases like IgA nephropathy, Alport's syndrome, etc. discussed above. Other features of these diseases may come up later in the course of disease. Therefore, with no additional information on examination, the earlier analysis stands; neither glomerular nor extraglomerular hematuria can be ruled out.

■ INVESTIGATIONS

Urine 150–200 RBCs, no casts   No pus cells   Proteins 30 mgm%   Urine culture negative
Urine Ca/creatinine ratio - 0.4
Abdominal USG normal

Analysis

Though there is a significant hematuria, absence of casts and the insignificant proteinuria rule out a glomerular disease. The urinary Ca/creatinine ratio suggests a diagnosis of hypercalciuria. It can be further confirmed by a 24 hours calcium excretion, which in this child exceeded 4 mg/kg/day.

■ FINAL DIAGNOSIS

Idiopathic hypercalciuria.

■ KEY MESSAGES

- Idiopathic hypercalciuria is a common cause of extraglomerular hematuria in children.
- The Ca/creatinine ratio, on a spot sample of urine, is a useful screening test to diagnose this condition.

■ RELEVANT INFORMATION

The classical symptom of idiopathic hypercalciuria is hematuria with or without dysuria and frequency of urination. Rarely, incontinence during the day or urinary tract infection may be the presenting symptom. It may present as irritability in infants. Other causes of hypercalciuria include vitamin D supplements, furosemide, and rarely malignancies. Nephrolithiasis is associated with hypercalciuria.

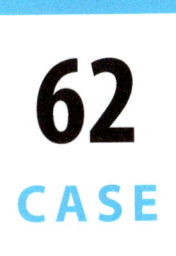

CASE 62

Recurrent Hematuria in a 10-year-old

■ HISTORY

A 10-year-old male child presented with recurrent episodes of hematuria and puffiness of face since the last 2 years. Each episode was preceded by a mild fever, cold and cough, and started with a painless passage of bright red urine without any clots, accompanied with a mild puffiness of face, lasting for 2–4 weeks and remitting on its own without any treatment. He suffered from 5 such episodes during the last 2 years. He remained apparently well in between the episodes and had a normal growth and activity.
- No history of oliguria, dysuria, fever
- No history of joint pain or swelling, skin rash, abdominal pain
- No relevant past or family history
- No history of deafness or visual problems
- No history of taking any drugs

Analysis

This "red" urine is likely to be hematuria (please refer to analysis of the history in the previous case of hematuria). It may be glomerular or extraglomerular. Painless hematuria favors a glomerular disease. **Extraglomerular hematuria** may be due to a surgical problem such as **urolithiasis**, in which case it is often accompanied with abdominal pain and/or dysuria. **Urinary tract infection** would also lead to fever, dysuria, frequency of micturition, etc. However, **tuberculosis** of the kidney may rarely present as painless hematuria (extraglomerular). On the other hand, a **glomerular** pathology manifests as edema or oliguria, with abdominal pain and dysuria being rare; though occasionally a "clot colic" may cause pain in a glomerular disease. As this child has presented with recurrent episodes of hematuria and each episode is associated with puffiness of face, it is likely to be a glomerular disease, i.e., **recurrent glomerulonephritis**. In view of a normal growth, he is unlikely to have a chronic progressive glomerulonephritis. There is no evidence of involvement of any other organ, in particular the skin, joints or the intestinal tract, even after 2 years of existence of the disease and hence a chronic glomerulonephritis associated with a systemic disease such as a collagen vascular disease is less likely. Other common causes of recurrent glomerulonephritis are **IgA nephropathy** and Alport's syndrome. The history of an apparent viral upper respiratory infection preceding each episode of hematuria may favor IgA nephropathy. However, such infections are even otherwise extremely common in children, and the association could as well be coincidental. Absence of family history and a history of deafness may not rule out **Alport's syndrome**.

■ PHYSICAL EXAMINATION

Fairly built and nourished	Weight 32 kg	Height 138 cm
Temp/pulse/RR normal	BP - 140/104 mm of Hg	
Mild puffiness of eyelids	No edema feet	No ocular abnormalities
Systemic examination normal		

Analysis

This child has definite hypertension. It may be renovascular or renoparenchymal. When associated with hematuria and puffiness of face, it clearly suggests **renoparenchymal hypertension**. This confirms that this is a recurrent *glomerulonephritis*. A systemic vascular disease may manifest with an isolated renal involvement initially, but generally it spreads to other organs over time. As this child has been suffering for 2 years without any suggestion of any other organ involvement, it is unlikely to be a generalized disease; however, he needs a close follow-up to watch for other organ involvement. Since, there are no other clinical findings, investigations may help to differentiate further, between the other possibilities discussed earlier.

■ INVESTIGATIONS

Urinalysis - proteins + +,	6–8 RBCs/hpf	No casts
24 hours urine protein - 396 mgm%	Urine vol. (24 hrs) 600 mL	
CBC/ESR/CRP normal	Serum creatinine normal	
Serum C3 normal	Abdominal USG normal	
Urinalysis of parents - Normal		

Analysis

When proteinuria is associated with hematuria, it strongly suggests a glomerular pathology. Though the presence of casts favor a glomerular disease, to demonstrate casts a fresh urine sample needs to be examined as the casts disintegrate with time. Normal CBC/ESR/CRP denotes absence of active inflammation; along with a normal C3 level it indicates that a systemic disease like SLE is unlikely. Since the parents do not show any urinary abnormality, Alport's syndrome is less likely. Renal biopsy is necessary for further evaluation of the glomerular pathology.

■ FURTHER INVESTIGATION

Renal biopsy - confirmed IgA nephropathy as demonstrated by immunofluorescence.

■ FINAL DIAGNOSIS

IgA nephropathy.

■ KEY MESSAGES

- Renal biopsy may be necessary in the evaluation of hematuria due to medical renal diseases while imaging studies are more important in surgical conditions. A biopsy sample should always be sent for light and electron microscopy, and immunofluorescence.
- Absence of casts in the urine does not rule out a glomerular disease.
- RBC morphology and RDW in the urine sample may help to differentiate glomerular from extraglomerular hematuria in case of doubt.

■ RELEVANT INFORMATION

IgA nephritis is seen in older children. It was considered to be a benign condition but extended follow-up has shown that 30–50% of the patients may develop end-stage renal disease over 10 years. Spontaneous remission is occasionally reported in children.

Five different clinical presentations are known.

Most common is asymptomatic microscopic hematuria with occasional gross hematuria (60–70%). The second most common is asymptomatic microscopic hematuria with or without proteinuria, hypertension and reduced renal clearance (20%). It can also present as acute nephritis with gross hematuria and hypertension (10%). Rarely it may present as a nephrotic syndrome or acute crescentic nephritis with oliguria, edema and hypertension.

CASE 63

Increased Precordial Activity Since Infancy

■ HISTORY

A 1-year-old male child presented with poor weight gain, feeding difficulty and increased precordial activity since early infancy. He was born after full-term and a normal delivery. The immediate neonatal period was uneventful.

At 2 months of age, he was hospitalized for high fever, cough and breathlessness and was treated with IV medications for 7 days. The treating doctor suspected a cyanotic congenital heart disease and advised further investigations. He continued to suffer from frequent episodes of fever, cough and breathlessness, which were treated with oral medications. However, cyanosis was never evident on subsequent examinations.

- On direct questioning, the parents had noticed "suck rest suck cycle" during feeding.
- H/o reduced activity as compared to children of his age
- H/o relative improvement in symptoms in the last 3 months
- History suggestive of a mild delay in gross motor milestones.

Analysis

Increased precordial activity, especially when noticed by the parents, feeding difficulty and a poor weight gain, clearly suggest a **congenital heart disease**. In this setting, an increased precordial activity also suggests an increased pulmonary blood flow (as against the silent precordium in Fallot's tetralogy, which is associated with a reduced pulmonary blood flow). When this child was admitted at 2 months of age, the treating doctor apparently noticed cyanosis; however, it was not evident thereafter. The subsequent history of repeated respiratory infections also indicates an increased pulmonary blood flow setting. Cyanotic heart diseases that present with an increased pulmonary blood flow, are usually complex malformations and in such cases, once the cyanosis manifests, it is usually persistent. So, it is **unlikely** to be a **cyanotic heart disease**. The mild cyanosis that was noticed only once may have been due to a severe respiratory infection and cardiac failure at that time. Increased precordial activity also signifies a hyperdynamic circulation as seen in conditions with a volume overload. Therefore, acyanotic heart defects that present with a *pressure* overload, such as congenital aortic or pulmonary stenosis and coarctation of aorta, seem unlikely. Lesions which cause a volume overload are left to right shunts, **regurgitant lesions**, and **cardiomyopathy**. As mentioned earlier, the history of repeated lower respiratory infections suggests increased pulmonary blood flow, in this setting. Therefore, we are probably dealing with a **left to right shunt**. Feeding difficulty and "suck rest suck" cycle are equivalent to exertional dyspnea in an older child. It suggests either left ventricular dysfunction (inability to meet the oxygen demands of the body) or pulmonary venous congestion secondary to raised pressures in the left atrium. Amongst the common shunts, an **atrial septal defect** is characterized by a volume overload of the *right* side of the heart, and is therefore less likely. Both a **patent ductus arteriosus** and a **ventricular septal defect** have a variable spectrum of presentation and are therefore likely in this child. The severity of symptoms suggests a large shunt. If this is a ventricular septal defect, though it is known to undergo a natural closure with age, this child is expected to have a large defect that is unlikely to close. Therefore, the apparent improvement in symptoms in the last 3 months in this child does not denote a closure of the defect. In fact, it may indicate an increasing pulmonary vascular resistance which can reduce the magnitude of the shunt, thereby temporarily ameliorating the symptoms. It may also mean successful anti-failure treatment.

■ PHYSICAL EXAMINATION

Poorly built and nourished
Weight 6.1 kg   Length 70 cm   Looks "sick"
Pulse 100/min   RR 30/min   Head Ⓞ 45 cm
No cyanosis   Moderate pallor   BP 90/46 mm Hg
No edema   JVP - Normal

CVS-
Mild precordial bulge
Apex beat in the left 5th intercostal space 1 cm outside the midclavicular line, forceful and ill sustained
Pulsations seen and felt in the left 2nd space in the parasternal region

Parasternal heave +, epigastric pulsations felt at the tip of the palpating finger
Systolic thrill in the 3rd and 4th space parasternally
P2 palpable

S1 N S2 narrow split, P2 component loud
Grd IV/VI blowing holosystolic murmur best heard parasternally in the 3rd and 4th space
Other systems   Normal

Analysis

The cardiovascular findings suggest *cardiomegaly* (apex beat outside the midclavicular line), *left ventricular hypertrophy* (character of the apex beat), *right ventricular hypertrophy* (parasternal heave, epigastric pulsations), *pulmonary artery dilatation* (left 2nd space pulsations) and *pulmonary hypertension* (loud and palpable P2, and a narrow split). The site of the systolic thrill and murmur suggest a septal defect at the ventricular level. The volume overloaded hypertrophied left ventricle suggests a large shunt.

So clinically this child probably has a **large ventricular septal defect** with elevated pulmonary vascular resistance, who is already developing pulmonary hypertension. This may have lead to a recent decrease in the shunt magnitude, thereby ameliorating the symptoms partially. Eventually, however this would lead to a reversal of shunt and cyanosis, if untreated.

■ INVESTIGATIONS

Hb 8 gm%   WBC 8,200/c. mm differential count- N
Chest X-ray – cardiomegaly with hyperemic lung fields
ECG – Biventricular hypertrophy with pulmonary hypertension
Echocardiogram – Large VSD with pulmonary hypertension

■ COMMENT

In large defects that are destined to shunt left to right, it is often the body's defense mechanism to delay the (natural) fall in pulmonary vascular resistance, thereby delaying the onset of shunting. This delayed fall of PVR as evident by the delayed splitting of S2, may be an important sign in the newborn period to predict a possible large left to right shunt in the near future.

■ FINAL DIAGNOSIS

Large ventricular septal defect with pulmonary hypertension.

■ KEY MESSAGES

- A single second heart sound after D3 of life may signify either pulmonary stenosis or a delay in the fall of pulmonary vascular resistance (thereby signifying a possible large shunt).
- Temporary alleviation of symptoms in large left to right shunts may falsely suggest an improvement, though in effect, it signifies worsening pulmonary hypertension.

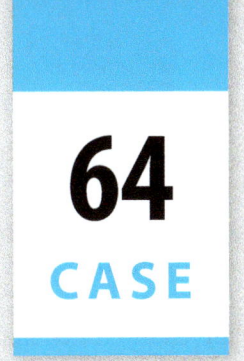

CASE 64

Incidentally Noticed Murmur in an Infant

■ HISTORY

A 1-month-old male infant is noticed to have a soft systolic murmur on routine examination. He was born after a full term normal delivery with no antenatal or perinatal problems. The birth weight was 3.2 kg. He was exclusively breastfed. He is the 2nd of 2 living children – the first daughter is 3 years old and is normal. There is no family history of any heart diseases.

■ PHYSICAL EXAMINATION

Weight 4.1 kg   Length 54 cm   Head ☉ 37 cm
Temp/pulse/RR normal
Comfortable   No distress
CVS - soft systolic murmur at the base, grade 2/6
P2 normal and split
No other abnormal findings

Analysis

Accidental detection of a soft systolic murmur without any other abnormal findings in an asymptomatic infant may be due to an **organic** defect or denote **"functional"** or "innocent" murmur. If the murmur in this infant represents an organic defect, it is unlikely to be a stenotic lesion such as **pulmonary** or **aortic stenosis** as these defects result in a harsh murmur (the only exception being a mild pulmonary stenosis which could produce a soft murmur). If it were a shunt murmur due to a **ventricular septal defect**, a soft murmur would suggest a large defect in which case it would have been symptomatic. On the other hand, if it were a small defect, the murmur would have been harsh. A **patent ductus arteriosus** would have resulted in a continuous murmur (the length of the murmur shortens only after development of pulmonary hypertension). An **atrial septal defect** causes an ejection systolic murmur of a scratchy quality, best heard at the pulmonary area with a widely split P2. Amongst cyanotic heart defects, **Fallot's tetralogy** may be asymptomatic in early infancy except for a soft pulmonary stenotic murmur. Occasionally, a myocardial disease may present with such a murmur; the disease may be otherwise well compensated and therefore asymptomatic. **Transient myocardial dysfunction** resulting from perinatal hypoxia may present with such a murmur. However, the infant will be often symptomatic; besides there is no such history in this case. **Mitral valve prolapse** may be asymptomatic and detected accidentally; a click may not be appreciated.

This infant may as well have an innocent murmur. **Hemodynamically benign murmurs** are not rare in healthy children. A peripheral pulmonic systolic murmur is heard all over the thorax and is not localized as in this infant. Venous hum is a continuous murmur and Still's murmur is generally heard in older children. Other conditions that can lead to functional murmurs like fever and anemia are not relevant here.

■ INVESTIGATION

2-D echocardiography showed hypertrophic cardiomyopathy.

■ FOLLOW-UP

Since there was no history of diabetes in the mother, or a family history of a similar disorder, this was feared to be due to an inborn error of metabolism. The patient was advised to investigate for the same, and a guarded prognosis was given. However, on follow-up, the infant remained asymptomatic and a repeat echocardiogram showed a marked improvement. It is well-known that infants of diabetic mothers may suffer from such a transient disorder. It is likely that the mother's diabetes was missed due to a single random blood sugar estimation done at any time during pregnancy.

■ FINAL DIAGNOSIS

Transient hypertrophic cardiomyopathy in infant of diabetic mother.

■ KEY MESSAGES

- It is important to assess the blood sugar of every pregnant woman at the beginning of the third trimester. At least a fasting and a postprandial level should be done, though a full fledged GTT over 3 hours is ideal.
- This would also ensure monitoring for a possible hypoglycemia at and shortly after birth, thereby preventing its disastrous consequences subsequently in terms of delayed neurodevelopment.

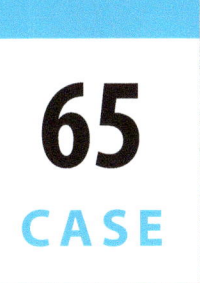

CASE 65

Failure to Gain Height

■ HISTORY

A 9-year-old female child born of a non-consanguineous marriage, presented with the complaint of not gaining height, noticed since the last 3 years. Ever since the parents perceived her short stature at 6 years of age, they have observed that she has been gaining around 3 cm in height every year. Prior to that, she was apparently growing normally, though the parents had not kept any record. She has been active, is developmentally normal and studies well. Her appetite has been normal and she consumes an average intake of calories and proteins. There are no other relevant symptoms and no other significant illness in the past. One paternal uncle is comparatively short.

Analysis

Since this child's height velocity has been recorded as only 3 cm per year, she definitely has growth failure. As she has been otherwise "well", a chronic **systemic disease** as the cause of her short stature is unlikely. Since there is no history of any other symptoms, a chronic infection is ruled out. **Chronic organ dysfunction** may sometimes present as short stature (as in renal tubular acidosis or malabsorption syndromes like gluten induced enteropathy). However, on direct questioning, usually some other symptoms will come forth. Since this child's mental development has been normal, disorders like **hypothyroidism** and **mucopolysaccharidoses** (except MPS IV and IX) are unlikely. A apparently normal growth in the early years makes **skeletal dysplasias** unlikely; besides, they would have presented with deformities also. **Turner's syndrome** should always be considered in a female child who presents as short stature. The other possibilities in this child could be **constitutional** or **familial short stature**, **growth hormone deficiency** and **idiopathic short stature**.

■ PHYSICAL EXAMINATION

Healthy child, normally nourished
Height 112 cm (height age 6 years)
Weight 26 kg (weight age 9 years)
US/LS – 1
No dysmorphic features   No infantile facies
No bony deformities   SMR prepubertal

Systemic examination normal

Mother's height 154 cm
Father's height 160 cm
Mid parental height 150.5 +/- 8.5 cm

Analysis

This child is more than 3 standard deviations short (the 50th centile for her age being 132 cm, the 5th centile being 122 cm) and therefore needs a proper evaluation. A normal weight for her age rules out systemic diseases. In chronic systemic diseases leading to short stature, the weight is affected much more than the height. Besides, a normal physical examination also goes against a chronic illness. Short stature in a child whose weight is normal, may be due to **chromosomal defects** or **skeletal dysplasias**. However, since there are no dysmorphic features or bony deformities, these are ruled out. In view of the history of short stature in an uncle, familial short stature may be considered. In these cases, the growth curve of the child runs parallel to, but at a lower centile, than the standard growth curve; however it is unlikely in this child since her height is significantly affected (more than 3 standard deviations). Clinically, constitutional short stature cannot be completely ruled out though in such cases, the height is not as markedly affected. There may be a family history of delayed puberty in such a patient who will eventually catch up in height. In this child, a history suggestive of significant faulting of height over the last 3 years favors a **growth hormone deficiency**. If this child's growth curve had been available, it would have been normal initially, with a downward crossing of centiles over the last few years, thereby strongly suggesting growth hormone deficiency.

■ INVESTIGATION

Bone age: 5 years and 2 months.

Analysis

This 9-year-old child has a height age of 6 years and a bone age of 5 years and 2 months. Since the bone age is equal to the chronological age in familial short stature, it is ruled out. A delayed bone age suggests constitutional short stature, growth hormone deficiency or hypothyroidism. In constitutional short stature, though the bone age may be delayed as compared to the chronological age at a given point in time, it corresponds to the height age at that time. In this child, since the bone age is delayed even beyond the height age, constitutional short stature is also ruled out. Thus, this child most probably has a growth hormone deficiency. Hypothyroidism is unlikely with this history and clinical findings. The diagnosis can be confirmed by hormonal assays.

■ FURTHER INVESTIGATION

Growth hormone assay confirmed a deficiency.

■ FINAL DIAGNOSIS

Growth hormone deficiency.

Failure to Gain Height

KEY MESSAGES

- Maintaining growth records (weight, length/height, head circumference) right since birth is important, and should be a part of the physical examination of every child who reports to the doctor for any illness. Unavailability of such records hampers clinical judgment.
- Growth charts help in the early diagnosis of malnutrition, short stature, microcephaly/ hydrocephalus, etc.
- Laboratory investigations are no substitute to growth monitoring.

RELEVANT INFORMATION

Wt	Ht	Wt/Ht	Inference
↓	N	↓	Acute PEM
↓	↓	N	Constitutional
↓	↑	↓↓	Constitutional + poor eating habits
↓↓	↓	↓	Chronic PEM
N	↓↓	↓	Endocrine (GH, Hypothyroid)

Chr age >Ht age >Bone age ---- Hypothyroid, GH def
Chr age >Ht age = Bone age ---- Constitutional delay
(Bone age = Chr age) >Ht age ---- Familial short stature

Bone Age

The bone age is one of the first investigations to be done in such cases. It is estimated accurately by comparing the shape of the small bones of the hands with an Atlas, as a part of a scoring system and **not** by looking at the number of carpal bones and ossification centers present, as is routinely done.

Constitutional Delay

In constitutional delay, though the child's growth curve is below normal, it is parallel to the normal curve, and there is usually a family history of delayed puberty. This child achieves puberty late, but due to a *delayed but normal* growth spurt, final height is normal. Though the bone age may be delayed as compared to the chronological age at a given point in time, it corresponds to the height age at that time.

Familial Short Stature

In familial short stature, the growth curve of the child runs parallel to, but at a lower centile, than the standard growth curve; however the height is usually not affected by more than 2 standard deviations. These children will have a normal pubertal development and though bone age need not be done at all, it is normal. Any child whose height is more significantly affected, is unlikely to be familial short stature.

Pitfalls in Lab Diagnosis

Definitive diagnosis rests on demonstration of absent or low levels of GH in response to stimulation with provocative tests. Peak levels below 7 µg/L are compatible with GH deficiency. But 20% of normally growing children, will fail to produce these levels on provocation with any one test; i.e., 4% will fail even two simultaneous tests.

Measurement of spontaneous secretion of GH is also unreliable.

CASE 66

Failure to Gain Height with Onset of Puberty

■ HISTORY

A 10-year-old female child presented with a failure to gain height since the last 3 years, breast development since the last 3 months, development of pubic hair since the last 2 months and menstruation since the last 1 month.

She is one of two children in the family, born of a non-consanguineous marriage, after a full term and a normal delivery. Her birth weight was average; the birth length was not recorded.

No previous height records are available, though for the first 7 years, the parents did not consider her to be short as compared to her peers. The mother had attained menarche at 13 years of age. There was no other relevant history.

Analysis

Short stature is best evaluated by a serial height record, with height velocity measured over time. Laboratory tests are no substitute for such a record. As this child does not have any record to fall back on, nor her length at birth is known, the next best is to compare the midparental height with a projection of her present height.

The normal sequence of sexual development starts with thelarche (breast development), is followed by adrenarche (pubic hair), which is finally followed by menarche. This child has gone through a similar sequence of events and hence her pubertal development seems to be normal. Therefore, her growth failure is **unlikely** to be due to **growth hormone deficiency** or **hypothyroidism**, as in both these conditions pubertal development is expected to be delayed. Since there are no other symptoms, a **systemic disease** is unlikely; physical examination will confirm the same. In primary malnutrition, puberty is often delayed. In normal pubertal development in girls, the pubertal growth spurt occurs before the onset of menarche in most of the cases. However, in this child menarche has already set in, thereby signifying that she may not gain much more in height. At the most she may gain 5–6 cm in height after the onset of menarche. **IUGR** babies have a poor catch up growth, early onset of puberty and low pubertal growth spurt. However, as per the history, this child was probably not an IUGR baby at birth. It is important to realize the difficulty in interpretation of such a history, when the past records are not available.

■ PHYSICAL EXAMINATION

Poorly built and nourished
Weight 14 kg (<5th centile) Weight age – 3 years
Height 114 cm (<5th centile) Height age – 7 years
US/LS - 1:1
Midparental height 152 cm SMR B3 P2
Temp./pulse/RR normal BP 90/60 mm of Hg

Systemic examination normal

Analysis

This child's weight is affected much more as compared to her height, though both are below normal (for her age). This may suggest **chronic malnutrition**. This may be **primary**, as is seen in children who were intrauterine growth retarded, or suffered from malnutrition in early infancy. Malnutrition **secondary** to systemic diseases or occult organ dysfunction is unlikely since there are no symptoms or signs to suggest the same. Clinically, though there are no signs to suggest growth hormone deficiency or hypothyroidism, they need to be ruled out by appropriate investigations. Being a treatable cause, hypothyroidism should always be looked for, irrespective of the clinical findings. Since this child has already achieved puberty and is still short, **constitutional delay** is **ruled out**. Since this child is considerably short, **familial short stature** is also **unlikely**.

■ INVESTIGATIONS

Bone age - 10.5 years TSH, T3, T4 normal
LH - 3.5 mIu/mL (normal pubertal levels - 5–10 mIu/mL)
FSH - 2 mIu/mL (normal pubertal levels - >1 mIu/mL)
S. Estradiol - 17 pgm% (normal pubertal levels - >15 pgm%)
USG pelvis - both ovaries show multiple follicles
Uterus size 37 mm (pubertal uterus size >35 mm)
Insulin like growth factor 3 - normal

Analysis

The bone age is equal to the chronological age. This rules out hormone deficiencies. While this may be seen in familial short stature, as discussed earlier, the degree of short stature rules it out. Therefore, this may be **idiopathic short stature**. Normal IGF 3 level is a screening test to rule out growth hormone deficiency; hormonal estimation is not necessary. The sex hormone levels are consistent with a normal pubertal development.

■ FINAL DIAGNOSIS

Idiopathic short stature with normal puberty.

KEY MESSAGES

- Every newborn's length must be measured accurately and recorded. (It is not easy to measure the length of the newborn due to a normally increased muscle tone).
- A serial record of height and weight must be maintained at periodic intervals. The pediatrician must measure these parameters at every visit as a rule and record them on a centile growth chart.
- Serial height record and bone age are enough to find the cause of short stature.
- With an appropriate growth record, growth hormone estimation can be done only for appropriate patients at the right time.

RELEVANT INFORMATION

MID PARENTAL HEIGHT

Mid parental height is calculated by:

Mother's ht + Father's ht   + 13 (in boys)   divided by 2
" "   – 13 (in girls)   "

The child's predicted height is mid parental height + or – 8 cm, e.g., in the above child it would be 154 + 160 – 13 = 301 div by 2 = 150.5 cm + or – 8 = 158.5 to 142.5.

Now if the child's current height as plotted on the growth curve is extrapolated to 18 years and falls within this range, it may be considered normal.

Height Velocity

More than a single ht reading, a series of readings over a period of time, at least 3 or 6 monthly readings, give us the velocity of height over a year, expressed as cm/yr. There are height velocity curves with percentiles, on which we can plot these values. A velocity less than 4–5 cm needs evaluation.

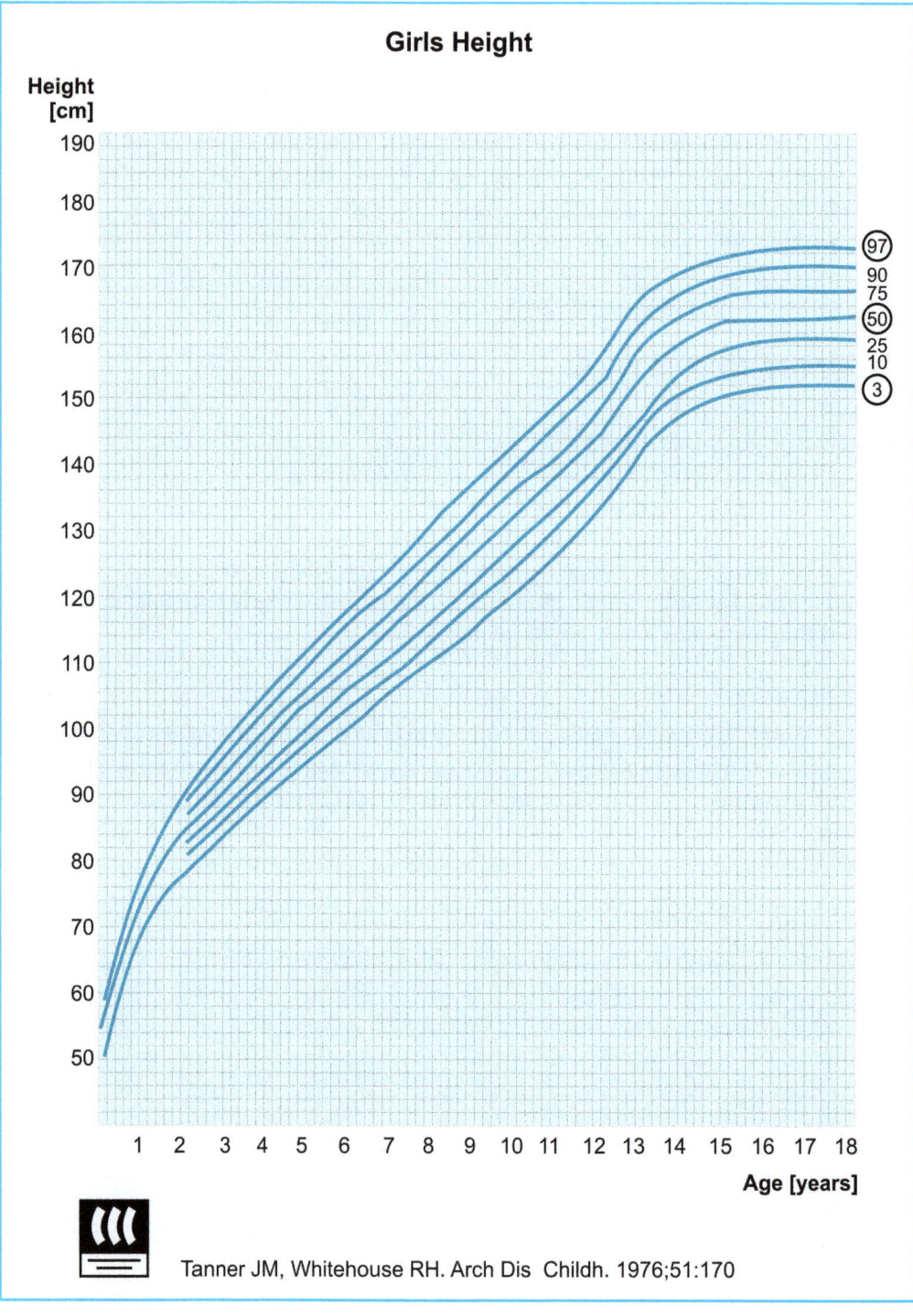

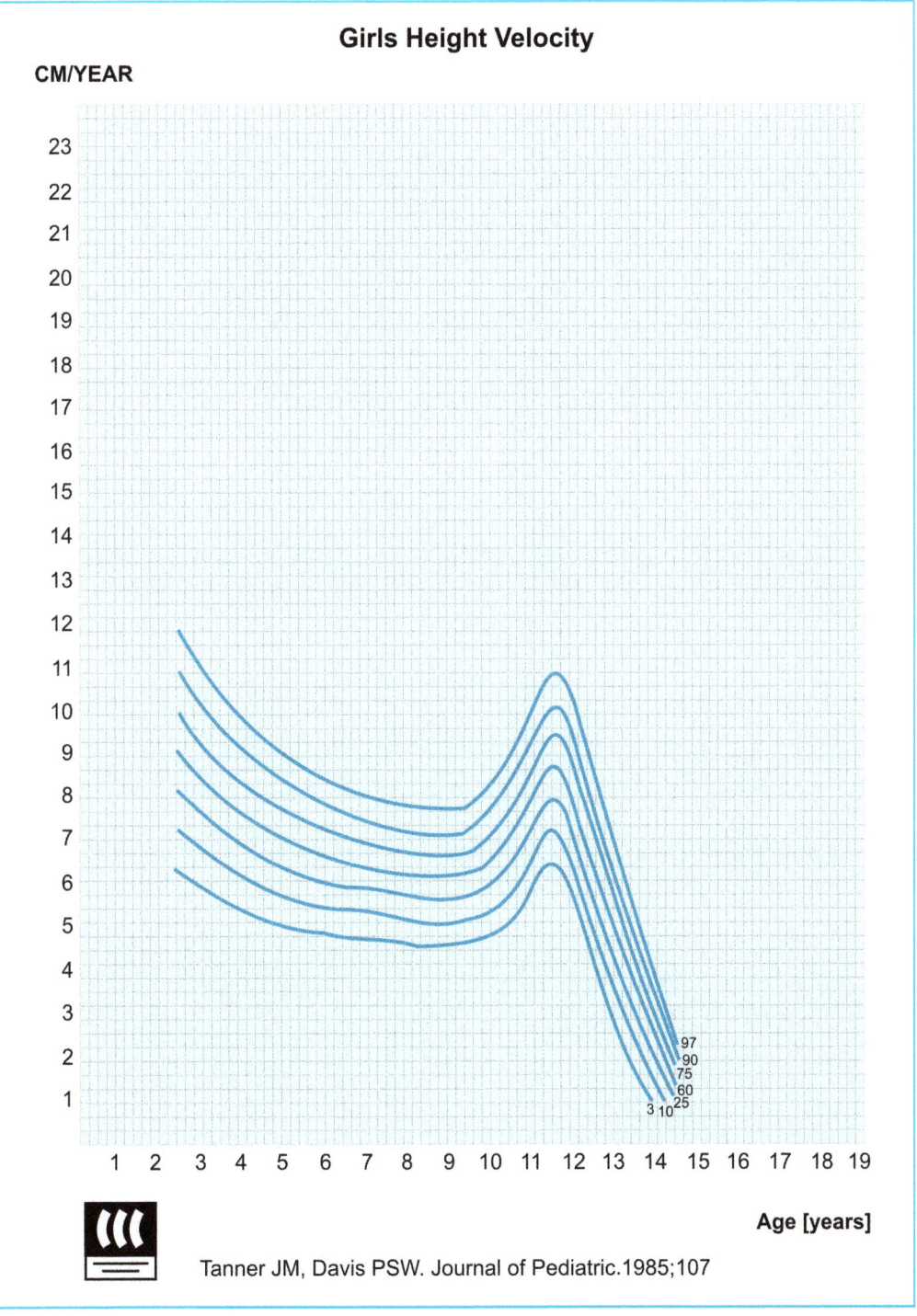

Tanner JM, Davis PSW. Journal of Pediatric.1985;107

67 CASE

Breast Development in an 8-year-old

■ HISTORY

An 8-year-old female child presented with breast development since the last 1 year, followed by pubic and axillary hair development since the last 6 months. On direct questioning, she reported a sudden increase in height over this period. She had not attained menarche yet.
    No past history of any head injury or CNS illness.
    No history of taking any medications or using skin creams.
    No history of noticing any excessive hair or deepening of voice.

■ PHYSICAL EXAMINATION

Fairly built and nourished
Height 130 cm   Wt 25 kg
SMR – 3 for both breasts and pubic hair
No signs of virilization
Rest of the examination normal

Analysis

Since this girl has started developing secondary sexual characteristics at the age of 7 years, her pubertal development is considered precocious (<8 years in girls and <9 years in boys). The order in which her pubertal development has proceeded, namely—premature thelarche followed by pubarche, coinciding with an increase in height before the onset of menstruation – simulates normal pubertal development. Therefore, this is likely to be **true** or **central precocious puberty** which is gonadotropin dependent. As there is no suggestion of virilization, it is *isosexual* precocity; true precocity is always isosexual. On the other hand, **pseudoprecocious puberty** (also known as peripheral precocious puberty or gonadotropin *independent* precocious puberty) is one where the cause is peripheral; it may or may not follow the normal pubertal pattern and it may be isosexual or heterosexual. In other words, this may as well be pseudoprecocious puberty.

    Since there is no history suggestive of virilization, there does not seem to be an abnormal androgen source such as androgen producing **adrenal/ovarian tumors** or **congenital adrenal hyperplasia**, or **exogenous androgens** in the form of anabolic steroids. Also, in such cases, one may expect premature pubarche (adrenarche) to precede thelarche; and (in tumors) the rate of progression of the pubertal changes may be more rapid. Autonomously functioning **ovarian cysts** act as abnormal sources of estrogens; they often lead to waxing and waning pubertal changes. **McCune-Albright syndrome** may present at an earlier age and there may be other features like abnormal pigmentation, other endocrine dysfunctions, or repeated fractures and pain. Precocious puberty may be the only presenting feature of some **CNS tumors** for as long as 1-2 years. Additional hypothalamic manifestations like appetite disorders, gelastic seizures or diabetes insipidus may point to a lesion in the brain. Therefore, in the absence of any history or signs to suggest any of the above causes, it is likely that this child has a **true idiopathic precocious puberty**, though a lesion in the brain cannot be clinically ruled out completely (and should be ruled out on investigations).

■ INVESTIGATIONS

Routine investigations normal
    Abdominal USG - ovaries and uterus enlarged for age, ovaries show multifollicular pattern
    CT scan of brain - normal

Analysis

The abdominal sonography findings are suggestive of a true precocious puberty that is gonadotropin mediated. Absence of any ovarian cysts or a brain lesion supports the diagnosis.

■ FINAL DIAGNOSIS

Idiopathic precocious puberty.

■ KEY MESSAGES

- Assessment of the sequence of sexual development is important, so also the timing of the growth spurt relative to the sexual development.
- True precocious puberty is isosexual and follows a normal pattern of sexual development.
- Pseudoprecocious puberty may be isosexual or heterosexual and may or may not follow normal pattern of sexual development.

■ RELEVANT INFORMATION

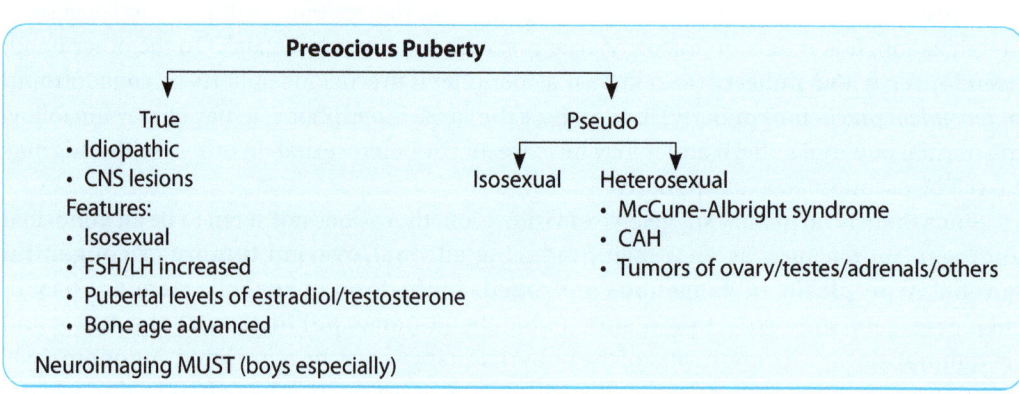

Premature Thelarche

Benign premature thelarche is characterized by unilateral or bilateral breast enlargement, usually before the age of 2 years. It resolves within 6 months to 3-5 years. It may be asymmetric, often fluctuates in degree, and is rarely progressive. No other signs of estrogenization are present. Laboratory studies are usually not indicated for premature thelarche. Clinical follow-up is adequate but mandatory to detect progression to precocious puberty or onset of virilization. Occurrence in children older than 3 years should prompt further evaluation.

Premature Adrenarche

Premature appearance of sexual hair, as an isolated manifestation, is the most common form of isolated precocious puberty. It is harmless, but a close follow-up is needed and a mild CAH should be kept in mind.

Premature Menarche

It is not so common, usually they have only 1-3 episodes of bleeding, but local causes should be carefully ruled out.

CASE 68

Pubic Hair Development in a 3½-year-old

■ HISTORY

A 3½-year-old child, born of a 3rd degree consanguineous marriage presented with vomiting for 2 days followed by recurrent attacks of short lasting generalized tonic/clonic seizures for the last 24 hours. The parents also complained that the child had developed pubic hair over the last 3 months.

This child was apparently alright 4 months ago when he started getting recurrent episodes of vomiting for which he was being treated with symptomatic treatment with temporary benefit. One such episode of vomiting during the last month needed hospitalization. He was treated with IV fluids. The vomiting was never bile stained, nor contained any blood. The routine investigations and the abdominal ultrasonography did not show any abnormality.

There was no history of diarrhea or fever, and he was apparently feeding well. There was no past history of convulsions. The developmental milestones were normal.

On direct questioning, the parents mentioned a darkening of skin color over the last 2 years and also reported that he craved for salt. On enquiring about the birth history, the parents mentioned that the doctors had noticed an ambiguity of genitalia at birth and were initially indecisive, but later on had declared this child as a male.

Analysis

Vomiting is a common nonspecific symptom in infants and toddlers that can accompany a variety of diseases. In such situations, vomiting is insignificant, occasional and never long lasting or recurrent. Thus, recurrent vomiting demands proper evaluation. **Recurrent vomiting** may be a result of repeated episodes of intestinal obstruction as in **volvulus**, which is accompanied by abdominal pain, bile stained vomiting and constipation. Absence of such symptoms rules out a surgical pathology. **Increased intracranial pressure** may present with repeated vomiting but would also have headache and other neurological symptoms. Recurrent vomiting may also represent **cyclical vomiting**. Recurrent vomiting is often the only manifestation of **metabolic or endocrine disorders**. Fluid and electrolyte disturbances may have caused the recurrent convulsions during the last episode of vomiting.

History of salt craving is unusual to come forth but whenever it is reported, it definitely suggests a **mineralocorticoid deficiency**. Darkening of skin color indicates melanocyte stimulation by ACTH. The logical stimulus for such an increased ACTH secretion is **glucocorticoid deficiency**.

Ambiguity of genitals in a newborn may mean one of two things – (a) *virilization* (masculinization) of external genitalia in a genetic female or (b) *incomplete masculinization* of external genitalia in a genetic male. The first situation occurs when the female fetus is exposed to excess of androgens. Typically, this is seen in **congenital adrenal hyperplasia (CAH)** due to 21-hydroxylase deficiency (the commonest) or 3 beta-dehydrogenase deficiency, where because of an enzymatic block in the synthesis of both glucocorticoids and mineralocorticoids, the precursors are shunted to the androgenic pathway. It can also be seen in situations where the mother has a **virilizing tumor**; however in that case, the mother would show signs of virilization herself, which is not so in this case. So if this child was incorrectly labeled a male, but is actually a genetic female, we need to consider a possibility of CAH due to either of these 2 enzyme deficiencies. On the other hand if this child was correctly declared a male, then it suggests that there is some incomplete masculinization, indicative of androgen deficiency.

Therefore, to sum up, this child definitely has a deficiency of mineralocorticoids (salt craving) and glucocorticoids (darkening of skin), and probably also has an androgen deficiency. This can happen in a congenital adrenal hyperplasia with a 3 beta-hydroxysteroid dehydrogenase enzyme deficiency because this is the only enzyme that is "shared" or needed in the first step of synthesis of all the above three hormones.

■ PHYSICAL EXAMINATION

Well built and fairly nourished
Weight 13 kg   Height 102 cm   US/LS - 1.3:1   TPR normal
BP 80/55 mm of Hg   Dark hyperpigmented skin
Bifid scrotum, hypospadias, phallic length 3.5 cm
Testes large in size with a volume of 6 mL   Pubic hair present
Systemic examination normal

Analysis

In any child with ambiguous genitalia, if one or both testis are palpable, it means there is definitely a Y component to the chromosome pattern and it is a **male genotype**. Inadequate masculinization, which gives the external genitalia their "feminine features" and hence the ambiguity, makes such a child a "**male pseudohermaphrodite**". So on clinical examination, we confirm the androgen deficiency. The glucocorticoid deficiency is also confirmed by the presence of dark hyperpigmented skin which is a sign of increased ACTH.

This child's height is almost above average, more so for a child who has been frequently unwell. This observation, and the development of pubic hair since the last 3 months suggests **precocious puberty**. Due to the enzymatic block, large amounts of precursor compounds like DHEA (dehydroepiandrosterone) accumulate over time, and may be peripherally converted to compounds with androgenic activity which can result in such premature isosexual development (precocious puberty). This is known as **pseudoprecocity** because it is not accompanied with the gonadal changes of puberty (increase in the size of the testis); the premature signs of puberty are driven by extragonadal hormones. A similar pseudoprecocity in the male and virilization in the female, is seen in other enzyme defects like 21 hydroxylase (most common form of CAH, more than 90% cases) and 11- hydroxylase, where the accumulated precursors are shunted to the androgen synthesis pathway.

However, this child's relatively large testicular volume (6 mL) suggests **true precocity**. But enlargement of testis is one of the earliest changes of puberty and we find that this child's pubic hair development is far advanced for this size of the testis. In other words, this child initially had a pseudoprecocity (tall child, advanced pubic hair, without enlargement of testis), and at a certain level of skeletal maturation, true precocity has been triggered off by gonadotropin releasing hormone (GnRH), so that he has now developed the earliest sign of puberty namely enlargement of testes.

■ INVESTIGATIONS

S. Cortisol (basal, 8 am) <8 mg%
S. ACTH (basal 8 am) 200 pg/mL
S. FSH 2.5 mIU/mL

S. DHEAS 600 mcg/dL
S. Testosterone 1.5 ng/mL
S. LH 1.5 mIU/mL

Analysis

The ACTH levels are high in response to the glucocorticoid deficiency. The high levels of androgenic compounds are consistent with the enzymatic block and a diversion of precursors to the androgenic pathway.

■ FINAL DIAGNOSIS

Congenital adrenal hyperplasia (CAH), with 3-beta-hydroxysteroid dehydrogenase deficiency, with pseudoprecocity, with recent onset of true precocious puberty.

■ KEY MESSAGES

- Recurrent vomiting demands proper evaluation.
- Complicated endocrine disorders can be clinically diagnosed if signs are carefully analyzed and hence absence of sophisticated laboratory facilities should not be a limiting factor especially when a disease can be a potential medical emergency.

■ RELEVANT INFORMATION

There are several aspects to the practical management of children with ambiguous genitalia.
1. The first step and the most important aspect of management is a constant dialogue with the parents and to ensure that they are adequately informed, both about the plan of action and the necessary investigations
2. The next step is to define the genotype. A karyotype is essential.
3. From a diagnostic standpoint what has to be decided is whether this is a virilized female or an inadequately masculinized male.
4. Evaluate ancillary problems, e.g., salt loss.

5. Discussing the above results with the parents and mutually deciding the sex of rearing is the most difficult. The issues involved are the wishes of the parents, the differing cultures, the (surgical) feasibility of assigning a particular sex, etc.
6. Implementing the gender confirming surgery.

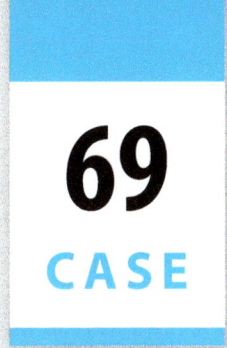

CASE 69

Excessive Weight Gain in a 10-year-old

■ HISTORY

A 10-year-old female child presented with an acute onset of high fever and a painful swelling of the left lower limb since the last 3 days. The parents also complained that she had gained excessive weight over the last 2 years.

- No history of trauma to the limb
- No history of headache or visual changes
- No history of any chronic drug ingestion
- No history of development of any secondary sexual characters yet
- No past history of any CNS disease
- No history suggestive of any muscle weakness
- No history of scholastic backwardness or deterioration of school performance
- No history suggestive of binge eating

She has a sedentary lifestyle with inadequate exercise and consumes 4,000 cal with 40 gm of protein

On direct questioning, the parents felt that she had not gained much height since the time she started gaining excessive weight, though they had not kept any height records.

Analysis

This girl has presented with obesity. History of excessive calorie consumption coupled with a sedentary lifestyle may suggest **nutritional** or **idiopathic obesity**. However, on direct questioning it has been noticed that her height gain has decelerated since the time she has started gaining excessive weight. Thus, it is likely that she is *short and obese*. Therefore, nutritional obesity seems unlikely in this child because these children are in fact tall for their age, i.e., tall and obese. If this child is short and obese, then the possible causes could be syndromic as seen in **Prader-Willi** or **Laurence-Moon-Biedl** syndrome; however, such children are mentally subnormal. Since there is no history of a prior CNS disease, a **hypothalamic** disturbance looks unlikely. **Turner's** syndrome is a possibility in any short girl, however obesity is not a prominent feature.

Though this child gives no history of somnolence or constipation, a decelerating growth may be the only indicator of **acquired hypothyroidism** initially. In such cases, school performance is known to be surprisingly preserved and the child may put on weight due to myxedema, reduced activity and lethargy. Therefore, acquired hypothyroidism may have to be considered, though it is rare in children.

Cushing's syndrome can also present as an obese short child. There is no history to suggest any exogenous source of steroids. So if it is Cushing's syndrome, at this age it is more likely to be Cushing's disease, i.e., primary pituitary adenomas causing bilateral adrenal hyperplasia rather than ACTH- independent functional adrenocortical tumors. This is so because adrenal tumors usually have a much shorter history whereas in this child the history dates back to 2 years. Besides, they are more common in infants. This girl has high fever and pain and swelling in the left lower limb since 3 days prior to presentation, which suggests local infection. Children with Cushing's syndrome are known to be more prone to infection.

■ PHYSICAL EXAMINATION

Pulse 110/m, all peripheral pulses well felt, no radiofemoral delay

RR 30/m	BP – 160/100 mm Hg	T – 101°F
Ht 123 cm	Wt 48 kg	No dysmorphic features
Moon facies, flushed face		Truncal obesity with buffalo hump
Knuckle pigmentation		Purplish striae on hips, abdomen and thigh

No abnormal pigmentation (acanthosis nigricans)

No skeletal abnormalities   No signs of virilization   Fundus – normal

Left lower limb – shiny, erythematous, edematous, tender below the knee, movements at the joints normal

Systemic examination normal

Mother's height 152 cm   Father's height 162 cm

Analysis

This girl's height falls below the 5th centile for her age (127 cm) and her weight is above the 95th centile for her age (47 kg). Therefore, this girl is short and obese, and she also has hypertension.

Nutritionally obese children may also be hypertensive. However, as discussed earlier, they are usually tall for their age. Besides, they have 'essential hypertension' i.e., they are mildly hypertensive to begin with (readings just above the 95th centile) and then slowly progress over time. On the other hand, significant hypertension as in this case is more likely to be secondary to disease. The truncal obesity with other physical features like striae, buffalo hump, in a short girl with secondary hypertension suggest Cushing's syndrome. Knuckle pigmentation suggests that it is an **ACTH dependent Cushing's syndrome**. Since ectopic ACTH secreting tumors are rare in children, it is likely to be an ACTH secreting pituitary tumor, leading to Cushing's disease. On examination, she seems to have a cellulitis of the left lower limb, though it could also be a pathological fracture.

Absence of any dysmorphic features and skeletal abnormalities and a normal fundus rules out syndromes like Prader-Willi and LMB. Girls with Turner's syndrome may have coarctation of aorta and may develop hypertension; however, this girl does not have the other clinical features of Turner syndrome or of coarctation.

■ INVESTIGATIONS

Hb - 15 gm%
Blood sugar
S. Cortisol (8 am and 8 pm) – increased,
Urinary free cortisol - 305 µg/24 hrs
Dexamethasone suppression test done after 120 mg/kg/day
Post test - urinary free cortisol - 40 µg/24 hrs
Bone age - 9 years

PCV - 55
Fasting 116 mg%

TLC - 12,400 N 70 L 29 E 0 M 1
Post prandial 172 mg%
No diurnal variation noted
Urinary 17 OHCS - 6 mg/m^2/24 hrs

urinary 17 OHCS - 2 mg/m^2/24 hr
MRI – normal

Analysis

In normal individuals, serum cortisol is normally elevated at 8 am but drops by more than 50% at 8 pm. The loss of this diurnal rhythm in this child favors Cushing's syndrome. Though elevated urinary 17 OHCS may be due to nutritional obesity itself, they are easily suppressed by a single dose dexamethasone administration which is not so here. Urinary free cortisol and 17 OHCS have been suppressed by more than 50% of baseline values following the high dose (120 µg/kg/day) dexamethasone suppression test. So this is an ACTH dependent Cushing's syndrome. The most likely source is a pituitary adenoma or microadenomas. However, the MRI was normal. In such cases the diagnosis may be confirmed by inferior petrosal blood sampling.

■ FINAL DIAGNOSIS

ACTH dependent Cushing's syndrome.

■ KEY MESSAGES

- A child who is tall and obese generally does not need to be investigated as the etiology is mostly nutritional or familial.
- A short and obese child must be investigated as it is almost always pathological.

■ RELEVANT INFORMATION

Obesity

Obesity is now an increasingly prevalent nutritional disorder among children and adolescents, threatening to be an epidemic in the next few years. It represents a serious concern and a challenge. Its major impacts include effects on blood pressure, intermediary metabolism, respiratory function, psychological well-being, social adaptation, and educational performance. Obesity is also associated with significant adult morbidity.

Definition of obesity in adults is derived from statistical data of body mass in relation to risk of acute and long-term morbidity and mortality. Because similar data in children is limited and difficult to interpret, no single definition of obesity in childhood has gained universal approval. A definition based on weight is misleading as weight is a variable parameter throughout the period of growth. The body mass index (BMI) is a continuous measure of body fatness. It corrects for body size and can be quantified readily and reliably in clinical settings. It correlates closely with total body fat as measured by DEXA scan. It is recommended that children be considered overweight if BMI exceeds 85th centile and obese if it exceeds 95th centile, (based on curves generated by NHS surveys in USA) or if it is more than 30 kg/m^2.

Energy imbalance from excessive energy intake or reduced expenditure results in obesity.

Most overweight children have a familial form of obesity that results from multiple environmental factors. The family patterns of food intake, exercise, selection of leisure activity (watching TV, etc.), and family and cultural patterns of food selection reflect prevalence of obesity. Genetic factors also play a considerable role in the development of childhood obesity.

Accumulation of body fat, particularly in a visceral distribution, produces a resistance to insulin action, which in turn predisposes to glucose intolerance, hypertriglyceridemia and hypertension. Resultant type 2 diabetes and cardiovascular disease reduces life-expectancy.

CASE 70

Progressive Deformity of Lower Limbs

■ HISTORY

A 4-year-old female Muslim child presented with a progressive deformity of both lower limbs noticed since the age of 2 years. According to the parents she has always been of a small build and a poor eater, but otherwise active and playful. She was weaned at 10 months of age, and had not received any vitamin supplements. Her milestones have been normal in infancy though she started walking at 16 months of age.

- No history of pain in the lower limbs or difficulty in getting up from squatting position.
- No history of delayed dentition.
- No family history of a similar illness.
- No history of any chronic drug intake or a past history of any significant illness.
- On direct questioning, no deformity was noticed in the upper limb, spine, or chest.

Analysis

History of deformity of both lower limbs in an otherwise playful active asymptomatic child suggests a **primary bony disorder**. In view of normal milestones in the first year but delayed walking, it seems that the disease has started sometime after infancy; this corroborates well with the history of noticing the deformity at about 2 years of age. As the deformity is progressive, it is unlikely to be a **chondrodystrophy** which is static deformity. Hence, it is suggestive of **rickets**. Since this child comes from a community where mothers may have less exposure to sunlight, has been weaned late, and did not receive any vitamin supplements, it may suggest **deficiency** rickets. However, though deficiency rickets may manifest in the first or second year of life, it is a **hypocalcemic** variety of rickets which is characterized by chest and upper limb deformities before developing lower limb deformities, muscle weakness and sometimes hypocalcemic tetany. Since these features are absent and this child has presented with lower limb deformities, clinically this is likely to be a **hypophosphatemic** variety of rickets. It may be **X-linked familial**, or as a part of **Fanconi's syndrome** or renal tubular acidosis. Even though there is no family history of similar complaints. Familial hypophosphatemia cannot be ruled out. Since this child is active and playful, **renal tubular acidosis** seems less likely though we can only be more certain after examination.

■ PHYSICAL EXAMINATION

Comfortable child, not "sick"
Weight 12.5 kg   Height 90 cm
Pulse 92/m   RR 24/m   BP 80/60 mm Hg   pallor +
Waddling gait, bow legs   double malleolus, minimal widening of wrists
No rickety rosary, no frontal bossing, no Harrison's sulcus
Spine normal
Systemic examination normal (specifically, muscle tone and power normal)

Analysis

Physical examination confirms rickets with signs seen predominantly in the lower limbs. This favors hypophosphatemic rickets. Besides, clinical signs consistent with a hypocalcemic rickets (as discussed earlier) are absent. Though this child's weight and height are less than the expected for his age, he may be of a small build rather than malnourished. He does not show any signs to suggest failure to thrive, nor is he clinically acidotic (tachypneic). Thus, renal causes of hypophosphatemic rickets are ruled out. Clinically, he is likely to be having **familial hypophosphatemia**, though **metaphyseal dysplasias** are also a possibility and need to be ruled out on investigation.

■ INVESTIGATIONS

Hb 10.5 gm%   CBC normal   Urinalysis normal
S. Calcium 9 mgm%   S. phosphorus 2.5 mgm%   Alk. Phos. 980 units
Renal profile normal
X-ray knee - active rickets

Analysis

Investigations confirm hypophosphatemic rickets.

■ FINAL DIAGNOSIS

Hypophosphatemic rickets.

■ KEY MESSAGES

- The time of onset of rickets offers a clue to the etiology
- Rickets with failure to thrive is always pathological.
- Hypocalcemic rickets presents with muscle weakness, while hypophosphatemic rickets with bony deformities.

RELEVANT INFORMATION

Renal Tubular Acidosis

The kidneys maintain acid-base balance by reclaiming bicarbonate and excreting acid. Glomerular dysfunction results in azotemia, anion retention and acidosis that is defined as uremic acidosis. Loss of tubular function prevents the kidneys from excreting hydrogen ions and thereby causing metabolic acidosis. Renal tubular acidosis refers to a diverse group of tubular disorders characterized by impairment of urinary acidification without urea and anion retention. These disorders are divided into two general categories, proximal (type II) and distal (type I and IV).

Proximal RTA (Type II - Bicarbonate-wasting Acidosis)

Bicarbonate reabsorption is defective in this condition. It rarely occurs as an isolated defect and is usually associated with multiple proximal tubular defects such as loss of glucose, amino acids, phosphates, uric acid and other organic anions such as citrate (Fanconi's syndrome). A distinctive feature of proximal RTA is that the urine pH can be lowered to less than 5.5 with acid loading.

Distal RTA (Inadequate Acid Secretion and Excretion)

It refers to metabolic acidosis occurring secondary to decreased renal acid secretion in absence of a marked decrease in glomerular filtration rate and characterized by a normal anion gap. They are further classified in hypokalemic (type I) and hyperkalemic (type IV) RTA. Urine pH cannot reach maximal acidity despite systemic acidemia, indicating low H^+ secretion in the collecting duct. Urinary pH is always above 5.5. Nephrocalcinosis, nephrolithiasis and bone disease are the typical complications of distal RTA.

HISTORY

5 years old male child born of 2ⁿᵈ degree consanguineous marriage presented with history of recurrent pain in joints for last 10 months. He was apparently well 10 months ago when he started with fever and pain in left shoulder. He was diagnosed as septic arthritis and treated with antibiotics for a week. He completely within 4-5 days and was well thereafter for ……… He presented involving right wrist and left ankle. ……… of ……… arthritis and treated with anti-inflammatory ……… week and treatment was discontinued after 2 ……… months. He developed acute pain in right hi……… result of laboratory tests was as follows.

HB 8 GM% microcytic hy………
WBC 6,500/CMM P 68 L 2………
PLATELETS ADEQUATE
ESR 25 MM

He was treated with anti-inflamm……… for next 6 weeks but without much change.

At that stage, he was subjected to radiolog……… examination. X-ray of right lower limb showed osteolytic ……… upper end of femur on right side.

……… ……… child was referred to a teaching ……… for further

the inconspicuous often makes the diagnosis obvious

Clinical Rheumatology

BACK TO BASICS

Detailed history is a prerequisite for diagnosis of rheumatic disorders as these disorders are syndromic in nature. A conglomeration of clinical patterns with carefully selected laboratory tests help make a diagnosis; the diagnosis often evolves over time. Besides the onset, duration and progress of the joint involvement, aggravating and relieving factors also offer a clue. For example, morning stiffness and pain that gets better as the day progresses indicates an inflammatory disease while aggravation on exertion and relief on resting suggests a mechanical problem. The site and the number of joints affected helps to classify the disease.

Classification Criteria for Rheumatoid Arthritis
1. Morning stiffness (1 hr)
2. Swelling (soft tissue) of 3 or more joints
3. Swelling (soft tissue) of hand joints (PIP, MCP, or wrist)
4. Symmetrical swelling (soft tissue)
5. Subcutaneous nodules
6. Serum rheumatoid factor
7. Erosions and/or periarticular osteopenia in hand or wrist joints seen on radiograph

PIP = proximal interphalangeal; MCP = metacarpophalangeal.

*Criteria 1 to 4 must have been continuous for 6 weeks or longer and criteria 2 to 5 must be observed by a physician. A diagnosis of rheumatoid arthritis requires that four of the seven criteria be fulfilled.

A history of skin rash, mouth ulcers, alopecia and nail abnormalities should be specifically enquired. A past history of any of these events, as well as any other manifestations affecting various organs must be carefully analyzed as many a times rheumatic diseases present with a sequential involvement of different organs, though they represent the same disease.

The physical examination of joints should be carried out in a systematic manner so as to pick up early signs of joint affection. Each joint must be thoroughly evaluated including the spine and the temporomandibular joints. Restriction of extreme movements may be the only clinical evidence of joint involvement. Joint effusion denotes active disease. Though most joints with long-standing affection demonstrate muscle wasting around the joint, it can also be seen in an acute arthritis (due to disuse, especially around the knee joint).

Clinical evidence of subtle affection of any organ must be carefully noted.

Laboratory tests for assessing various organ involvement are necessary even in absence of clinical signs. However, many investigations can be falsely positive in many unrelated disorders; therefore, one needs to ask for specific investigations focused towards a probable clinical diagnosis to avoid confusion.

As far as therapy of rheumatic disorders is concerned, symptomatic relief is not the only goal, proper management is necessary to prevent long-term disability.

71 CASE

Limb Pain with Difficulty in Walking

■ HISTORY

A 6-year-old male child presented with pain in the legs off and on for the last 12 months. He was apparently well 1 year ago when he started complaining about pain in the legs, which was intermittently severe, incapacitating him to an extent that he would find difficulty in walking. He would cry with pain when it was unbearable. There were no apparent aggravating factors, but it was at times relieved by massage. He was initially treated with analgesics and anti-inflammatory drugs, with temporary relief. Several tests were carried out and at one stage, he was diagnosed as polymyositis. Considering it to be an inflammatory disorder, he was treated with oral prednisolone for 4–6 weeks during which period he felt relieved and had no pain. After the steroids were discontinued, he had a recurrence of symptoms and the pain had now gradually involved the upper limbs as well. Another course of oral steroids failed to relieve him and he was getting worse. Hence, he was referred for further evaluation.

No h/o any diurnal variation in the pain.
No h/o any color or temp changes in the limbs.
No history of fever.
No history of joint pains or swelling.
No other symptoms.
No relevant past or family history.

Analysis

This child's complaint is "limb pain" as against joint pains. When severe limb pain is the presenting complaint, the anatomical origin of such a severe pain could be muscle, bone, or nerves. If it is the **bone**, the possible pathologies could be osteoporosis, periosteal involvement as in leukemia or scurvy, or vaso-occlusive crisis of sickle cell disease. In this child there is no background history to suggest development of **osteoporosis**, and the illness is spanning over too long a period for **leukemias** to be otherwise asymptomatic and without any deterioration in the general condition. In the absence of an exceptionally poor nutritional history, **scurvy** is unlikely at this age. Vaso-occlusive crisis (as seen in **sickle cell disease**) would usually affect specific parts of the limbs and would affect other organs as well. So while it cannot be ruled out completely, it is less likely.

Relief of pain on massage may suggest a **muscular** origin. Generalized muscle pain may be in the form of so called **"growing pains"** (now believed to be associations of hypermobility syndromes) which can also occasionally be severe enough to make the child cry; however, they occur after a period of exertion, i.e., at the end of the day, and rarely occur in the upper limbs. However, other **musculoskeletal pain syndromes** could be considered. **Fibromyalgia** is one such condition; however, because of the absence of a history of obvious tender points, it is less likely. Pain without a history of fever and swelling is less likely to be inflammatory, and therefore **myositis** is unlikely. Since the pain increases in severity intermittently, it may be ischemic muscular pain. Such **ischemia** could be due to vasospasm, or arterial or venous thrombosis. Involvement of both upper and lower limbs may also suggest a generalized disorder affecting the blood vessels such as **vasculitis**. However, generalized vasculitis is usually a part of a systemic inflammatory disorder; one expects some constitutional symptoms which are lacking.

Neurogenic pain due to irritation of the nerve roots as in polyneuritis or cord compression is localized to a dermatome; over time the pathology would progress leading to other neurological symptoms. Therefore, it is unlikely to be neurogenic. **Reflex sympathetic osteodystrophy** can also be a possibility though it is usually characterized by color and temperature changes in the limb.

■ PHYSICAL EXAMINATION

Fairly built and nourished

Weight 20 kg	Height 108 cm	Temp. normal
Pulse 90/min	Peripheral pulses well felt	BP 150/100 mm of Hg
RR 28/min	Macular skin rash scattered over legs	

Left ring finger was cold as compared to other fingers. It was pale with a black area at the tip
Limbs were apparently normal, though restriction of movements of both limbs due to pain

No redness, warmth, swelling or tenderness
Spine and skull normal   Central and peripheral nervous system- normal
CVS normal   Other systems normal

Analysis

A cold and pale left ring finger with a black area at the tip suggests **impending gangrene** of the finger, which is definitely indicative of an **arterial block**. In the absence of any bony abnormality on examination, the pain in the limbs could be explained on the basis of ischemic muscular pain. The skin rash may denote an affection of arterioles in the skin. Since there is definite evidence of arterial involvement, it is likely that the systemic hypertension may be the result of involvement of the renal artery. Thus, it seems that small and medium sized arteries are involved. An arterial block can be caused by **thrombosis** or inflammation of the vessel wall. Thrombosis may result from a **hypercoagulable state** such as protein C or protein S deficiency, or antiphospholipid antibody syndrome (APLA). It could also be a part of systemic **vasculitis**; the disease is probably yet evolving.

INVESTIGATIONS

Hb 9 gm%
ESR 90 mm
Urine routine normal
ANA negative
Anti-smooth muscle antibody negative
APLA +ve

WBC 8,000/cmm   P 60 L 36 E 2 M 2
CRP strongly positive
S. Creatinine 0.3 mg%   Blood urea 25 mg%
c-ANCA and p-ANCA negative
Anti-mitochondrial antibody negative
Anticardiolipin antibody +ve

Analysis

The high ESR and a positive CRP denote that this is an **inflammatory disease**. The presence of antibodies suggests an **immune mediated** disorder. Since the renal parameters are normal, there is no renal dysfunction. In this setting, the **hypertension** is **renovascular** and not renoparenchymal. Since ANA is negative, SLE is almost ruled out (though it is presumed that the ANA test has been done by indirect immunofluorescence, which is the reliable and ideal method). The presence of antiphospholipid and anticardiolipin antibodies in a setting of an inflammatory disorder suggests a **secondary APLA syndrome**. The exact nature of the primary inflammatory disease is as yet undefined. Primary APLA syndrome is characterized by non-inflammatory thrombosis and is therefore ruled out.

FINAL DIAGNOSIS

Secondary APLA syndrome.

FOLLOW-UP

This child was treated with warfarin and low dose aspirin. Within 3 days of warfarin therapy, the left ring finger regained color and warmth. He was also put on a calcium channel blocker for hypertension.

KEY MESSAGES

- Musculoskeletal pain needs to be analyzed with proper logic. While inflammatory pain is not difficult to diagnose, non-inflammatory pain may be ischemic, neurogenic or psychogenic. A specific diagnosis is possible only by evaluating the further progress of the illness.
- Rheumatological disease evolves over time before it can be labeled as a specific entity. In this case the diagnosis evolved after the development of gangrene and hypertension. Prior to that, correct analysis of the history helped to narrow down the possibilities to be kept in mind. Based on these, one could anticipate or look out for relevant findings on subsequent examinations till the diagnosis evolved.
- While the blood pressure is routinely recorded in obvious renal and cardiac cases, it should also be done in undiagnosed cases, as also in every case of headache.

■ RELEVANT INFORMATION

Antiphospholipid syndrome can occur within the context of several diseases, mainly autoimmune (secondary antiphospholipid syndrome), or it may be present without any recognizable disease, so-called primary antiphospholipid syndrome. It is the most common cause of acquired thrombophilia associated with either venous or arterial thrombosis or both. According to the International Consensus Statement, a diagnosis of antiphospholipid syndrome requires the presence of at least one each of the following clinical and laboratory criteria:

Clinical Criteria

1. One or more episodes of vascular thrombosis
2. Complications of pregnancy – unexplained fetal death/repeated abortions or premature delivery

Laboratory Criteria

1. Detection of anticardiolipin IgG or IgM antibodies in moderate or high titers on 2-3 occasions at interval of 6 weeks.
2. Detection of lupus anticoagulant antibody on 2-3 occasions at interval of 6 weeks.
   Other laboratory abnormalities that may be seen in this syndrome include thrombocytopenia, hemolytic anemia, proteinuria or hematuria.

Management

Prophylaxis against thrombosis in patients with antiphospholipid syndrome demands lifelong warfarin treatment, maintaining INR between 3 and 3.5.

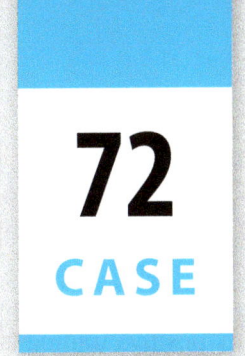

CASE 72

Limb Pain for a Year

■ HISTORY

An 8-year-old female child presented with pain in the legs mainly in the evenings for the last 1 year. The pain was severe at times making her cry and she found it difficult to fall asleep. It was relieved by massage. She was quite normal through the day and was able to go through strenuous physical activities. Though the pain was mostly in the legs, sometime it used to involve upper limbs as well, especially the small muscles of the hand.

No history of worsening of symptoms over a year.
No history of any other major symptoms.
No relevant past or family history.
She had been taking analgesics frequently when the pain became intolerable.
Routine investigations were normal including X-rays and serum calcium.

Analysis

This child seems to have a non-progressive or a slowly progressive disorder which is intermittent, with periods of normalcy in between. Pain appearing mainly in the evening without affecting her physical activities through the day suggests a **mechanical** problem rather than an inflammatory disease. Inflammatory pain is worst early in the morning and then it eases over the day as activity increases. Further, inflammatory pain will worsen on pressure/massage. Therefore, this is a noninflammatory pain, which could have arisen from either the muscles, or the **bones** as in periosteal involvement in **leukemia** or **osteopenia**. However, the bony pain of leukemia is a vague pain, usually constant, worsened by pressure/massage, and it does not have a diurnal variation. Similarly osteopenic pain is a vague generalized pain, which though noninflammatory is also worsened by pressure so that use of the limb/walking, etc. is painful. On the other hand, pain in the evening after the day's exertion denotes tired muscles with accumulation of metabolites, which are cleared away by massage thereby relieving the pain. Such **musculoskeletal** pains are known to be associated with hypermobility syndrome. Since, this child is young enough not to expect mechanical problems like degenerative changes, a diagnosis of hypermobility syndrome is favored.

■ PHYSICAL EXAMINATION

Well built and nourished child Healthy and comfortable
Weight 28 kg Height 128 cm Arm span 125 cm BP normal

Excessive mobility of joints demonstrable at wrists, knees, elbows and spine.
Skin and subcutaneous tissue normal
Other systems normal

Analysis

A healthy comfortable child rules out a progressive disease. The only positive finding is hypermobile joints. Absence of any abnormality like hyperelasticity or abnormal stature (marfanoid features) rules out syndromic hypermobility.

■ INVESTIGATION

Hypermobility syndrome is a clinical diagnosis and does not justify any investigations.

■ FINAL DIAGNOSIS

Hypermobility syndrome.

■ KEY MESSAGES

- Earlier dubbed as "growing pains", this is due to hypermobility of joints.
- It is a connective tissue disorder, not so uncommon in the community and it is benign.
- Treatment is symptomatic and heat in any form applied to the painful areas relieves pain.

■ RELEVANT INFORMATION

The hypermobility syndrome presents with arthralgias due to increased joint laxity in the face of muscle disuse. Hypermobility may be a part of many syndromes.

The Ehlers-Danlos family of disorders is a group of related conditions that share a common decrease in the tensile strength and integrity of the skin, joints, and other tissues.

Other syndromes may mimic hypermobility syndrome and they include Marfan's syndrome/Menkes kinky hair disease/William syndrome/Stickler syndrome/cutis laxa.

CASE 73

Joint Pains—Recurrent

■ HISTORY

A 5-year-old male child born of a 2nd degree consanguineous marriage presented with a history of recurrent pain in the joints for the last 10 months. He was apparently well 10 months ago when he started with fever and pain in the left shoulder. He was diagnosed as acute septic arthritis and treated with antibiotics for a week. He improved completely within 4–5 days and was well thereafter for 2 weeks. A similar episode occurred again this time involving the right wrist and the left ankle. Hence, he was diagnosed as reactive arthritis and treated with anti-inflammatory drugs. He improved over a week and treatment was discontinued after 2 weeks. After an interval of 2 months, he developed acute pain in the right hip joint and was investigated. The results of the laboratory tests were as follows:

Hb 8 gm%, microcytic hypochromic anemia   WBC 6,500/c.mm   P 68 L 28 E 4
Platelets adequate   ESR 25 mm

He was treated with anti-inflammatory drugs but without much relief. At that stage, he was subjected to a radiological examination.

The X-ray of the right hip showed an osteolytic area at the upper end of femur. Further X-rays revealed a similar area at the lower end of tibia on the left side.

At this juncture the child was referred to a tertiary center for further management.

No history of a similar disease or any other complaints prior to the onset of these complaints

No relevant family history.

Analysis

This child started with fever and pain in the shoulder joint. However, when the complaint of pain pertains to deep-seated joints like the shoulder and hip, and no definite swelling is documented, it may or may not be a joint pathology. Further, though he was diagnosed as an acute septic arthritis, it is unlikely to improve within a few days of antibiotic therapy. Therefore, it is likely that this was a self-limiting disease of an acute onset, affecting the **joint or** the **periarticular** structures (including the bone), which was **not infective**. That it may be non-infective is further corroborated by the fact that in the subsequent episodes, pain has been the prominent complaint and not fever. Reactive arthritis is often a self-limiting disease that is seen after viral or bacterial infections, may involve multiple joints, and may appear "migratory". However, a clinical course spread over 10 months with periods of normalcy in between, rule it out. Specific syndromes of reactive arthritis that can persist for so long and then evolve into spondyloarthropathies are characterized by enthesitis and a definite history of a GI or GU infection. A non-infective disease causing recurrent bone or joint manifestations may be related to a **malignancy**, vasculitis, or hematological disorders. A local **bony** malignancy is ruled out as the symptoms have recurred and that too, at different sites. A **systemic** or a **hematological** malignancy should have led to other manifestations by now. A **systemic vasculitis** (Henoch-Schönlein purpura) is possible, though one expects some other symptoms affecting other organs as well, over a period of 10 months. **Scurvy** is seen in severely malnourished children whereas there are no other symptoms to suggest **hemophilia**. **Sickle cell disease** may be associated with bony infarcts and could be considered.

Osteolytic areas on the X-ray may suggest chronic infections like TB, local bony tumors or cysts, eosinophilic granuloma, secondaries from systemic malignancies or bony infarcts (as in ischemia). Multifocal lytic areas are unlikely in TB and local tumors; an aneurysmal bone cyst can be multifocal and so also eosinophilic granulomas, secondaries and ischemia. Since secondaries from systemic malignancies are unlikely as discussed above, these may be **eosinophilic granulomas**, **bone cysts**, or **bony infarcts**.

■ PHYSICAL EXAMINATION

Poorly built and nourished	Weight 16 kg	Height 97 cm
Not sick looking	Moderate pallor present	No lymphadenopathy
Joints normal	No restriction of movements	

Soft tissue swelling over left ankle and right wrist but free from joints
Mild tenderness present, not warm or inflamed

Liver 3 cm +, firm, not tender	Spleen 2 cm +, firm

Other systems normal

Analysis

Growth failure, moderate anemia with mild hepatosplenomegaly and bony lesions in a child with 2nd degree consanguinity favors the diagnosis of **sickle cell anemia**. Secondary spread from **neuroblastoma** may lead to multiple bony lesions with hepatosplenomegaly and anemia but such lesions would not recover and then recur, and growth failure is not explained. **Leukemia** may have similar manifestations but the disease has gone on for 10 months and hence unlikely.

■ INVESTIGATIONS

Hb 8 gm%   WBC 12,000/c mm   P 70 L 24 E 3 M 3
Microcytosis, hypochromia, anisocytosis, poikilocytosis, normoblasts and target cells
ESR 10 mm   Hb electrophoresis - HbS 60%
Sickling test was initially –ve but on rechecking (with a *freshly prepared* reagent) it was positive. Both parents were carriers.

■ FINAL DIAGNOSIS

Sickle cell disease.

KEY MESSAGES

- Soft tissue or bony lesion around the joint is easily mistaken as joint disease. Restriction of movements, joint effusion, synovial thickening and swelling of the joint with obliteration of joint space are the manifestations of joint pathology.
- Multiple bony lesions due to acute bacterial infections are rare, and may be seen only in newborns or immunocompromised patients; such lesions are never recurrent.
- Scurvy and hematological diseases like leukemia, hemophilia, Henoch-Schönlein purpura and sickle cell anemia may mimic bone or joint disease.

RELEVANT INFORMATION

Skeletal Manifestations of Sickle Cell Disease

The skeletal manifestations of sickle cell disease are the result of changes in bone and bone marrow caused by the chronic tissue hypoxia that is exacerbated by episodic occlusion of the microcirculation by the abnormal sickle cells. The main processes that lead to bone and joint destruction in sickle cell disease are infarction of the bone and bone marrow, compensatory bone marrow hyperplasia, secondary osteomyelitis, and secondary growth defects such as bone shortening (premature epiphyseal fusion), epiphyseal deformity with cupped metaphysis, peg-in-hole defect of distal femur and decreased height of vertebrae (short stature and kyphoscoliosis).

CASE 74

Joint Pains with Constitutional Symptoms

■ HISTORY

An 8-year-old female child presented with a low grade fever and generalized weakness and fatigue since the last 3 months. She was apparently alright 3 months ago when she started getting a low grade fever which was accompanied by a feeling of weakness and fatigue. As a result, she stopped playing and going to school. When taken to the local doctor after a month, nothing specific was detected on clinical examination, so she was investigated. The results were: Hb 10 gm%, WBC count 9800 N 54 L 42 E 4, ESR 98 mm at the end of 1 hour, Mantoux test positive 12 × 12 mm, and X-ray of the chest normal. Based on these reports, she was put on antituberculous treatment. Two weeks later, she developed a rash on the face, which was initially apparent only when she went out in the sun, but was later persistent. From about the same time she also started getting pain in both her knees and ankle joints. The pain was not associated with any swelling of the joints but was sufficiently severe to incapacitate her. The rash was attributed to the drugs and the joint pains were taken as part of her generalized "weakness". She was additionally treated with analgesics and some skin creams without any sustained relief. Meanwhile, there was no response in her primary symptoms either and she now reported a weight loss of 2 kg. At this point she was referred for further evaluation.

On direct questioning, there was
No history of a contact with tuberculosis.
No history of puffiness of face, edema, or hematuria.
No history of a rash elsewhere in the body, or petechial spots.
No history of any major illness in the past.

Analysis

Constitutional symptoms for 3 months may denote a chronic infection like tuberculosis, systemic inflammatory disorders or a malignancy. While a high ESR and a positive Mantoux test may support the diagnosis of tuberculosis in this setting, antituberculous treatment should be based on more definitive proof. Such a high ESR could also denote malignancies or systemic inflammatory disorders, and a positive Mantoux test at this age is not uncommon in the community in otherwise asymptomatic children. In the light of a normal chest X-ray and no history of a contact with tuberculosis, this could also have been a malignancy or systemic inflammatory disease in evolution. Though the leukocyte counts have been reported as normal in the beginning of the illness, a hematological malignancy cannot be ruled out and needs to be investigated for. A drug related rash may not specifically involve the face alone, and generalized debility (unless severe) would rarely give rise to *incapacitating* joint pains. Such pains are more likely to indicate a primary inflammatory involvement of the joints. Therefore, the subsequent development of a facial rash, in association with joint pains could point to an evolving inflammatory disorder. In a girl, systemic lupus erythematosus is a strong possibility.

■ PHYSICAL EXAMINATION

Averagely built and nourished
Weight 19 kg   Height 121 cm
Pulse 84/min   RR 24/min   Temp. 100°F   BP 92/58 mm Hg
Erythema over the bridge of the nose and malar areas with periorbital edema, without any thickening or scaling of the skin

No other skin rash	No petechial spots	Nails normal
No telangiectasia	No oral ulcers	No alopecia
Mild pallor	No lymphadenopathy	No pedal edema

Bones and joints normal (no swelling, deformity)
CNS
Higher functions, cranial nerves normal
Tenderness of quadriceps and calf muscles
Gower's sign positive
Power Grade IV in shoulder flexors, extensors, abductors in hip flexors, calf muscles
Deep tendon reflexes normal   Sensory system normal
Other systems normal   No hepatosplenomegaly

Analysis

The physical findings suggest inflammation of various muscles with muscular weakness. In view of the facial rash, it denotes a possibility of juvenile dermatomyositis. While a similar rash may also be seen in SLE, the muscular involvement favors dermatomyositis. There is no clinical evidence of tuberculosis or a malignancy.

■ INVESTIGATIONS

Hb 9 gm%   WBC 6,400   P 64 L 32 E 4   Pl count 1.8 Lacs/c.mm
ESR 72 mm at the end of 1 hour   Urine routine - normal
AST – 320 units   LDH –elevated   CPK – 400
S. Creatinine 0.4 mg%
ANA – positive, speckled pattern   Anti-dsDNA negative
X-ray chest normal   ECG normal

Analysis

A positive ANA may be seen in SLE and JDM. However, anti-dsDNA being negative rules out SLE. There is definite laboratory evidence of inflammation of muscles. The anemia may be a combination of chronic illness and a resultant poor nutrition. The high ESR is unusual; it is usually reported to be normal in JDM. There is no other evidence of renal or any other system involvement.

■ COMMENT

After clinical examination, certain details in the history were again asked. The parents now mentioned that they had noticed a difficulty in getting up from the squatting position since the last 2 months. The child also found it difficult to comb her hair; however, all these symptoms were attributed to her general weakness.

■ FINAL DIAGNOSIS

Juvenile dermatomyositis.

■ KEY MESSAGES

- Constitutional symptoms often represent a disease in evolution. A careful examination and a follow-up is necessary to detect subtle abnormalities which may offer a clue to the diagnosis.
- Anti-TB treatment should be started only if there is reasonable evidence in favor. If started empirically, failure of an expected response should prompt a search for alternative diagnosis.

CASE 75

Acute Onset Multiple Large Joint Swellings

■ HISTORY

A 12-year-old healthy child presented with acute onset of pain and swelling involving both knee and ankle joints for the last 3 days. No other joints were involved and there were no other symptoms. There was a history of (H/o) a recent viral upper respiratory tract infection (URTI). There was no family history of any rheumatological disorders.

Analysis

The acute onset of symmetrical affection of four large joints with swelling and pain suggests noninfective inflammation. **Acute septic arthritis** is a monoarthritis presenting with high fever and so, ruled out in this child. Similarly, **trauma** and **hemophilia** are also ruled out because they would not involve four large joints at the same time. Periarticular diseases may mimic arthritis and need to be considered. **Leukemia** may present with bony pain (slightly different from joint pain) but would have systemic symptoms, such as fever; hence, it is unlikely in this child. This could be an evolving **juvenile idiopathic arthritis**—oligoarticular at this point in time. It is possible that the patient may not have noticed small joint involvement; this needs to be confirmed on direct questioning and later, on examination. Further, one must be careful not to miss any involvement of the eyes in particular. The H/o of a recent viral infection preceding the onset of this illness may suggest that this is **reactive arthritis** without any organ involvement. It is important to follow the progress of the symptoms to define a probable diagnosis.

■ PHYSICAL EXAMINATION

Not sick looking pGALS ruled out the affection of other joints
Wt 35 kg Ht 150 cm
TPR normal No skin rash or glossitis
Swelling, tenderness and restricted movements of both knee and ankle joints
Other systems normal.

Analysis

The findings suggest symmetrical arthritis involving the large joints of only the lower limbs in an otherwise comfortable child. At this stage, possibilities include **reactive arthritis** or evolving **juvenile idiopathic arthritis** (JIA) syndrome that may unfold over time to enable us to label the disease. Moderate pain and swelling may favor reactive arthritis; in JIA, there is often moderate swelling and minimal pain. However, this cannot be a strong differentiating point. At this stage, one must use only symptomatic therapy and watch carefully for progress and repeat a periodic detailed physical examination.

■ INVESTIGATIONS

Hb 13 g%   WBC 12,000/c.mm   P 72 L23 M 2 E 3 PC 2.1 L/cmm
ESR 35   No other tests were ordered.

Analysis

There is possibly a mild inflammatory response but there are no other clues.

■ PROGRESS

This child was treated with ibuprofen and improved over the next week completely without any residual joint damage.

■ FINAL DIAGNOSIS

Reactive arthritis.

■ KEY MESSAGES

> While evaluating any child with arthritis, the first step is to confirm "arthritis" and rule out periarticular connective tissue disorders. In periarticular pathology, restriction of movements is not throughout the range of movement and passive movements are not painful. Arthritis presents with restriction of movements throughout the range and both active and passive movements are painful. The next step is to consider whether it is a standalone joint disease or if other organs are affected. Then one focuses on the number of joints affected, whether small or large or both, symmetrical or asymmetrical, whether the spine is affected or not, whether the tendon insertions around the joints are painful or not (enthesitis), and whether the swelling extends beyond a joint line or not (to decide whether there is a joint effusion).

■ RELEVANT INFORMATION

Reactive arthritis is an inflammatory condition triggered by infection and may present as standalone arthritis or also involve other organs. Symptoms generally start 1–4 weeks after infection and present as pain, swelling, and stiffness of lower limb joints. Other sites may also be involved. Occasionally, reactive arthritis may also present as monoarthritis or arthralgia. It may be triggered by viral infections or streptococcal group A bacterial infection (different from acute rheumatic fever which presents as migratory arthritis, usually involving large joints and responds very well to aspirin). Several bacterial infections can also trigger such a reaction, especially intestinal and genitourinary organisms including *Campylobacter, Yersinia, Chlamydia, Escherichia coli, Salmonella, Shigella,* and *Clostridium difficile*. Risk factors include age (older children and adults) and genetic susceptibility. Reactive arthritis resulting from such infections may last for a much longer period and need long-term management.

CASE 76

Joint Stiffness and Pain with Short Stature

■ HISTORY

A 5-year-old child was presented with stiffness in the morning and pain affecting multiple joints for the last 2 years. He was also noticed to be awkward in walking and running. Born after full-term normal delivery (FTND), the child appeared normal through the first 2 years. By the third year, his parents thought that he was short for his age, but his weight was average. They also noticed an awkward gait and stiffness at various joints after waking up in the morning—they felt that he had pain and mild swelling in multiple joints. There were no other symptoms or any family history of (H/o) similar problems. The parents were of average height, and this was their only child.

Analysis

Joint stiffness in the mornings and pain favors a generalized inflammatory joint disorder. But since parents have noticed short stature at around the same time as the onset of these complaints, it is unlikely to be **juvenile idiopathic arthritis**, because stature would get affected after years of chronic inflammation. So, it is likely that a **primary skeletal disorder** that can also cause joint stiffness and pain, is leading to short stature. Based on history alone one may keep **non-nutritional rickets** in mind, though joint pain and stiffness are unusual complaints in rickets. Rickets due to **renal tubular acidosis** is unlikely as he has not presented with failure to thrive and general systemic symptoms. Thus, it looks like a slowly worsening generalized bone and joint disease, but probably a congenital disorder. One should keep in mind a type of skeletal dysplasia—may be a **chondrodysplasia**.

■ PHYSICAL EXAMINATION

Not sick though irritable
Wt 17 kg   Ht 92 cm
TPR Normal   BP Normal

Mild swelling at various joints with painful restriction of movements (at the extremes of range) of many big and small joints, some of them are deformed, dynamic contractures at few joints, bow legs+
Chest, spine and skull normal.   Gait clumsy but stable
Other systems normal.

Analysis

Generalized arthritis with few deformed joints and dynamic contractures at an early age suggests a progressive epiphyseal disorder resulting in damage to joints over time. It favors the diagnosis of epiphyseal dysplasia.

■ INVESTIGATIONS

X-rays showed a flattened and squared epiphyses with delayed and irregular ossification centers. Biochemistry and radiology ruled out rickets. Genetic study showed mutational changes specific to the diagnosis of multiple epiphyseal dysplasia.

■ FINAL DIAGNOSIS

Multiple epiphyseal dysplasia.

■ KEY MESSAGES

> Arthritis may result from many causes other than inflammatory disorders including infections, autoimmune diseases, malignancy, and metabolic disorders. Early onset arthritis is typical of genetically determined chondrodysplasia that may mimic rheumatological diseases.

■ RELEVANT INFORMATION

Cartilage matrix protein accumulates in the cartilage and causes premature destruction and early arthritis. Symptoms are joint pain after activity and joint stiffness after prolonged rest. As the disease progresses, joints are destroyed. Metabolic bone diseases may mimic skeletal dysplasias that are genetic in origin—both may lead to generalized bony involvement.

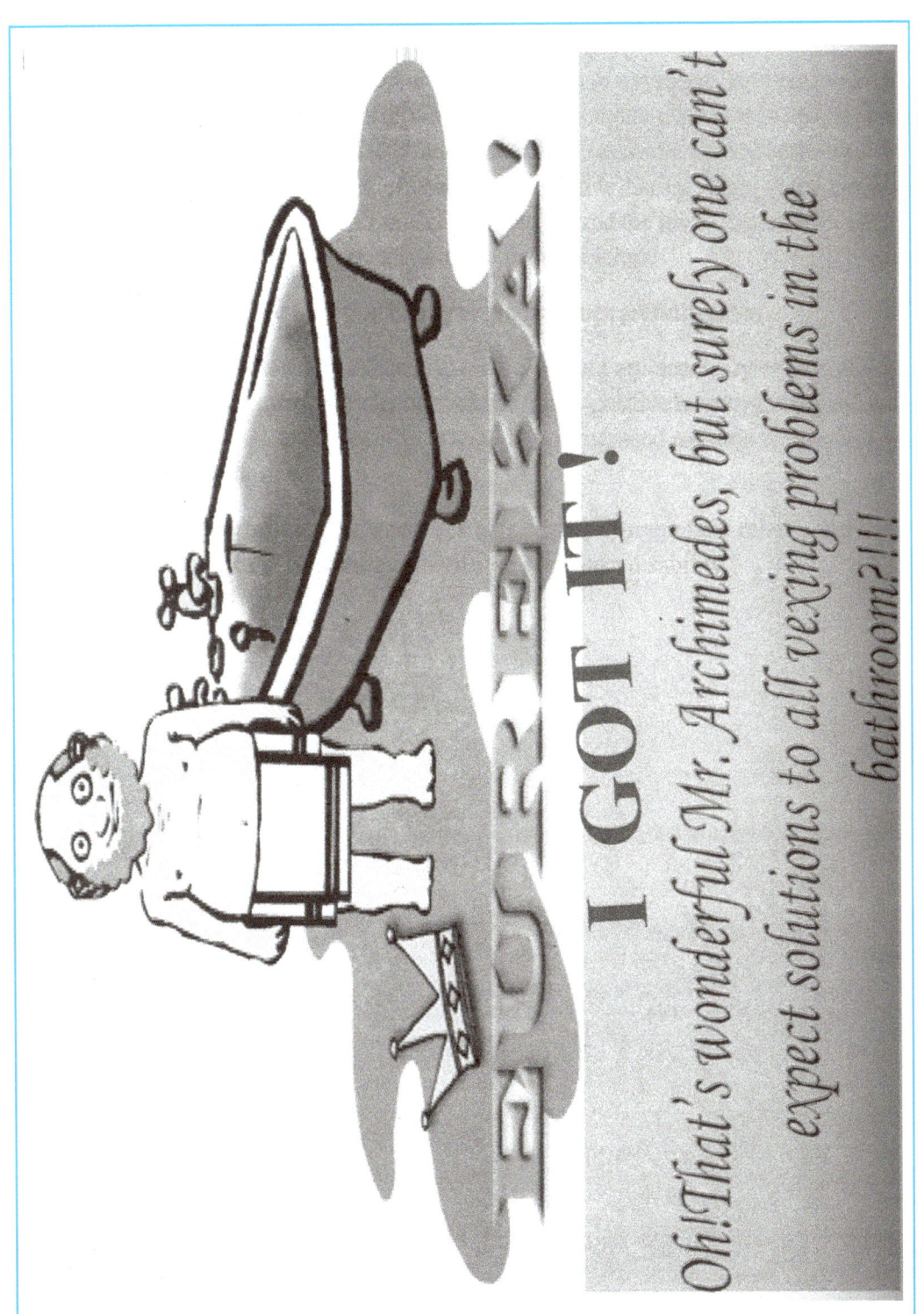

Clinical Neurology

BACK TO BASICS

Neurological Examination

Initial Screening

Observation and play techniques are essential means of monitoring intellectual, behavioral and motor functions, especially in infants and younger children. Beyond 4-5 years of age, neurological examination is more conventional and routine. Gross motor function can be screened by simple maneuvers such as hopping on each foot, tandem walking forwards and backwards, toe walk and heel walk. Subsequently the child should be asked to stand with his feet together, eyes closed and hands outstretched. This maneuver allows simultaneous assessment of abnormal movements and Romberg sign. Finger-nose test adds further information.

Developmental Reflexes

These are patterned responses that help assessment of general development of the nervous system in the first-2 years of life. Abnormality may be in the form of a continued presence of a reflex that should have disappeared, absence of expected response or asymmetric response. Usually they do not have any localizing value. However, the abnormal persistence of reflexes (e.g., persistent ATNR) may be an early sign of cerebral palsy. Similarly an asymmetric response may indicate a unilateral lesion. Absence of expected responses may indicate depressed cerebral function.

Most commonly evaluated developmental reflexes

Reflex	Age of appearance	Age of disappearance
Truncal incurvation	Birth	1-2 months
Rooting	Birth	3 months
Moro	Birth	4-5 months
Palmer grasp	Birth	3-4 months
Tonic neck response	Birth	5-6 months
Plantar grasp	Birth	9-10 months
Parachute	8-9 months	Persists for life
Landau reflex	10 months	24 months

Developmental Assessment—Rapid Screening

Moderate developmental delay resulting from prenatal or perinatal insults is obvious by 3 months of age, though it may be suspected earlier in life (but needs confirmation). Milder forms of delay may be apparent much later.

Thus, if an infant has a normal development at 3 months of age, normality may be nearly assured.

Every infant at 3 months of age must be evaluated for normal developmental by rapid screening.

Check head holding, recognition of mother, focusing on face, watches own hands follows objects through full arc, social smile, vocalizes when talked to, holds objects momentarily when offered, puts fingers to mouth. Mild variation in achieving age appropriate milestones may be acceptable and so also lagging behind in a single milestone. However, careful evaluation is mandatory.

Further development must be monitored at every visit and any deviation from the expected pattern deserves close follow-up.

Beware of Abnormal Development

Early head control–may denote spasticity.

Cooing is not a guarantee of normal hearing.

Failure to recognize strangers by 6-7 months of age is abnormal though often considered by parents as "socially good" behavior.

If speech is not developed by 18 months of age, relevant investigations for the delay are mandatory.

Hypotonia

This may be non-neurological (nonparalytic) or neurological (may be nonparalytic or paralytic).

Nonparalytic-malnutrition, chromosomal defects, congenital syndromes, systemic diseases, benign congenital hypotonia, hypotonic CP, myopathy (IEM, renal, endocrine).

Paralytic-LMN type of disorder.

Gait Disturbances

Before assessing a gait abnormality, it is essential to examine for contractures at various joints and scoliosis of the spine. Any pain associated with movements should be evaluated. In infants, congenital dislocation or subluxation of hip should be ruled out. Abnormal movements are often accentuated by walking and must be carefully observed.

Spastic hemiplegic gait-The classic circumduction gait where the child uses a circular motion to clear the ground with the "longer" spastic limb (because it is in plantar flexion) is appreciated in older children; the spastic upper limb "swings" comparatively less.

Spastic paraplegic gait-Toe walking may be the only manifestation of early spastic paraplegia. However, toe walking during the first few years of life may be familial and not pathological or indicative of future developmental problems. Close assessment for upper motor neuron signs is necessary.

Ataxic gait-Unsteady wide based gait resembling a drunken man's gait.

Extrapyramidal gait-Shuffling with Short and slow steps, rigidity, decreased automatic movements and abnormal posturing.

High steppage gait-Seen in peripheral nerve, muscle or anterior horn cell disease.

Broad based waddling gait with Lordosis-Seen in muscular dystrophies and spinal muscular atrophy.

Involuntary Movements

INVOLUNTARY MOVEMENTS					
SLOW		RAPID (JERKY)		RHYTHMIC (OSCILLATORY)	
DYSTONIA	ATHETOSIS	TICS	CHOREA	TREMORS	MYOCLO
Abnormal posturing of limbs, face and trunk	Restricted to limbs, associated with chorea	Voluntarily Suppressible	Incorporated into voluntary action	Continuous oscillating	Oscillations with pause

Ballismus: It can be likened to a high amplitude violent chorea occurring at shoulder and hips.

Bladder Disturbances

Uninhibited neurogenic bladder occurs with bilateral involvement of the frontal lobes. Frequency and urgency of urination may ultimately lead to automatic bladder emptying; however, the bladder sensation is preserved. Lesions of the spinal cord above lumbar segments are accompanied with urgency, increased frequency, incontinence and nocturia. Lesions of the spinal cord between L4-S2 segments result in a small constricted "spastic" bladder with loss of voluntary control with incontinence. Lesions below S3 segment, cause incontinence of urine with hypotonic distended bladder.

Vertigo

Acute paroxysmal
        with hearing loss   - Labyrinthitis
        without hearing loss - Vestibular neuronitis/benign paroxysmal vertigo (<4 years)/migraine/seizure disorder

Unremitting
        with hearing loss   - Acoustic neuroma/cerebello-pontine angle tumor/posterior fossa tumor
        without hearing loss - Metabolic abnormality

Vertigo is an altered feeling of rotation or whirling. It results from alteration in vestibular function either due to peripheral vestibular dysfunction (otitis or cholesteatoma) or central abnormalities of vestibular nuclei and/or their brainstem or cerebellar connection. Examination of tympanic membrane would differentiate these conditions. Benign paroxysmal vertigo is seen in children between 1 and 3 years of age. Viral labyrinthitis occurs in older children and resolves in 2-3 weeks. Benign positional vertigo results from sudden change in head position. Drugs may cause vertigo (toxic labyrinthitis)-aminoglycosides, quinine, salicylates.

Increased Intracranial Pressure

Pressure-volume relationship of intracranial contents is not a straight line. At the lower end of the curve, changes in volume are accompanied with only small changes in pressure. As the volume increases, intracranial pressure rises more rapidly; at higher pressures, a small increase in volume produces a marked increase in pressure. When intracranial volume increases very slowly as happens in tumors, compensatory mechanisms postpone the manifestations of raised intracranial pressure. With increasing intracranial pressure, cerebral perfusion pressure is reduced which produces serious consequences.

Continuous monitoring of intracranial pressure and appropriate treatment is most important to "improve survival in severe head injury", Grades 3-4 Reye's syndrome and coma due to hypoxia or meningoencephalitis.

Coma

It results from inadequate interaction between cerebral cortex and reticular activating system of diencephalons, midbrain and pons. Involvement of cerebral hemispheres and basal ganglia leads to delirium associated with a normal breathing pattern, normal pupillary reaction, roving eye movements and spontaneous movements of extremities.

Diencephalic dysfunction result in stupor with periodic or Cheyne-Stokes breathing, positive oculocephalic, (doll's eye movements) and oculovestibular reflexes, small reacting pupils and decorticate posturing.

Signs of midbrain and upper pons involvement include hyperventilation dilated pupils, dysconjugate gaze with loss of oculocephalic and oculovestibular reflexes and decerebrate posturing.

Disturbance of lower pons and medulla present "with fixed and dilated pupils", shallow and irregular breathing pattern and absent eye movements.

Rapid nostrocaudal deterioration suggests central tentorial herniation. Unilateral pupillary dilatation with midbrain dysfunction denotes uncal herniation. Supratentorial mass lesions may cause central or uncal herniation on presentation.

Coma vigil is a vegetative state in which the child appears conscious but is totally unresponsive, with persistence of primitive functions (such as breathing, swallowing, etc.). It may be occasionally seen in severe brain damage as in TB meningitis.

Cerebral Edema

Brain swelling is catagorized as cytotoxic (disruption of intracellular metabolism as in Reye's syndrome, viral encephalitis, HlE, SJADH), vasogenic (disrupted blood-brain barrier as in trauma, infarcts, tumors, abscess) and interstitial (acute hydrocephalus forces CSF to pass through ependymal linings of ventricles).

Dexamethasone is the preferred steroid in the management of vasogenic cerebral edema. It was well known that the use of mannitol in cytotoxic edema should be restricted to the first few days. Recent consensus is in favor of smaller doses, administered just once or twice.

CASE 77

Developmental Delay Since Birth

■ HISTORY

A 7-month-old female child born of a 3rd degree consanguineous marriage was for two episodes of generalized tonic-clonic convulsions on the day of admission. Both convulsions lasted for about 25–30 minutes each and occurred about 10 hours apart. In the intervening period, the infant was apparently normal and feeding well.

No history of fever   No history of trauma   No past history of convulsions

Birth history: Term LSCS for breech presentation.   Birth wt. 1.75 kg.

She was admitted in the NICU on day 2 for respiratory distress and bluish discoloration of soles. She was treated with IV fluids and IV mediations for 10 days and then discharged.

Developmental history:
- Does not hold head well
- Does not focus on mother's face
- No history of roving eye movements
- Does not roll over
- No eye contact
- Does not reach for objects
- No history of rubbing of eyes

Social smile in response to mother's voice and touch since 5 months of age

Cooing since 6 months of age

History of pulmonary TB in her father, diagnosed 1 yr ago and on treatment since then.

Analysis

Since this infant does not focus on her mother's face and there is no eye contact, it denotes an **impairment of vision**. This may result from a lesion anywhere in the visual pathways, from the cornea to the visual cortex. A lesion in the anterior visual pathways (cornea, lens or retina) before fixation develops usually gives lise to searching nystagmoid movements. Absence of such movements suggests that the lesion is in the optic nerve or beyond. This child also has **delayed development**. Assessment of development in an infant with visual impairment has to be based upon the responses to nonvisual inputs. Such inputs are auditory and tactile stimuli. Based on such an assessment (as per the history), this infant's gross motor development is around 3 months, fine motor around 4 months and cognitive and preverbal speech around 3 months of age. Thus, this 7-month-old infant has a global developmental delay with a DQ of around 50%. The history suggests that this is a **static disorder**, as there has been no regression or deterioration of previously achieved milestones.

Developmental delay in this child may be related to the problem that led to the **NICU admission** on day 2 of life. This has been an IUGR baby and such a neonate is prone to metabolic abnormalities (hypoglycemia hypocalcemia), polycythemia and sepsis. Alternatively, the intrauterine growth retardation may be the result of a **prenatal** pathology such as chromosomal abnormalities, intrauterine infections or CNS malformations. Other causes of delayed development such as inborn errors of metabolism and storage disorders are unlikely as this is mostly a static disorder.

As this infant developed two episodes of generalized seizures without any accompanying symptoms or provocation, these are likely to be "**remote symptomatic**" **seizures** and not "acute symptomatic" seizures. (An acute symptomatic seizure is one where an acute brain insult occurs around the time of seizure and hence it is a provoked seizure and does not denote epilepsy. In a remote symptomatic seizure the insult would have occurred sometime prior. Therefore, it is an unprovoked seizure and denotes epilepsy).

Thus, this infant has a static, global developmental delay with a seizure disorder, due to either a prenatal or a perinatal insult.

The history of TB contact has no relevance in this infant as she has not presented with acute symptoms of an infection referable to the central nervous system.

■ PHYSICAL EXAMINATION

Weight 6.7 kg   Length 63 cm   Head Ⓞ 43 cm   Chest Ⓞ 44 cm
Temperature normal   HR 108/min   RR 28/min
No dysmorphic features   No neurocutaneous markers
Anterior fontanelle 2.5 × 2.5 cm   Posterior fontanelle closed

Developmental examination:
When pulled to sit, holds head momentarily, but wobbles
In prone position, lifts head but not chest, off the bed

Does not hold object in hand	Sucks fist but not fingers
Does not focus on the face	No roving eye movements or nystagmus
Smiles in response to voice or touch	Cooing in response to voice
CNS examination: symmetrical posture	Spontaneously moves all four limbs
Pupil not reacting to light	Bilateral optic atrophy
Muscle tone normal DTR normal	No abnormal neonatal reflexes
No involuntary movements	
Liver just palpable, soft Spleen not palpable	Other systems normal

Analysis

This child has a **global developmental delay** involving all aspects of development (i.e., gross and fine motor, cognitive and language milestones) nearly equally. The optic atrophy confirms the visual impairment. Remote symptomatic seizures are likely to be due to an epileptic disorder. There is no active neurological disease and hence these neurological abnormalities must have resulted from a significant brain insult that occurred either prenatally or perinatally and has left behind a static damage.

Considering the NICU admission on D2 of life, a **perinatal** cause is possible. However, a perinatal insult leads to cerebral palsy and in the absence of a change in tone or posture, this is not cerebral palsy. Hypoglycemia is known to give rise to developmental delay without any tone abnormality. However, the optic atrophy cannot be explained. Besides, a normal head circumference is unlikely in hypoglycemic brain damage. Thus, this is unlikely to be due to a perinatal cause.

Amongst the prenatal conditions, **intrauterine infections** would have resulted in a poor postnatal growth, hepatosplenomegaly and either microcephaly or hydrocephalous. The head ☉ in this child is within normal limits as compared to her length, though it is smaller than her chest ☉ (though only by 1 cm). A storage disorder is unlikely because there is no neuroregression and organomegaly. A syndromic disorder or **chromosomal disorders** are the likely diagnostic possibilities though the latter are often associated with dysmorphic features. So, it is quite likely that a **genetic** cause is responsible for this developmental delay. History of consanguinity may favor such a possibility.

■ INVESTIGATIONS

EEG – abnormal epileptogenic foci
Karyotype – normal
MRI – normal
Thyroid profile – normal

■ FINAL DIAGNOSIS

Global developmental delay with optic atrophy with remote symptomatic seizures, probably genetic in etiology.

■ COMMENTS

In such cases, investigations must be prioritized. Treatable causes should always be ruled out even if the clinical profile is not suggestive. Thus, it is always worth doing thyroid function tests (TSH). A baseline metabolic screen may be considered on clinical judgment. The yield of MRI is rather low in such cases. EEG may be important as specific abnormal patterns may forewarn the possibility of severe epilepsy to follow. Karyotype is useful from the point of view of genetic counseling. ERG may be useful in such a case to evaluate visual impairment. Though at the end of such investigations, etiological diagnosis is often elusive.

■ KEY MESSAGES

- Developmental delay should be clearly differentiated as static or progressive.
- Change in tone and posture is a prerequisite to the diagnosis of cerebral palsy.

■ RELEVANT INFORMATION

Static versus Progressive Neurological Disorder

At time it is not easy to differentiate a static neurological disorder from a slowly progressive one. In cases of developmental delay, developmental quotients obtained at intervals of every

3 months, either retrospectively based on the history and previous records or evaluated prospectively, would spell out the difference. In case of a very slowly progressive disorder, it may take a year or even longer to be same about the static or progressive status.

Similar problems may be faced in the case of muscle or nerve disorders. Periodic charting of individual muscle function over a long time would make the distinction clear.

CASE 78: Regression of Milestones

■ HISTORY

A 9-year-old male child born of a non-consanguineous marriage was brought for gradually diminishing vision since the last 4 years, inability to speak and decreased interest in routine activities since the last 3 years and inability to walk since the last 6 months.

He was absolutely alright 4 years ago. The illness started with an intermittent squint noticed by the parents, which was initially ignored. Subsequently, there was a gradual diminution of vision. Consequently, he had repeated falls and sometimes he banged into objects. For the last 2½ years he had been almost blind. There had also been a slowing down of speech with a diminished content, beginning about 3 years back. More or less from that time he had not been taking interest in day-to-day activities nor interacting and playing with friends. There had also been a deterioration in intellectual function to a point that lately he could understand only simple commands. He developed toe-walking a year back; his gait difficulty increased and for the last 3 months he was confined to bed. He had difficulty in feeding as well as sphincter incontinence. There had been a gradual loss of hearing over the last 1 year and he was deaf for the last 3 months.

He had been taking treatment from many doctors but the illness had progressed relentlessly and new symptoms had been developing.

No history of seizures or abnormal movements.
No history of recurrent ear discharge.
Birth history–normal.
No family history of similar disorder.

Analysis

This child has regression of milestones after having achieved them normally. The deterioration has been gradual in onset but has progressed fairly rapidly. It has affected his vision, intelligence, speech and motor function. In other words, though the pathology does not seem confined to any particular anatomical region, it seems to have affected both gray as well as the white matter over time. However, if we were to analyze the events as they occurred, we realize that the illness started as an *intermittent strabismus*. This can occur in **ocular myasthenia**; in which case it would be associated with ptosis and there would be a diurnal variation. If the strabismus was due to **ophthalmoplegia**, it would not be intermittent. It could also be an initial manifestation of gradual deterioration of vision; the subsequent history of banging into objects and the eventual development of blindness confirm the same. This gradual **diminution of vision** culminating in blindness could be due to a lesion anywhere from the cornea to the visual cortex.

Slowing down of speech could be due to **cerebellar** involvement or as a result of corticospinal tract involvement. The history of dysphagia (feeding difficulty) later in the disease supports the latter, while there is nothing else to suggest cerebellar involvement. While a *diminished content* of speech as well as a decreased interest in day-to-day activities and play could also be a manifestation of **psychosis** or a **behavior disturbance** when interpreted in isolation, in view of the above features it suggests **intellectual deterioration**. Subsequent deterioration in functions like swallowing and control of sphincters confirms a progressive organic disease.

Toe walking suggests **spasticity** or a disparity in the power of ankle flexors and extensors.

Complete deafness (acquired) can either be due to bilateral **cochlear** damage (as a complication of otitis media) or due to a **retrocochlear** pathology like demyelination of auditory radiations. Since there is no history of recurrent ear discharge, it is likely to be due to a lesion of the auditory radiations.

History thus suggests that this child has a progressive disease characterized by blindness (a lesion affecting cornea/lens, or the visual pathways from the optic nerve, retina to the occipital cortex), **deafness** (central lesion in auditory radiations), **motor regression** (a peripheral pathology of muscles or a central lesion in corticospinal pathways) and **dementia** (cortical lesion). Since multiple peripheral lesions due to one pathological process are unlikely, a central but **diffuse neurological lesion** is most likely. This lesion presently involves **both** the **gray** and the **white matter**. However, since visual impairment was the *initial* manifestation, it suggests a white matter disease to begin with (other *presenting* manifestations of white matter disease being focal neurodeficits or spasticity, while those of gray matter disease being personality change, seizures and dementia), which has subsequently progressed to extensively involve gray and white matter both. Such a disease could be a leukodystrophy. Amongst the childhood onset (5-15 years) rapidly progressive leukodystrophies, the commoner ones are adrenoleukodystrophy, childhood onset varieties of metachromatic leukodystrophy (MLD), Krabbe's disease and Leigh's disease.

■ PHYSICAL EXAMINATION

Poorly nourished	Average build	
Weight 19 kg	Height 126 cm	Head ⊙ 52 cm
Pulse 90/min	RR 23/min	BP 110/60 mm Hg
Generalized hyperpigmentation		
Vacant look	Smiles without interaction	
Eardrums–normal	Does not respond to any auditory or visual stimulus	
Strabismus present	Pupils dilated sluggishly reacting to light	
Bilateral optic atrophy		
No speech	Pooling of saliva in mouth	Soft palate not moving
Spasticity in all 4 limbs	Blinks on glabellar tap	Jaw jerk brisk
Brisk tendon reflexes	Plantar extensor	
Power grade 4-5 in all limbs		
No abnormal movements	No myoclonus	
Cerebellar functions could not be tested		MacEwen's sign - ve
Liver/spleen not palpable		Other systems–normal

Analysis

Physical examination reveals signs of corticospinal tract involvement at the subcortical level (spastic quadriparesis, pseudobulbar palsy), blindness (due to optic atrophy), and dementia (primitive reflexes). There is no clinical evidence of peripheral neuropathy. Thus, this 9-year-old boy has a rapidly progressive neurological disease which began at 5 years of age and is characterized by diffuse white and gray matter degeneration.

It could be an acquired disease like **SSPE** or HIV encephalopathy or it could be a genetically determined leukodystrophy like adrenoleukodystrophy, late childhood onset variety of **metachromatic leukodystrophy** or **Krabbe's disease**. SSPE has in addition to dementia, myoclonic seizures and extrapyramidal signs and is therefore unlikely. The median age of onset of **HIV encephalopathy** is 19 months, it is often characterized by intermittent "plateaus" in the clinical progression and is not characterized by blindness or deafness (focality). Therefore, it is unlikely. As discussed earlier, since the illness *began* with a manifestation of white matter involvement, it suggests a *primary* white matter disease. Presence of generalized hyperpigmentation clinches the clinical diagnosis of **adrenoleukodystrophy**.

■ INVESTIGATIONS

MRI of brain: suggestive of leukodystrophy
Very long chain fatty acids show abnormally high levels.

■ FINAL DIAGNOSIS

Adrenoleukodystrophy.

■ COMMENTS

Most of the genetic metabolic neurodegenerative disease with onset in late childhood (after 2 years of age) have neurological abnormalities more or less restricted to particular systems of neurons, e.g., extrapyramidal, spinocerebellar. As against that, in those disorders with onset in late infancy and early childhood (before 2 years of age) there is diffuse neurological involvement so that, often there is no characteristic clinical neurological picture. Most of them have many clinical features, which are common and overlap; a precise clinical diagnosis is therefore difficult.

■ KEY MESSAGES

- In a neurodegenerative disorder the age of onset and the initial presenting manifestation gives a clue to the probable diagnosis, though eventually there may be features of widespread involvement.
- Adrenoleukodystrophy may present to an endocrinologist with only adrenal manifestations and should be watched for neurological involvement.

CASE 79

Differential Developmental Delay

■ HISTORY

A 2-year-old female child, 2nd by birth order, born of a non-consanguineous marriage, presented with delayed milestones. The parents attributed it to the generalized weakness of the child, arising out of frequent illnesses. The child was hospitalized at 8 months of age and again at 18 months of age for febrile illnesses, and has apparently lost weight since the last illness. Her birth history was normal; her birth weight was 2 kg. She was breastfed for the first 2 months and thereafter was on diluted milk feeds. Semisolids were introduced at 10 months of age.

History of pulmonary TB in the mother since the last 1 month.

Developmental history:

		DQ
Gross moto:	partial head holding – 3 months, stable head control – 7 months	40%
	prone to supine – 11 months, supine to prone – 1 year	40%
	sitting with support – 15 months, sitting without support – 18 months	40%
	walking without support – 20 months, cannot run/climb	60%
Fore motor:	spontaneous head opening – 6 months	50%
	reaching for objects – 9 months	60%
	ulnar grasp – 8 months, radial grasp – 11 months, pincer grasp 1 year	75%
	drank from a cup – 20 months	60%
	could feed herself with spillage and help in undressing – 20 months	75%
Social:	social smile – 3 months	50%
	recognized mother – 5 months	40%
	stranger anxiety – at 1 year	60%
	stranger anxiety disappeared at – 18 months	50%
	used to enjoy mirror image – 18 months	50%
	used to play with sibling – 20 months	60%
	bladder bowel control (dry by day) not achieved	<75%
Language:	auditory expressive—	
	cooing – 6 months	25%
	laughing – 24 months	16%
	raspberry speech (preverbal rasping sounds) – 12 months	25%
	monosyllables – 24 months	25%

vocalizing sounds – 24 months	25%
auditory receptive—	
responding to sounds – 6 months	33%
recognized mother's voice – 6 months	50%

Analysis

This child is delayed in all fields of development as indicated by her developmental quotient (DQ) of 60% in gross motor development, 60–75% in fine motor/adaptive functions, 60% in social development and only 25% in language/speech development. Thus, there is a **differential delay in development** with the speech and language functions being affected *more* than the others. Since her early milestones (like social smile) are also delayed, the problem is present from birth. However, there is no history of a **perinatal** insult to account for the same. Since she had a low birth weight, a poor gain in weight with a history of improper feeding practices and illnesses needing hospitalization, it may appear that **nutrition, systemic** diseases and **environmental factors** may have led to her delayed development. However, her delayed development was manifest ever since she was one and a half to 2 months of age, much before these factors were operative. Moreover, they give rise to a significant delay in motor development, but a much less delay in adaptive, social and language achievements. A DQ of less than 70% in all fields of development is unlikely to be *entirely due to* such factors and an organic cause for the same is also present. Since the birth history is normal, it could be due to a **prenatal** cause.

Language delay may be due to a receptive or expressive language disorder. Receptive language may be defective because of impaired hearing and/or a cognitive disorder. Expressive language is bound to be affected if there is a receptive disorder. In this child impaired hearing must be ruled out by appropriate investigations even though the history suggests a response to sound and the mother's voice. If the hearing is normal, the additional affection of language (as compared to other spheres of development) could be due to either a cognitive defect or an expressive defect, but it is part and parcel of the global developmental delay. However, if the hearing is abnormal, it explains the additional delay in language.

■ PHYSICAL EXAMINATION

Weight 5.5 kg   Length 75 cm   Head ⊙ 42 cm   Chest ⊙ 42 cm
Temp. normal   Pulse 100/min   Resp. 30/min   BP 90/70 mm Hg
pallor +, hair coarse. dry lusterless   BCG scar seen
no edema   loss of subcutaneous fat +
bilateral axillary lymph nodes 1.5 cm in diameter. not matted ENT - normal
Developmental examination of gross motor, Fine motor, social and language milestones confirms the DQ obtained earlier on history.
CNS –   vision normal
    generalized hypotonia, muscle power and reflexes normal, no focal signs.

Analysis

This child has a **grade IV PEM, growth failure** and **microcephaly** without dysmorphic features, cutaneous abnormalities or organomegaly. Her vision is normal, she can hear (to be confirmed due to limitations of clinical assessment) and has no local neurological signs.

Developmental examination confirms the gross motor DQ to be 60%, fine motor/adaptive between 60-75%, social DQ of around 60% and language/speech DQ of 33%. Therefore, there is a **global** and **differential developmental delay** as was earlier analyzed on history. Since there are no pointers to the etiology on examination, in the absence of any significant perinatal insults, it is likely to be **prenatal** in origin. A history of consanguinity would have favored, though its absence does not rule out a genetic etiology.

■ INVESTIGATIONS

BERA and Impedance audiometry – normal
HIV + ve (ELISA)   Mantoux test – negative   Chest X-ray – normal

Analysis

Even though this child's hearing is normal, the disproportionate language development can be explained on the basis of differential involvement of different aspects of development in a case of global delay.

■ FINAL DIAGNOSIS

Global developmental delay with additional receptive language disorder, probably due to HIV encephalopathy, with severe PEM.

■ KEY MESSAGES

- Developmental evaluation of any child should be separately done for each individual sphere of development, namely – gross motor, fine motor/adaptive, social and speech/language.
- A disproportionate lag in any sphere should be further evaluated for any specific additional etiological factor contributing to it.
- Vision and hearing should be objectively tested in a child with delayed development.

■ RELEVANT INFORMATION

Developmental delay may be uniformly global or differential in various combinations.

Disorder	Gross motor	Fine motor	Social	Language
Mental retardation	Delay +	Delay + to + +	+ + to + + +	+ + +
Cerebral palsy with mild MR	Delay + + +	Delay + +	+	+

Contd...

Contd...

Disorder	Gross motor	Fine motor	Social	Language
CP with MR	Delay +++	+++	+++	+++
Hearing impairment	No delay	No delay	No delay	+++
Impaired vision	No delay	Delay ++	No delay to delay +	No delay
Spinal muscular atrophy	+++	Delay + to ++	No delay	Receptive normal, Expressive may be delayed

CASE 80

Delayed Speech in a 2½-year-old

■ HISTORY

A 2½-year-old male child was brought by the parents because he could not talk as yet. He was a product of a non-consanguineous marriage, born after a normal pregnancy and delivery. His birth weight was 3.2 kg. He had maintained normal growth and development through infancy and early childhood and had no significant past history. One of the paternal uncles had developed speech after 3 years of his age and he was reported to be normal thereafter.

As he was not able to speak at all, the parents had sought advice from a doctor at about 2 years of age. As the parents were sure that he was able to hear well and also had age appropriate understanding, the doctor had assured them that he would start talking over time. But as he did not develop any speech over another 6 months, they were referred for further evaluation.

On direct questioning, the parents considered him to be moody and often engrossed with his toys, which according to them was nothing abnormal.

Analysis

This child has been reported to have a normal hearing and also normal cognitive function. Even then, it is important to evaluate hearing objectively and also to confirm normal cognitive function. Many a times, the parents' perception of normal hearing or normal cognitive ability may not be reliable and must be always confirmed by physical examination and relevant investigations. If we consider the history to be accurate, it is likely that his behavior may not have been normal and the delayed language development may have resulted from **auditory inattention**. However, it may also be just a **familial trait** as one of the uncles had delayed language development, but it should never be taken for granted.

■ PHYSICAL EXAMINATION

Well built and nourished	Weight 13 kg	Height 90 cm
Head ⊙ 50 cm	TPR normal	BP 90/55 mm of Hg
Hearing apparently normal	General exam normal	Systemic exam normal

Gross motor and fine motor milestones within normal limits
Hyperactive child   No eye-to-eye contact   Lack of concentration
Stereotyped behavior   Impulsive   Unpredictable response
Speaks incoherently and repeats words, at times

Analysis

This child has obviously abnormal behavior–typical of autism. It is the auditory inattention that is the cause of delayed language development. There is no evidence of any other abnormality. It is most likely that this child has a normal hearing and also cognitive development. However, it must be confirmed by appropriate tests.

■ INVESTIGATIONS

BERA and impedance audiometry normal.
DQ within normal limits.
Developmental and behavioral analysis confirmed autism by standard criteria.

Analysis

With a normal hearing and cognitive function, receptive language disorder is ruled out. Developmental and behavioral analysis confirms autism.

■ FINAL DIAGNOSIS

Autism.

■ KEY MESSAGES

- Absence of language development by 18 months of age demands urgent evaluation of hearing ability, cognitive function and behavior pattern.
- Delay in diagnosis and therefore management of autism increases the risk of a poor outcome.

Delayed Speech in a 2½-year-old

■ RELEVANT INFORMATION

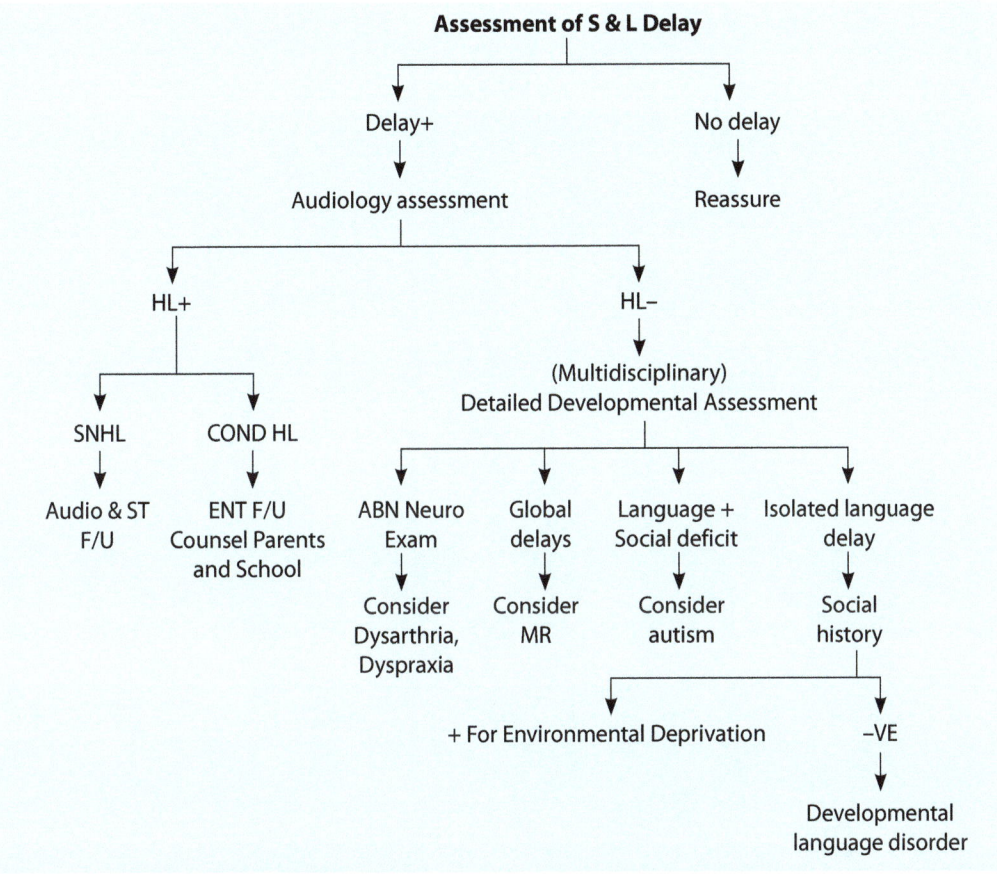

81 CASE

Focal Convulsion in a 2-month-old

■ HISTORY

A 2-month-old infant presented with a focal convulsion a day prior to admission to the hospital. He was reported to be apparently well until then. He was exclusively breastfed. There was no history of fever or refusal of feeds. He used to vomit off and on and it was considered to be regurgitation. His bowel movements and urination were normal. He could focus on the mother's face but she was not sure about a social smile.

He was born after a full-term by a vaginal midforceps delivery. The delivery was difficult but he cried immediately and had an uneventful postnatal course. He weighed 3.5 kg at birth.

No significant illness in the mother during pregnancy.

Analysis

A sudden onset focal convulsion in an apparently normal infant suggests a metabolic seizure most probably due to hypocalcemia. However, it may be important to assess the growth and development of this infant to consider other probable causes of this convulsion. **Hypocalcemic convulsions** are typically seen in otherwise normal infants who have gained good weight as they may develop early rickets. The vomiting could be physiological if the infant has gained weight adequately but if not, the vomiting could very well be pathological. Since accurate developmental assessment is difficult on history alone at 2 months of age, other possible causes of this convulsion include **congenital malformations** and **birth injuries**. It could also be the first manifestation of an **oncoming progressive neurological disorder**. Behavior abnormalities or feeding disturbances are the initial manifestations of a birth injury; when reported, they help in the diagnosis. However, these are often overlooked by the mother.

■ PHYSICAL EXAMINATION

Irritable
Weight 4.2 kg   Length 54 cm   Head ☉ 40 cm   Chest ☉ 34 cm
Temp normal   Pulse 120/min   RR 35/min
Moderate pallor   No icterus   No respiratory distress
No other abnormal findings on general examination
CNS - conscious, cry and activity normal, fundus normal
Anterior fontanelle wide open and boggy, nonpulsatile   Posterior fontanelle closed
Metopic suture open   Other sutures within normal limits
Tone mildly increased   No motor deficit   Neonatal reflexes normal

Development: Focuses momentarily on the face, head control corresponds to 6 weeks,
No signs of cardiac failure   Liver 1 cm soft, spleen not palpable
Other system normal

Analysis

This infant has **failed to thrive** as he has gained only 700 grams over 2 months in spite of exclusive breastfeeding. He is also moderately pale. His head Ο is large as compared to his chest Ο and length, fontanelle is bulging and nonpulsatile, and metopic suture open. This suggests **increased intracranial pressure** due to hydrocephalus or a space-occupying lesion. **Hydrocephalus** is the commonest cause of such a lesion. However, a seizure rules out a hydrocephalus due to a congenital malformation of CSF pathway. Hydrocephalus due to a **congenital infection** such as toxoplasmosis is possible; the seizure. failure to gain weight and the presence of moderate pallor may be explained. In view of the focal seizure, it could be an **intracranial space-occupying lesions** or a **malformation** such as hydranencephaly or porencephaly. (Cranial transillumination may help to detect such a lesion). However, pallor remains unexplained on the basis of such a malformation. Correlating the pallor, the space-occupying lesion may be a **subdural hematoma**. A case of child abuse can also present this way; there may be intracranial bleeding which can explain these features.

If one analyses pallor in this infant presenting at 2 months of age, it could have been a late manifestation of **ABO blood group incompatibility** provided there was a history of neonatal jaundice. **Hemolytic anemia** rarely manifests at this age. Other causes of pallor at this age include red cell aplasia or leukemia. While **red cell aplasia** is possible, a seizure cannot be explained: **leukemia** is extremely rare at this age. Hemorrhage may result in anemia at this age; since there is no history of any manifest bleeding it may be an occult hemorrhage. Since other causes of anemia seem less likely in this infant, **occult bleeding** could be the likely cause and in that cause it is obviously in the intracranial compartment in view of the focal seizure. The absence of cardiac decompensation suggests that this anemia must have developed slowly and hence it is likely to be due to birth injury with slow accumulation of blood in the subdural space. A late manifestation of **hemorrhagic disease of the newborn** is also a possibility.

It is interesting that clinical analysis with either seizure or pallor as a leading point, leads one to the same conclusion that it must be a subdural hematoma.

■ INVESTIGATIONS

Hb 6 gm%   WBC count normal   Platelet count 85,000/c.mm   Retic count 2%
Serum bilirubin 2.1 mg%   Indirect 1.9 mg%   Direct 0.2 mg%
Cranial USG -   subdural hematoma, no evidence of any other bleed
                no hydrocephalus

Analysis

Retic count is normal and suggests normal functioning of the bone marrow. Obviously, the low platelet count is not due to low production of platelets but due to peripheral consumption. Similarly, mild increase in serum bilirubin is not indicative of hemolysis in the presence of a normal retic count. A mild increase in serum bilirubin and the low platelets are due to consumption of RBCs and platelets in a hematoma.

Of course, cranial USG proved the diagnosis.

■ FINAL DIAGNOSIS

Subdural hematoma.

■ KEY MESSAGES

- When the presenting symptoms pertain to more than one system. It is important to lead the analysis with each of the major symptoms. It is still possible to arrive at the same probable diagnosis, as exemplified in this case.
- Cranial transillumination may be a helpful bedside screening test in the evaluation of a large skull.

CASE 82

Headache and Vomiting for a Year

■ HISTORY

A 10-year-old child presented with recurrent episodes of headache and vomiting for the last 1 year. He was apparently well 1 year ago when he started suffering from severe headache. It would come on mainly early in the morning and many a times he would get up from sleep with headache. It would last for a few hours and then subside with analgesics. This was accompanied with vomiting, which often relieved the headache. Such attacks would come on erratically and there would be pain-free intervals for a while but he was never absolutely comfortable.

No history of fever, behavior change, visual disturbance, loss of appetite or weight.
No history of otitis media, head injury, or drugs.
No history of migraine in the family.   No past history of any significance.
He was investigated, the details of which are not known. However, the parents were informed that the tests were normal.

Analysis

This child has symptoms suggestive of **raised intracranial pressure** in terms of typical morning headache and vomiting. Though the headache apparently came in attacks, the child was never absolutely comfortable. This indicates that though the severity of the headache fluctuated, it must have been due to a persistent pathology. This rules out migraine, as there are always symptom free periods between two attacks of migraine. Thus, this child definitely has raised intracranial pressure. As the headache has existed for a year without any other symptoms, it is unlikely to be any **inflammatory** pathology. **Space-occupying lesions** leading to raised intracranial pressure are commonly infratentorial tumors. They are likely to present with symptoms related to the involvement of many structures including cranial nerves. As against this, supratentorial tumors rarely *present* with raised intracranial pressure; they usually manifest with focal seizures or neurodeficits. Thus, a space-occupying lesion is less likely in this child. However, **midline tumors** may lead to obstructive hydrocephalus without any other involvement and may present with headache as the only manifestation. **Pseudotumor cerebri** may be another possibility, which can explain increased intracranial pressure without any other pathology evident on history. **Systemic hypertension** may be a cause of headache though it is unlikely to exist for a year without other manifestations of the primary disease leading to hypertension. Psychogenic headache may be another consideration if there are no abnormal positive findings.

■ PHYSICAL EXAMINATION

Averagely built and nourished Weight 28 kg Height 118 cm
Pulse 70/min RR 20/min BP 125/80 mm Hg
No significant abnormality on general examination
CNS – No neurodeficit Fundus–papilledema
Other systems normal

Analysis

Papilledema confirms the presence of **raised intracranial pressure**. A relatively low pulse rate and a mildly increased blood pressure may have resulted from raised ICP. There is no systemic hypertension of significance. In the absence of any other abnormal physical finding there is no clue to the probable cause of raised ICP, though intracranial infections and space-occupying lesions can be almost ruled out. As discussed in the analysis of the history, **midline tumors or pseudotumor cerebri** should be considered.

■ INVESTIGATIONS

MRI – Chinky ventricles/no evidence of any other pathology
CSF – Opening pressure high Cells – 2, lymphocytes
     Proteins 10 mg Sugar – 50 mg

Analysis

Pseudotumor cerebri is confirmed by these characteristic findings - high opening CSF pressure, normal CSF cytology and chemistry, normal brain and ventricles on MRI.

The cause of pseudotumor is not evident and may need further investigations for an endocrinopathy.

■ FINAL DIAGNOSIS

Pseudotumor cerebri.

■ KEY MESSAGES

- Recurrent headache due to migraine should be clearly differentiated from the fluctuating severity of a persistent headache as seen in raised intracranial pressure.
- Migraine is essentially a diagnosis made on the pattern of headache with a positive family history to support it.

■ RELEVANT INFORMATION

The precise underlying mechanism of increased CSF pressure resulting in pseudotumor cerebri (PTC) is unknown. Several hypotheses have been put forth based on our understanding of CSF dynamic. In general, elevated CSF pressure may arise from a number of different mechanisms including: (1) obstruction or resistance to CSF outflow at the level of the arachnoid granulations,

(2) increased rate of CSF formation, (3) alteration in the elasticity of the brain parenchyma and intracranial blood vessels, (4) obstruction to the venous outflow at the level of the superior sagittal sinus, and (5) reduction in the capacity of the cranial and spinal subarachnoid space to expand.

Endocrine abnormalities, certain antibiotics, autoimmune disorders and steroids have been implicated as etiologic agents. Unlike in adults, causative agents are often identified in pediatric patients.

Diurnal variations in CSF pressure are seen and hence pressure measured at a single time may not reflect the peak. Thus, CSF pressure may be recorded as normal in patients suspected to have PTC. If the diagnosis is strongly suspected, repeat or prolonged measurement should be considered.

Migraine

Migraine is a recurrent, intermittent headache syndrome which does occur fairly commonly in young children. The headache is severe and throbbing; during episodes, the child often looks ill and pale. Typically, sleep relieves the headache. Initial evaluation focuses on excluding other serious diseases or conditions. Treatment consists of identifying trigger factors in the environment, providing acute pain relief, and considering prophylaxis.

Migraine presents with various neurological and non-neurological symptoms that are exacerbated with routine physical activity and relieved by sleep. Recurring spells of vomiting, abdominal pain, or dizziness may be juvenile forms of migraine. Two most frequent forms are classic migraine (with aura) and common migraine (without aura). Complicated migraine may present with sudden development of focal features and neurodeficit lasting for 24 hours. Familial hemiplegic migraine is an autosomal dominant disorder. Any clinical feature in neurology may be a manifestation of migraine; the diagnosis should be considered based on the pattern of evolution and progress of the disease.

Headache

A detailed history and physical examination facilitates ideal management and helps to avoid unnecessary neuroimaging studies.

In general, headaches are divided into two groups—primary and secondary. Primary headache is due to temporary or recurrent changes in the brain's chemical, physical or electrical makeup without any brain disorder. Secondary headache results from diseases of the brain.

The onset, duration and progress of any headache provides clues to its probable cause. An acute onset severe headache (occurring for the first-time) with fever suggest probable intracranial infection. Early morning headache, slowly progressive over weeks denotes probable space-occupying lesion. It is often accompanied with vomiting. A detailed neurological examination is vital to pick up subtle abnormalities in both these conditions.

Recurrent episodes of acute headache interspersed with asymptomatic periods (lasting for days) indicates migraine, especially in presence of a family history of similar disease. Low grade persistent headache with intermittent acute episodes is characteristic of tension headache and a headache due to sinusitis. Neurological examination is normal in these conditions and the diagnosis rests on a detailed history.

A refractive error does not cause a headache, though this is a common misconception. Patients with refractive error often misinterpret heaviness of the head or eye strain as a headache.

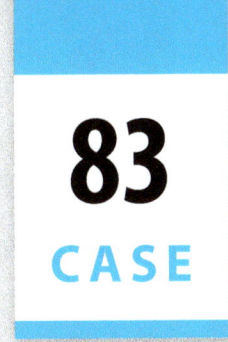

CASE 83

Gradually Progressive Hemiparesis

■ HISTORY

A 6-year-old male child presented with paucity of movements of the right upper and lower limb since 1 month. The patient was apparently alright 2 months back when he started getting a headache. It was moderately severe, generalized, more or less throughout the day, but particularly pronounced in the morning. There were no aggravating factors but it was relieved by vomiting at times. It was associated with non-bilious, non-projectile vomiting off and on.

A month later, he developed a gradual onset weakness of the right upper limb. It started as just a weakness of the fingers which gradually progressed to involve the whole limb over a week, so that he had a difficulty in holding objects. This was followed by a weakness of the right lower limb over another week, resulting in difficulty in walking. For the last 2 weeks, the weakness has been static, so that at present, though he can move both the right upper and lower limbs, using them is difficult.

A fortnight back he developed 3 episodes of generalized tonic clonic convulsions lasting 5–10 minutes each, spread over 7 days, without any focal onset or postictal paralysis.

No history of any behavior change noticed by the parents.
No history of diplopia, blurring of vision.
No history suggestive of a cranial nerve palsy.
No history of any change in speech.
No history or sensory disturbances.
No history of fever.

Analysis

This child has a recent onset, persistent headache which gets worse early in the morning, strongly suggestive of **raised intracranial pressure**. Migraine may closely mimic such a headache, except that it is episodic and interspersed with an absolutely normal period in between and hence unlikely in this child. At this juncture the etiology of the headache is difficult to judge, though in the absence of fever or any other symptoms, an acute infective intracranial pathology is unlikely. Subsequently, this child has developed a gradual onset, slowly progressive hemiparesis. A gradually progressive *unilateral* focal neurodeficit with increased intracranial pressure denotes a **supratentorial space-occupying lesion**. This hemiparesis could not have originated in the internal capsule as it would have been an acute onset dense hemiplegia. Similarly an origin in the motor cortex would have presented with a focal seizure and/or neurodeficit *before* the development of raised intracranial pressure.

Hence, this space-occupying lesion must have started in the subcortical area and then spread to involve the motor cortex. Occurrence of a seizure corroborates such a lesion, even if the seizure is generalized (focal seizures may spread rapidly to the reticular formation thereby clinically manifesting as generalized seizures). Since this non-infective space-occupying lesion is progressing rapidly, it is likely to be a **malignancy**.

■ PHYSICAL EXAMINATION

Averagely built, poorly nourished
Weight 14 kg   Height 108 cm
Pulse 80/min   RR 24/min   Temp. normal   BP 86/54 mm Hg
MacEwen's sign +ve   Fundus - papilledema
Rest of the general examination normal
CNS-
Higher functions normal   No cranial nerve palsy
Right upper and lower limb - hypertonia, power Grd 3/5 in all muscles
Left side tone and power normal
Deep tendon reflexes brisk bilaterally   Plantars extensor bilaterally
Sensory system normal   Coordination normal

Analysis

This child has a raised intracranial pressure (MacEwen's sign and papilledema) with a right upper motor neuron hemiparesis without cranial nerve involvement suggestive of a cortical/subcortical involvement. However, as analyzed in the history the origin of this lesion is likely to be in the subcortical area.

■ INVESTIGATION

MRI showed a large space-occupying lesion in the left parietal lobe.

■ FINAL DIAGNOSIS

Malignant astrocytoma.

■ KEY MESSAGE

> Supratentorial space-occupying lesions present as focal seizures (unilateral manifestations) with a later onset of raised intracranial pressure. On the other hand, infratentorial space-occupying lesions present with early onset of raised intracranial pressure, bilateral signs, and seizures are uncommon.

■ RELEVANT INFORMATION

Though this child did not have a facial nerve palsy, it usually goes hand in hand with upper motor neuron lesions like a hemiplegia/hemiparesis.

When there is a slight asymmetry of the face and there is a doubt about the presence of any facial weakness, it is best to test the upper face. If eye closure is quite normal and symmetrical, there is no facial weakness.

If there is apparently an upper motor neuron type of facial weakness, but there is no ipsilateral/contralateral hemiparesis, it is likely that the facial weakness in this case is actually of the lower motor neuron type. Such a (LMN) facial palsy is either an incomplete one, or there has been an early recovery of upper facial muscles.

If there is a significant weakness or the entire half of the face as is seen in a lower motor neuron palsy and it is associated with an ipsilateral hemiparesis, then the facial palsy is likely to be of the upper motor neuron type. Some patients have a greater than usual upper motor neuron control over the opposite cranial nerves. Hence, a UMN palsy gives rise to weakness of the upper face as well. The lower weakness is always much more pronounced in this case.

Hence, any facial weakness can be more correctly evaluated by taking into consideration the nature of involvement of the upper face and the associated hemiparesis.

CASE 84

Paucity of Left Sided Movements for 5 Days

■ HISTORY

A 2½-year-old male child, 2nd of twins, born of a non-consanguineous marriage was brought with the chief complaints of a convulsion 5 days back and paucity of movement of the left upper and lower limbs since then.

The child was apparently alright 5 days back when he developed a left sided tonic clonic convulsion, lasting for 2 hours, which subsided after medications given at a local hospital. Later the parents noticed that the child was not moving his left upper and lower limbs. However, over the next 2–3 days, he was gradually able to move his upper limb but was unable to grasp objects. He also started moving his left lower limb at about the same time.

No history of facial asymmetry, involuntary or movements, altered sensorium, headache, vomiting, visual disturbances, fever or speech involvement.

He was a preterm, one of twins, his birth weight being 2 kg. He was hospitalized in the NICU ror 5 days for low birth weight.

Developmental history normal.

Immunized completely for his age.

Analysis

This normal child had a sudden onset seizure involving the left half of the body, followed by hemiparesis which is gradually improving. Acute hemiparesis in a child can be with or without a seizure. When it occurs without a seizure it is usually **vascular** in origin (as happens in an infarct). When it is in association with a seizure it may be vascular or **epileptic** in etiology. There is no personal or family history of a seizure disorder in this child. However, its absence does not rule out an epileptic etiology. This was a preterm baby, one of the twins, who was in the NICU for 5 days. These babies are prone to birth injury, hypoglycemia, sepsis, etc. whose subtle manifestations may go unrecognized. They may present later as **remote symptomatic seizures**. However, these would give rise to a transient hemiparesis if at all (after the seizure), and not persistent, as in this case.

Vascular lesions giving rise to acute hemiplegia are usually infarcts secondary to thrombosis (hypercoagulable states), vasculitis (Henoch-Schönlein purpura, SLE), vasculopathies such as MELAS, Moyamoya, homocystinuria, embolism (heart disease), sickle cell disease, other disorders like hemorrhage into an intracranial vascular malformation, trauma to carotid/vertebral arteries and idiopathic cerebral artery infarction. Amongst these, the history may help to rule out vasculitis, heart disease and carotid trauma. However, the other conditions cannot be ruled out on history.

PHYSICAL EXAMINATION

Well grown for age
Weight 11.5 kgLength 88 cmHead Ο 47 cm
AfebrilePulse 80/minRR 26/minBP 90/66 mm Hg
No meningeal signsNo pallor, cyanosis, clubbing or lymphadenopathy
Skin, skull, spine normalNo neurocutaneous markers
Conscious, well-oriented, interested in surroundings
Cranial nerves normalPupils bilaterally equal, reactive to light
Hypertonia in left upper and lower limb
Power grade III/V in the left upper and lower limb, normal on the right side
DTR brisk on the left side, no clonusPlantar extensor on the left side
Sensations normalNo cerebellar signs
Other systems normal

Analysis

This child has a left sided spastic hemiparesis, no cranial nerve palsy, no signs of raised ICP, no sphincter disturbances and no clinically detectable sensory loss. Other systems are normal. A **recovering spastic hemiparesis** without cranial nerve involvement can occur in subcortical lesions (corona radiata). It is possible that it may be due to an internal capsular lesion in which the ipsilateral facial palsy has already recovered. Being a vascular lesion, this is most likely to be an infarct. However, **hemorrhage** cannot be ruled out. The underlying etiology of the infarction (or hemorrhage) is not clear from the examination.

INVESTIGATIONS

Hb 12 gm%WBC and platelet counts normalESR 14 mm at the end of 1 hour
Sickling test negativeMantoux test negativeUrine routine normal
APLA negativeANA negativeX-ray chest normal
CT scan of the brain—Hypodensity in the right frontal and parietal areas, involving the anterior and middle cerebral artery territory suggestive of an infarction.

Analysis

Investigations confirm an infarct, and rule out hemorrhage. However, no etiology could be established.

FINAL DIAGNOSIS

Left sided hemiparesis due to an infarction in the territory of anterior and middle cerebral arteries.

KEY MESSAGE

It is difficult to prove the etiology of an acute hemiplegia in spite of extensive investigations in most of the cases. However, investigations to rule out treatable causes must always be done.

RELEVANT INFORMATION

Acute Hemiplegia

While upper motor neuron lesions are characterized by loss of power with an increased tone, there are certain special situations.

Damage to pyramidal pathways gives rise to a particular pattern of weakness, i.e., weakness primarily in the gravity muscles. The residual power (better maintained in the antigravity muscles), in the affected area is maintained through extrapyramidal tracts under the influence of a *normal cortical function.*

If the whole area of cortex supplying a limb is damaged, the extrapyramidal fibers cannot maintain the strength, and *flaccid* paralysis of the limb takes place. At first it may be associated with depressed/absent tendon reflexes and no clear plantar response. Later the reflexes return and the plantar becomes extensor, but the flaccid paralysis remains.

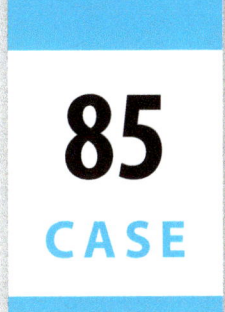

CASE 85

Irritability with Refusal to Walk

■ HISTORY

An 18-month-old child presented with excessive irritability and reluctance to walk for the last 2 weeks. He was apparently well prior to the onset of these symptoms and had achieved milestones normally. He had been walking without support since the last 6 months. The symptoms started insidiously and have been worsening since then. his sleep has also been disturbed. Initially the parents thought that he was behaving stubbornly but when he got worse and refused to stand, they sought medical advice. As there were no abnormal findings on physical examination, he was prescribed analgesics but without any relief. On direct questioning, he could move his legs when lying down though he was reluctant to do so. He continued to use his upper limbs without any problem.

No history of a fall or injury.
No history of a swelling noticed by the parents anytime.
No history of fever.
No bladder or bowel disturbances.
No relevant past or family history.
He was on a normal diet, taking family food.

Analysis

Excessive irritability in association with refusal to stand and walk, is mostly due to **pain** in the lower limbs, with or without an associated weakness. Since he was moving his legs in bed, if there was an element of **muscular weakness** it was likely to be minor. Pain may be commonly inflammatory in origin but may also be neurogenic, ischemic or psychogenic (though the parents initially thought so, psychogenic pain is uncommon at this age and the disturbed sleep rules it out).

Inflammation in the lower limbs may be due to trauma, infection or malignancy in which case, it is fairly localized to a particular part of the limb. Inflammatory conditions are usually associated with fever, and the pain is aggravated by touch or pressure. Therefore, inflammatory pain seems to be less likely in this child. **Ischemic** pain as in deep vein thrombosis is rare in children. It is mostly episodic in nature and aggravated by exercise. Thus, this child probably has **neurogenic** pain. As he has difficulty in standing and walking, the pain seems to be in *both* lower limbs. Hence, the anatomical site of the disease must be the spinal cord with involvement of the nerve roots. In fact, if pain is the more dominant complaint as compared to the weakness, the **involvement of roots** must be more than that of the cord. As the disease started insidiously and gradually worsened, it must be a progressive pathology affecting the nerve roots, either in isolation or as an extension from the cord or vertebral bodies. A cord lesion will usually give rise to sphincter disturbances also (though such changes may develop later). Thus, this child is probably refusing to walk due to neurogenic pain resulting from a progressive lesion involving the nerve roots innervating the lower limbs. The lesion could be related to an **unreported trauma** to the spine, or a **low grade infection** (spinal meningitis, TB spine) in which fever may not be obvious. It could also be a **space-occupying lesion**, or due to mechanical stretch as in **spinal dysraphism**.

■ PHYSICAL EXAMINATION

Fairly built and nourished
Weight 10 kg   Length 81 cm   Head ⊖ 47 cm
Temp. normal   Pulse 110/min   RR 28/min   BP 85/55 mm Hg
No pallor   No lymphadenopathy

Irritable and uncomfortable

No swelling, edema, rash or tenderness of legs; range of movements full at both knees and ankle joints. Passive flexion at the hip joints as in SLR test was painful suggestive of a nerve root lesion.

Spine normal, no paraspinal muscle spasm
CNS -
Higher functions normal   No signs of meningeal irritation
No signs of raised intracranial pressure   Cranial nerves normal
No cerebellar signs (such as truncal ataxia, titubation, past pointing and nystagmus).
Motor system - tone and power *apparently* normal (difficult to examine in view of initability)
Nutrition - mild wasting of calf muscles on right side
No abnormal movements
DTR - ankle jerk on right side absent   Other reflexes elicited normally
Superficial reflexes normal   Plantars - flexor response
Bladder not palpable   Anus not petulant
Other systems normal

Analysis

Physical signs reveal a lower motor neuron lesion involving the spinal roots (root pains, positive SLR test) at the level of S1, S2 on the right side as depicted by wasting of the calf muscles and the absent ankle jerk on that side.

■ INVESTIGATIONS

CBC normal   X-ray spine normal
MRI (plain and contrast) revealed a tumor of the cauda equina involving S1, S2 on the right side. This child had to be operated and the histopathology revealed an undifferentiated malignancy.

FINAL DIAGNOSIS

Undifferentiated cauda equina tumor.

KEY MESSAGES

- Pain may be inflammatory, neurogenic, ischemic or psychogenic. Each type of pain has its own characteristics for possible identification.
- A dull continuous pain in a young child may present with irritability, while an acute severe pain may present with excessive crying.
- SLR test (active or passive) is a good test for demonstrating root pains related to the legs. Its counterpart in the upper limbs (flexion of an arm at the shoulder joint) demonstrates root pains related to the upper limbs.

RELEVANT INFORMATION

In localization or lower motor neuron lesions, it is worth remembering that
"*anterior horn cell*" **atrophies**, "*root*" **pains**, and "*nerve*" **tingles**.

Clinical Manifestations of Spinal Tumors

Extramedullary tumors (e.g., cord compression due to TB spine) present early in the course of the illness.
1. Root pains may give rise to unexplained irritability and refusal to walk in a small child. An older child may be able to localize the pain.
2. Corticospinal tracts are the most sensitive to external pressure probably because of venous blockage. Hence, pyramidal tract symptoms will appear first, e.g., frequent falls, gait disturbance, etc.
3. Bladder and bowel dysfunction is the next to appear and will be noticeable early in a continent child.
4. Sensory disturbances will occur the last; they are difficult to detect in a small child.

On the other hand, in intramedullary tumors presentation of the child will be late in the course of illness.
1. Since sensory tracts carrying pain and temperature are located centrally in the cord, loss of these sensations occur early. However, it is asymptomatic and difficult to detect in a child.
2. Bladder and bowel dysfunction is the next to occur. In a previously continent child it will be noticed by the parents.
3. Atrophy of muscles of the lower limb may be detected.
4. Pyramidal tract involvement resulting in spasticity of the lower limb is the last to occur. It results in gait disturbances and frequent falls.

Thus, most of the children with intramedullary tumors present for the first-time with a bladder disturbance and pyramidal tract involvement, by which time it is often too late.

86 CASE

Difficulty in Walking for 5 Years

■ HISTORY

A 9-year-old boy presented with a difficulty in walking and frequent falls for the last 5 years and difficulty in getting up from the sitting position for the last 4 years. The child was apparently well until 4 years of age and was able to walk and run well. Around that time, the parents noticed that he was not able to run smoothly and used to fall frequently. Thereafter he was observed to get up awkwardly from the lying down or the sitting position. He would need to take support of railings while climbing up and down stairs. The difficulty went on increasing to an extent that since the last 1 year, he found it difficult to comb his hair or wear a shirt. He had been taking some treatment but had no relief.

- No history of intellectual deterioration
- No visual or auditory disturbances
- Bladder and bowel functions normal
- Developmental history: Standing at 2 years
- No history of abnormal movements
- No history of seizures
- No history of headache or vomiting
- Walking at 3 years

Fine motor, social and adaptive milestones achieved within normal limits
He went to school for 2 years but dropped out due to difficulty in walking.
- Birth history normal
- No family history of a similar illness

Analysis

This boy has a slowly progressive deterioration of motor function of the arms and legs without any intellectual deterioration, seizure disorder or symptoms of raised intracranial pressure.

This would rule out a cerebral cortical lesion. **Congenital progressive hydrocephalus** can give rise to a difficulty in walking but would have resulted in symptoms of raised ICP over the last 5 years. An isolated degeneration of the pyramidal fibers as in **hereditary spastic paraplegia** can result in progressive motor dysfunction of the lower limbs but this child has also weakness of the upper limbs and there is no family history of a similar illness. A **compressive myelopathy** of the cervical cord (basilar impression or Arnold-Chiari malformation) would present with sphincter disturbances and sensory changes. However, sensory changes may not be complained of and sphincter disturbances may occur later. Progressive anterior horn cell degeneration as in **juvenile spinal muscular atrophy** results in progressive motor dysfunction of limbs as an isolated abnormality and is a distinct possibility. **Hereditary sensory motor neuropathy** may also present in a similar way. In myoneural junction disorders like **myasthenia gravis**, the weakness is episodic with a diurnal variation, rather than progressive. However in one variety of myasthenia (Limb-girdle myasthenia), the weakness is progressive rather than episodic, and involves the muscles of the limbs especially the girdle. A similar clinical picture can be seen in muscle disorders like **muscular dystrophies** and in inflammatory and metabolic myopathies.

■ PHYSICAL EXAMINATION

Averagely built and nourished Weight 22 kg Height 130 cm
Lordotic stance Waddling gait
Higher functions normal Cranial nerves normal Speech normal
Power - Grades 3-4 in most of the limb muscles except wrist and fingers (normal)
Generalized hypotonia Calf muscle hypertrophy No fasciculations
Prominent deltoid and infraspinatus muscle with a groove in between (Pradhan sign)
Mild head lag DTR absent except ankle jerk (present)
Plantars flexor response Sensory system normal No cerebellar signs
Gower's sign positive Heart normal Other systems normal

Analysis

Hypotonia, areflexia (except ankle jerk) and flexor plantar response suggests **lower motor neuron** involvement. Waddling gait, Gower sign and assessment of power suggests that the weakness is **more proximal** than distal. In addition there is a weakness of the paraspinal and neck flexor muscles. Facial and external ocular muscles are spared. There is also marked hypertrophy of calf muscles.

A neuropathy is unlikely as it would have led to distal weakness and wasting with the ankle jerk lost early in the course of the illness. Juvenile spinal muscular atrophy (type 3) may present with a similar clinical picture; however the deterioration is very slow and the hypertrophy is never marked. In limb girdle myasthenia, there is progressive proximal weakness but the onset of symptoms is usually after 10 years of age and tendon reflexes are preserved.

Thus this child has a muscle disease. The distribution of weakness, absence of tendon reflexes and marked hypertrophy of calf muscles favors the diagnosis of **Duchenne** or **Becker** muscular dystrophy. Onset at 4 years of age and rapid progression of weakness suggests Duchenne muscular dystrophy. Other types or muscle disorders such as inflammatory, metabolic or endocrine myopathies are ruled out.

■ INVESTIGATIONS

S. CPK 13040 U/L X-ray chest normal
ECG and 2 D Echocardiography - suggestive of early cardiomyopathy
EMG - suggestive of muscle disease, no evidence of denervation
Nerve conduction velocity normal
PCR - intragenic deletions identified at Xp21 locus
Muscle biopsy demonstrated dystrophin levels of less than 3% of normal

Analysis

The investigations rule out a neuropathy and confirm the diagnosis of muscular dystrophy. Becker muscular dystrophy is the same fundamental disease as Duchenne with a genetic mutation at the same site. However, the clinical course and the dystrophin levels of less than 3% confirm classic Duchenne's muscular dystrophy.

■ FINAL DIAGNOSIS

Duchenne's muscular dystrophy.

■ KEY MESSAGE

Though the diagnosis of Duchenne's muscular dystrophy may be clinically obvious, it should always be confirmed by a muscle biopsy (dystrophin analysis) and genetic analysis, especially if it is the first case in the family. This is necessary for genetic counseling.

CASE 87

Difficulty in Walking, "Head Nodding" for 8 Days

■ HISTORY

A 2½-year-old male child born of non-consanguineous parents, 2nd by birth order, was brought with the chief complaints of difficulty in walking for 8 days, and inability to stand or walk for the last 2 days.

The child was apparently alright 8 days back, when the parent noticed that he had a difficulty in walking. The parents were not able to exactly define the nature of the problem; they just said that he could not walk properly. For the last 2 days he was unable to stand, had a difficulty in maintaining his balance in the sitting position and he also had "head nodding" movement. The upper limbs were normal. Apparently there was no pain anywhere. His understanding and memory were unaffected. There was no history suggestive of disturbances of speech, cranial nerves, bladder or bowel. There was no history of any convulsions.

Analysis

An acute onset of a painless difficulty in walking could be due to affection of power, tone, or due to ataxia or dystonia. "Head nodding" movements indicate titubation, suggestive of **cerebellar dysfunction**. Therefore, the imbalance in the sitting position may be due to truncal ataxia and the difficulty in walking due to ataxia of gait. This denotes that this child has a cerebellar dysfunction in the form of an acute cerebellar ataxia. There may also be an additional neurological involvement of the **motor** and/or **extrapyramidal systems** (which cannot be clearly deduced from the history available), though the ataxia seems to be a major complaint. In children, acute ataxia is most commonly due to acute **postinfectious cerebellitis** or **drugs**. Though he was given some medicines for the first 2 days after the onset of symptoms, drug induced ataxia is not likely to be persistent and progressive, more so when the offending drug is no longer continued. Similarly, acute cerebellar ataxia due to post-infectious cerebellitis has an explosive onset, the symptoms are maximal in the first few hours of onset, and they do not progress over a week. Therefore, this child is unlikely to have a drug induced ataxia or postinfectious acute cerebellitis. **Acute brainstem encephalitis** is unlikely because there is no suggestion of involvement of cranial nerves or a diffuse brain involvement (including the cerebral cortex). **Miller Fisher syndrome** is also unlikely because there is no history to suggest ophthalmoplegia. In children, acute cerebellar ataxia can also be due to a **cerebellar tumor**. Primary brain tumors normally present with a gradual onset of symptomatology. However, a rapid growth of the tumor, hemorrhage into a tumor or development of acute hydrocephalus can lead to an acute presentation. Moreover, the initial subtle clumsiness of gait may not be noticed by the parents and thus, an *acute* ataxia may seem to be the *presenting* manifestation of cerebellar tumors. Rarely, an acute ataxia may be the first episode of a **recurrent ataxia** (usually a genetic cause or migraine). However, the ataxia subsides in hours or a couple of days and is never progressive.

Thus, this child has an acute onset, rapidly progressive cerebellar ataxia, may be with an additional motor/extrapyramidal system involvement (to be determined on examination). As discussed above, though an intracranial space-occupying lesion is a possibility, there is no history to suggest raised intracranial pressure. Physical examination will help to analyze further.

■ PHYSICAL EXAMINATION

Irritable child
Weight 10 kg   Length 79 cm   Head ⊙ 48 m   Mild pallor
Anterior fontanelle closed, sutures normal.   MacEwen's sign +ve
No meningeal signs   No papilledema
Cranial nerves normal   Speech normal   Hypotonia of all four limbs, no wasting
Power grade III to grade IV in all limbs   DTR exaggerated R>L, plantars extensor
No intention tremor, dysmetria of upper limbs   Titubation and truncal ataxia present
Other systems normal

Analysis

This child has bilateral pyramidal tract signs, midline cerebellar signs and signs of raised intracranial pressure suggestive of an **intracranial space-occupying lesion,** which could be supra-tentorial or infra-tentorial. **Supra-tentorial** tumors usually *present with* unilateral focal neurological signs; though they can also cause a gait disturbance and ataxia, these do not have an acute onset and are not the *presenting* symptoms. **Infratentorial** tumors may present acutely and have bilateral, pyramidal and cerebellar signs with raised ICP. In view of midline cerebellar signs, this is likely to be a midline cerebellar tumor. Common cerebellar tumors at this age are astrocytoma, ependymoma and medulloblastoma.

■ INVESTIGATIONS

Routine investigations normal
   CT scan of brain—midline mass in the pineal region, cystic in consistency, compressing on the cerebellum, suggestive of medulloblastoma.

■ FINAL DIAGNOSIS

Medulloblastoma.

COMMENT

After physical examination revealed signs of raised intracranial pressure, on questioning the parents again it was revealed that the child did vomit off and on in the last 8 days. They had also noticed his irritability but had attributed it to his inability to walk and unsteadiness.

KEY MESSAGES

- It is important to consider a diagnosis of a space-occupying lesion even in a case of acute ataxia.
- At times, certain important details in the history are brought out only after the parents are requestioned on the basis of physical findings.

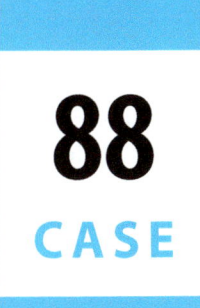

CASE 88

Clumsiness of Gait Since Last 4 Years

■ HISTORY

A 6-year-old male child presented with clumsiness of gait from the age of 2 years. He started walking at the age of 2 years and ever since then his gait was clumsy. For the last 2 years it had perhaps become slightly worse, but he could walk without support and climb, though he could not run. They also report some clumsiness of the hands over these 2 years though this did not come in the way of his daily routine. His speech had become indistinct from about the same time. There was no intellectual deterioration, headache, vomiting, seizures, impairment of vision or hearing.

On detailed questioning, the "clumsiness" was likened by the parents to a drunken man's gait. There was also a history of involuntary movements at rest, which used to disappear in sleep. There was a history of swaying of the bands on attempting any action. He is the first child, born of 3rd degree consanguineous parents, birth history being normal. He started walking late at about 2 years, but his other milestones were within normal limits. He goes to school and is in the first standard but is apparently not coping up in his studies as compared to his peers.

History of hospitalization 4 months back for pneumonia.

No family history of any similar illness.

Analysis

Shortly after any child starts walking, his gait may appear to be "clumsy" for a few weeks before he stabilizes. Persistence of gait disturbance beyond this period needs to be looked into; it may be due to a **neurological** or a **skeletal** problem (such as congenital dislocation of the hip or rickets). In this child, the presence of other neurological feature, i.e., clumsiness of hands and a speech disturbance rules out a skeletal problem.

Clumsiness of gait can occur in **disorder of the motor unit** (power, tone), **cerebellum** (ataxia, dysmetria), or **extrapyramidal** system (truncal dystonia. involuntary movements). However, since he can walk and climb, a significant disturbance of tone and power seems unlikely. Involuntary movements suggest extrapyramidal involvement. A gait akin to that of a drunken man and the reported swaying of hands on attempted movement denotes a cerebellar ataxia. Therefore, this child has a disorder with both cerebellar and extrapyramidal components. Since these complaints have been noticed ever since the child started walking, it may be a static developmental disorder like an **ataxic cerebral palsy, dystonic (akinetic) cerebral palsy** or a congenital malformation like **Arnold Chiari** or **Dandy Walker**. However, there is also a *suggestion* on history that this disorder may be progressive in which case it could be a very slowly progressive neuroregression like ataxia telangiectasia. Though this child may be having a mild scholastic backwardness, ataxic and dystonic cerebral palsies arising out of perinatal insults are usually associated with a significant mental retardation and are therefore unlikely, Therefore this child has an early onset, static or a very slowly progressive disorder involving the cerebellum as well as the extrapyramidal system without significant mental subnormality.

■ PHYSICAL EXAMINATION

Weight 18 kg   Height 105 cm   Head ☉ 49 cm
No dysmorphic features, cutaneous abnormalities or skeletal deformity
No pallor clubbing, or lymphadenopathy   MacEwen's sign negative
No cataract   Nystagmus present   Fundus - normal
Higher functions normal   Gait - wide based, ataxic.
Slurred speech   No cranial nerve palsy   No ophthalmoplegia
Ocular movements slow on lateral gaze; head moves first, eyes follow slowly
Power, tone - normal   DTR - sluggish   Plantars - flexor
Choreo- atheoid movements of upper limbs   Dysmetria present.
Sensory system normal   Romberg's sign negative
Other systems normal

Analysis

This child is confirmed to have a cerebellar disorder as suggested by the ataxic gait, dysmetria of hands, slurred speech and nystagmus. He also has a peculiar abnormality of gaze, viz. oculomotor apraxia. There is extrapyramidal dysfunction in the form of choreoathetosis, but no rigidity or dystonia. There are no signs of raised intracranial pressure or pyramidal tract involvement.

Ataxic cerebral palsy is characterized by hypotonia, brisk tendon reflexes, and is usually associated with significant mental retardation. In cerebellar ataxias due to malformations like Dandy Walker, etc. there *would* be no oculomotor apraxia. Hence, this is unlikely to be a static disorder of the cerebellum.

In view of a cerebellar ataxia associated with extrapyramidal manifestations and oculomotor apraxia, this is likely to be **ataxia telangiectasia**. Though the progressive nature of this child's illness is not certain, ataxia telangiectasia is known to be slowly progressive. Even though there is no ocular telangiectasia on physical examination, it is known to develop later. Ataxia telangiectasia is also characterized by immunodeficiency. However, the severity of the immunodeficiency may vary; this child has already been hospitalized once for a pneumonia.

Ataxia-oculomotor apraxia syndrome is another disorder that presents in this manner with an early onset and a slow progress. It differs from ataxia telangiectasia by way of absence of ocular telangiectasia and immunodeficiency, and is therefore possible.

Other progressive ataxias include **abetalipoproteinemia**, which is characterized by steatorrhea, failure to thrive, retinitis pigmentosa, etc. and is therefore ruled out. Spinocerebellar ataxias including **Friedreich's ataxia** may begin early in life and progress slowly: but they do not have choreoathetosis and oculomotor apraxia and they also develop skeletal changes, and are therefore ruled out.

■ INVESTIGATIONS

CBC - normal
Serum IgA levels were markedly low.

Analysis

Even in the absence of a gene diagnosis, markedly reduced serum IgA strongly supports the diagnosis of ataxia telangiectasia, in this setting.

■ FINAL DIAGNOSIS

Ataxia telangiectasia.

■ KEY MESSAGES

- It is difficult to differentiate a static from a very slowly progressive disorder, particularly when the manifestations begin early in infancy.
- In very slowly progressive disorders, the diagnosis may only evolve over time with the appearance of new symptoms and signs.

■ RELEVANT INFORMATION

Three basic control mechanisms are established in the first few months of life, provided the child has normal vision.
1. The ability to look in any desired direction until an object of interest is found. These movements occur as little flick of the eyes called "saccadic movements".
2. The ability to hold the object on the same spot on the retina in spite of any movement it may make. These movements of the eyes are known as pursuit movements and are smooth to avoid jerky vision.
3. In order to keep the eyes in a straight ahead (midline) position most of the time, continual adjustments are made in the eye position in relation to the position or the head in space.

Oculomotor Apraxia

When the child is asked to turn his head suddenly to one side, the eyes do not follow; instead they rotate to the opposite side and then slowly return to the midline. While doing so they overshoot and there is a compensatory head thrust. When the head is held in midline and the child is asked to look to the side without moving the head, he can initiate the eye movements only after a long lag (latent period) and the movements are grossly saccadic. This difficulty in voluntary movements results in a fixed gaze though there is no ophthalmoplegia. This is known as oculomotor apraxia.

CASE 89

Fever Followed by Prolonged Seizures

■ HISTORY

A 10-year-old female child presented with uncontrolled seizures and unconsciousness. She started with fever and cough 6 days back, for which she received paracetamol and some cough syrup, but without any benefit. On day 5, she developed some macular rash and was diagnosed as "measles". Her cough subsided but the fever continued. At this juncture, her CBC and chest X-ray was normal. On day 6, she suddenly developed generalized seizures that lasted 8–9 hours in spite of drugs administered, details of which are not known. Prior to the seizure he was neurologically normal and had no symptoms other than fever and cough. She was admitted at this stage for uncontrolled seizures and unconsciousness. There was a past history of generalized seizures at the age of 4 years accompanied with fever, diagnosed at that time as febrile seizures. She remained seizure free thereafter, till the present episode. She was not on any anticonvulsants.

Past history of measles at the age of 2 years.
No other significant illness in the past.
No family history of seizure disorder or any other neurological disease.
Developmental history was normal. She attends school and has an average performance.

Analysis

This child has developed **status epilepticus** on day 6 of a febrile illness. It is unlikely to be **acute bacterial meningitis** or **TB meningitis**. At this age, these should have *presented* with symptoms of raised intracranial pressure and then progressed over a few days to develop a seizure, i.e., they would have *presented primarily as meningitis* rather than generalized seizures. (As against this, a seizure may be the first manifestation of an intracranial infection *in infants*). **Viral encephalitis** usually presents early in the course of a viral illness and a change in the sensorium would have *preceded* the generalized seizures. Thus, it is unlikely to be an intracranial bacterial or viral infection. **Cerebral malaria** normally has encephalopathic manifestations, which are usually followed by a convulsion with in a short period (in 2–3 days), but it has a varied presentation. It is possible that this child is suffering from cerebral malaria. **Metabolic encephalopathies** may be triggered by fever but again, there should have been a prodrome of altered sensorium and vomiting preceding the seizures. Moreover, it is unlikely to present for the first time at 10 years of age. Sudden occurrence of seizure without any prior neurological symptoms can occur in a vascular or an epileptic disorder. Amongst vascular disorders, an arterial pathology would have resulted in a focal deficit due to an infarct. On the other hand, a venous pathology (as in **venous sinus thrombosis**) may result in passive cerebral edema with or without a focal neurodeficit and symptoms of raised ICP, before the occurrence of a generalized seizure. Therefore, it is possible in this child. Since there is a history of a convulsion at 4 years of age, it could be a primary seizure disorder triggered by a febrile illness. The earlier convulsion was diagnosed as a simple febrile seizure at that time, but it is unlikely to be so, because the first episode of a febrile convulsion mostly occurs earlier in childhood. However in **Generalized Epilepsy Febrile Seizure plus (GEFS +) syndrome**, the first febrile seizure could occur late as in this child. This is a genetic disorder in which there are febrile seizures in the child and generalized epilepsy in a parent. There is no such history here. The febrile illness in this child may be a viral exanthematous illness, but is unlikely to be measles as she had already suffered from measles at 2 years or age. Besides, in measles the fever declines within 48 hours of appearance of the rash, though the cough persists for a longer duration. Thus in this child, the likely diagnosis is an intracranial vascular pathology, an epileptic disorder or cerebral malaria.

■ PHYSICAL EXAMINATION

Averagely nourished, heavily sedated child
No dysmorphic features or markers of neurocutaneous syndromes
No skin rash   No papilledema   MacEwen's sign negative
Liver 1 cm +, soft   Spleen not palpable

Analysis

Physical examination rarely helps in the diagnosis in such a child. Either the further course of the illness or the investigations will guide further.

■ INVESTIGATIONS

CBC normal   Peripheral smear for malaria - negative
CSF examination normal   Anti-measles IgM antibody negative.
CT scan of brain (plain and with contrast) normal

Analysis

Investigations have ruled out an intracranial infection as well as focal neurological lesions.

■ FURTHER PROGRESS

The convulsions were controlled over half an hour. Over the next 2 days, she started responding to painful stimuli and thereafter was easily arousable. At that stage, she had no neurodeficit. Hence, this could have been cerebral malaria or a primary epileptic disorder. Hence, an EEG was ordered after 2 weeks.
    EEG - suggestive of a primary generalized epileptic disorder.

FINAL DIAGNOSIS
Primary generalized epilepsy.

KEY MESSAGE

> In an intracranial infection, a seizure is always preceded by headache, vomiting, or change in behavior or sensorium, *however subtle*. In newborns and young infants, however, this is not true.

RELEVANT INFORMATION

Febrile Seizures and Epilepsy

About 80% of children with febrile seizures will experience only one or two seizure episodes. The risk factors for recurrent febrile seizures are occurrence of the seizure below 1 year of age or at a low degree of fever, history of febrile seizures in parents or sibs, or a brief duration between the onset of fever and occurrence of the seizure. With no risk factors the risk of recurrence is 20% and with all risk factors it is about 70%.

Children with simple febrile seizure have no greater risk of later epilepsy than the general population. The factors that are associated with increased risk of later epilepsy are complex febrile seizures and a positive family history of epilepsy in which case with two risk factors the risk of developing epilepsy is 10%.

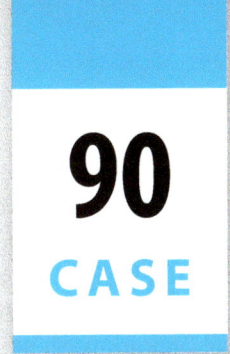

CASE 90

Unusual Case of Altered Sensorium

■ HISTORY

A 6-year-old child presented with high fever for 3 days followed by drowsiness and abnormal movements. For the first 3 days, the fever was rhythmic every 8–10 hours, responding to paracetamol, and the child looked normal during the interfebrile period. By day 4, fever was less but the neurological symptoms came up. He was absolutely normal prior to the onset of present illness. His growth and development were normal. There was no significant past or family history.

Analysis

High fever at onset, rhythmic, with normal interfebrile period would suggest an **acute viral infection**, even though accompanying symptoms such as cold and cough are absent. This illness localized to the nervous system on day 4 and hence one may think of **viral encephalitis**. However, typical viral encephalitis is a primary neurological disease in which neurological symptoms present early in the course of illness and mainly affect bilateral cerebral cortex. This child developed neurological symptoms not only late in the course of illness but also involved basal ganglia as evident by abnormal movements, besides cerebral cortex. Hence, it may have resulted from **complications** triggered by probable viral infection. Such complications are either **immune mediated** or **metabolic.** Inborn errors of metabolism are rare at this age and do not present with sudden onset of cerebral cortical and basal ganglia lesions. So, this may be an immunological complication of infection or an immune mediated disease itself, like **ADEM**.

■ PHYSICAL EXAMINATION

Drowsy but responds to painful stimuli

Weight 19 kg	Height 108 cm	Temp normal
Pulse 72/min	RR 18/min	BP 90/55 mm Hg

No other abnormality on general examination

CNS examination

Drowsy	No meningeal signs	Moves all limbs
Tone increased	Dystonia	Choreoathetosis +
Cranial nerves normal	DTR brisk	Plantar extensor
Fundus normal	Other systems normal	

Analysis

Physical examination has confirmed involvement of bilateral cerebral cortex with upper motor neuron signs and affection of basal **gangila** in the form of choreoathetosis. So, this child has diffuse cortical lesion along with basal gangila. Such a combination of signs may be seen in **TB meningitis,** which would have been a subacute presentation with signs of meningeal irritation, hydrocephalus and a chronically ill child prior to the onset of neurological symptoms. Hence, it is unlikely. Thus, this may be **immune mediated encephalitis.** Further tests would define the nature of the immune mechanism.

■ INVESTIGATIONS

CBC normal ESR 35 mm
CSF—clear fluid, Cells 45, P35 L65, Proteins 70 mg%, Sugar 50 mg%, Globulins increased
Culture no growth
Anti-NMDA receptor antibody +ve

Analysis

Mild cellular and protein response in CSF suggests inflammatory process. It may be compatible with viral infection. However, presence of anti-NMDA receptor antibody denotes antibody related encephalitis.

■ FINAL DIAGNOSIS

Anti-NMDA receptor antibody encephalitis.

■ KEY MESSAGE

Clinical pattern of presentation differed from typical viral encephalitis and hence one had to think about another cause. This is certainly not a common disease but is an example of how one should consider causes beyond the usual when clinical presentation differs from the standard.

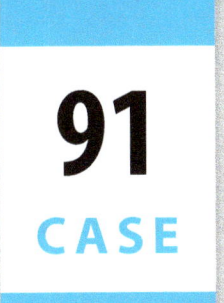

CASE 91: Sudden Onset Hemiplegia with Seizures in the Recent Past

■ HISTORY

A 10-year-old child presented with a history of (H/o) inability to move one side of the body noticed on waking up in the morning. He was completely alright the night before. There is a past H/o of two separate episodes of seizures 2 months apart, 6 months ago—it was labeled as idiopathic epilepsy. He is regular at school and his school performance is good.
No H/o any significant events in the past
No H/o consanguinity
No family H/o any neurological disease.

Analysis

This healthy child has developed an acute onset of left hemiplegia, though since it happened during sleep, we are not sure whether it developed in minutes or hours. Obviously, it is a **vascular event** affecting either the subcortical area or the internal capsule. There is no history suggestive of any risk factors for embolism, so it may be due to thrombosis. A hemorrhage would have been a catastrophic onset and **vasculitis** is an inflammatory disorder; so, without any other symptoms, unlikely in this child. **Vasospasm** is a possibility that results from a metabolic disorder that may evolve further. Two separate episodes of seizures suggest a preexisting neurological condition. In every seizure, we must enquire about the onset. On direct questioning, it was realized that both seizures were focal in onset with secondary generalization at different sites. This means that there was more than one abnormal focus. Considering the present event as of vascular origin, these two focal seizures also could have been the result of two separate focal vascular lesions. Thus, we may conclude that there have been three vascular events at different sites, and one disorder that can lead to these is moyamoya disease.

■ PHYSICAL EXAMINATION

Comfortable
Wt 30 kg Ht 135 cm HC 50 cm
No dysmorphism No neurocutaneous markers
Signs of left UMN dense hemiplegia
Other systems normal.

Analysis

The findings indicate an acute infarct in the territory of the middle cerebral artery. Coupled with the earlier two focal seizures, and the discussion above, this may be moyamoya disease.

■ INVESTIGATIONS

Cerebral angiography proved the diagnosis.

■ FINAL DIAGNOSIS

Moyamoya disease.

■ KEY MESSAGES

When a patient presents with a seizure, the first step is to confirm that it is a seizure, ruling out a pseudo-seizure. Once a seizure is confirmed, we must assess the onset and events before, during, and after the seizure. A focal seizure with impaired awareness and with secondary generalization can be easily mistaken for a generalized seizure. Most generalized seizures are followed by a postictal phase with the exception of a hypocalcemic seizure.

■ RELEVANT INFORMATION

Moyamoya means "puff of smoke" in the Japanese language, and it is used to describe the tangled appearance of tiny collateral vessels compensating for a vascular blockage. In this disease, there is a narrowing of some blood vessels in the brain, probably genetic in origin. Trauma may be a trigger factor. Angiography can differentiate these conditions. Surgical revascularization can help moyamoya disease and the outcome may be good. Prevention of strokes may be partly possible by reducing the risk factors, such as hypertension and obesity. The use of aspirin is hypothetical in such cases.

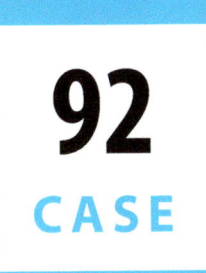

CASE 92: Irritability and Seizure in an Afebrile Infant

■ HISTORY

A 3-month-old infant presented with irritability for the last 2 weeks followed by a generalized seizure lasting for 2 minutes, for which he was hospitalized. Born after full-term normal delivery (FTND), he was feeding and growing well in the first 2 months. Around that time, he started becoming irritable and started craving for breastfeeds all the time. He would remain a little quiet while breastfeeding and seemed to be never satisfied. The mother was sure she had enough breast milk, and the infant was passing urine well. The treating doctor thought it to be either an intestinal colic or inadequate breast milk.

Analysis

Superficially this story may look like that of inadequate breast milk, but the mother was quite sure that she had enough breast milk, and the baby was passing urine very well. Once hunger is ruled out at this age, irritability usually suggests **pain** or **CNS irritation**. It is not an **intestinal colic** as that would have been episodic, for a short time, and with quite normal periods in between. It could be periosteal pain as in **scurvy**, but breastfed infants do not get scurvy and that too at this age. Similarly, **congenital syphilis** causing periosteal pain is ruled out because this irritability started after 2 months of age. Pain due to any other cause would be usually acute and would be followed by other manifestations. Thus, pain is not the cause of irritability in this child, and it is likely to be neurological in origin. **Raised intracranial pressure** would have presented with an acute onset of encephalopathy and seizures and the infant would be usually febrile. So, the irritability could be due to **metabolic** disturbances. In this context, if we go back to the history of (H/o) craving for breastfeeds all the time and not being satisfied, we realize that this baby could be thirsty and therefore asking for continuous feeding. A thirsty baby who is passing urine well would suggest **diabetes insipidus** and the subsequent seizure could be due to hypernatremia.

■ PHYSICAL EXAMINATION

Drowsy infant
Wt 4.3 kg (birth weight 2.5 kg) Length 57 cm HC 40 cm
HR 125/m RR 28/m Temp. N
Signs of severe dehydration and shock
No focal neurological signs Fundus N
Other systems normal

Analysis

The onset of the disease is around 2 months of age as suggested by weight and length; weight is more affected while the length is just below the lower end of the normal range. The head circumference is normal. Signs of severe dehydration and shock despite a good volume of urine indicate polyuria. Had it been due to a renal tubular disorder, one would have noticed fast acidotic breathing. Diabetes mellitus often presents with an acute onset of diabetic ketoacidosis and coma. So, one may consider the possibility of diabetes insipidus in this infant.

■ INVESTIGATIONS

Serum Na was 176 mEq/L
Serum osmolality 325 mOsm/kg (high) and urine osmolality 30 mOsm/kg (low)
Magnetic resonance imaging (MRI) did not reveal any evidence of inflammation or tumor in the hypothalamus/pituitary.
A genetic study proved the diagnosis of diabetes insipidus. Water-deprivation tests can be performed in milder cases but not in this child who had been presented with acute hypernatremia and cerebral irritation.

■ FINAL DIAGNOSIS

Congenital diabetes insipidus.

■ KEY MESSAGES

> Polyuria is difficult to evaluate, especially in early infancy. Usually, one tends to ask for oliguria but not polyuria. Irritability may be due to pain or cerebral irritation due to a variety of causes. Cerebral irritation may result from raised intracranial pressure or due to metabolic disorders without raised intracranial pressure (ICP).

■ RELEVANT INFORMATION

Diabetes insipidus is rare in infancy. It may result from a structural or functional disorder of the hypothalamic-pituitary axis either due to trauma, radiation, inflammation, or tumor. It may also be due to a congenital functional defect that can be proved by mutational analysis. Treatment in such a child consists of a gradual reduction of serum sodium over the next 24–48 hours (to prevent cerebral edema) by using initial fluid containing normal sodium. After normalization of hydration and electrolyte balance, desmopressin is required to maintain an adequate level of homeostasis, replacing the deficient natural vasopressin.

Index

A

Abdomen 15
Abdominal distension 7, 15, 19, 27, 51, 143
   progressive 16
Abetalipoproteinemia 352
ABO blood group
        incompatibility 324
Abscess 306
   intraspinal 165
   retropharyngeal 215
Acidosis, metabolic 58, 77
Acyanotic congenital heart
        diseases 106
Adenoiditis 58
Adrenal hyperplasia,
        congenital 263, 268, 269
Adrenarche 257
   premature 265
Adrenoleukodystrophy 230
   clinical diagnosis of 313
Airway disease 57
   generalized 57
   signs of 236
Akinetic cerebral palsy 351
Alkaline phosphatase 41, 52
Alkalosis, metabolic 163
Allergic alveolitis, probability of 106
Allergy 62
Alport's syndrome 243
Altered sensorium 359
Alveolar collapse 58
Alveolar disease, disseminated 162
Amikacin 61, 165, 183
Aminoglycosides 305
Ampicillin 61
Androgens, exogenous 263
Anemia 115, 128, 135
   acquired hemolytic 135, 143
   aplastic 128
   chronic 135, 143, 144
      deficiency 143
      hemolytic 140
   congenital hemolytic 136, 139, 143
   deficiency 136, 139, 140
   hemolytic 3, 33, 135, 324
   macrocytic normochromic 40
   microcytic hypochromic 122, 289
   moderate 145
   pre-existing chronic 139
   severe 67, 74, 139
Angiography 105
   cerebral 362
Anorexia 111
Anterior horn cell 341
Antiepileptics 123
Antihistamines 123
Antineutrophil cytoplasmic
        antibodies 41
Anti-NMDA receptor antibody
        encephalitis 360
Antiphospholipid syndrome 286
Antipyretics 181
Aortic regurgitation,
        rheumatic 85
Aortic valve involvement 84
Apex beat 248
Apla syndrome, secondary 285
Aplasia, causes of 136
Appetite 111
Arnold-Chiari malformation 343
Arterial block 284
Artery
   pulmonary 111, 112
   vertebral 335
Arthritis 73, 131, 300
   acute septic 297
   early onset 300
   generalized 300
   juvenile chronic 73, 75, 166
   rheumatic 131
   traumatic 131
Ascites 3, 7, 15, 19-21, 70, 71
   acute onset of 20, 21
Ascitic fluid 21
Aspiration syndrome 157, 161, 235, 236
Aspirin 123
Asthma 57, 58, 65, 235-237
Asthmatic attack 77
Astrocytoma 348
Ataxia 347, 351
   acute 348
   oculomotor apraxia
        syndrome 352
   telangiectasia 352, 353
Atelectasis 66, 90, 188
Atopic dermatitis 163
Atopy 65, 235
Atresia
   biliary 118
   pulmonary 101
Atrial septal defect 248, 251
Atrophies 341
Auditory
   impairment 228
   inattention 319
   radiations 312
Autism 320
Autoantibodies 41
Autoimmune disorders 53, 146
Autonomic dysfunction 181
Autosomal recessive disorder 163
Azure lunulae 33

B

Bacteria 63
Ballismus 305
Basilar impression 343
Battered baby syndrome 117
B-cell immune deficiency 161
Becker muscular dystrophy 344, 345
Behavior disturbance 312
Bicarbonate-wasting acidosis 277
Bicytopenia 127, 146
Biliary tract
   abnormality 54
   disease 1
Bilirubin, serum 8, 32
Bilirubinemia, direct 119

Biopsy, renoparenchymal 244, 245
Birth injuries 323
Bladder 341
    disturbances 305
    neurogenic 305
Bleeding
    disorder 11, 115, 123, 133
    episode, treatment of active 133
Blindness, development of 311
Blood
    backflow of 112
    brain barrier, disrupted 306
    obligatory complete
        mixing of 101
    pressure 285
Body fat, accumulation of 274
Bone 287
    age 255
    cysts 290
    diseases, metabolic 300
    malignancy, primary 154
    marrow
        aplasia 118, 129, 135, 136, 139
        disease 122, 139
        disorder 127
        failure syndromes 117
        hypoplasia 170
        infiltration 3, 143, 144
        transplant 146
Bony disorder, primary 275
Bony lesion 291
    multiple 291
Bowel dysfunction 341
Brain
    abscess 173, 191, 211, 212
        diagnosis of 213
        multiple 213
    swelling 306
Brainstem 305
    encephalitis, acute 347
Breast development 257, 263
Breathing 215
Breathlessness 15, 44, 57, 61, 65, 69, 73, 79, 83, 235
    complains of 187
    episode of acute 187
    gradually progressive 79
    recent development of 73
    sudden onset of 77

Brisk pulse 84
Bronchiectasis 97, 187
    extensive 188
Bronchiolitis 57
    obliterans-organizing pneumonia 75
Bronchoalveolar
    disease 187
    lavage 158
Bronchopneumonia 158
Bronchoscopy 110, 185
Brucellosis 146, 153
Budd-Chiari syndrome 17
Bull's neck 215

C

Calf muscles, marked hypertrophy of 344
Campylobacter 298
Candida albicans 189
Capillary leak syndrome 62
Caplan's syndrome 75
Cardiac catheterization 105
Cardiac disease 19, 43, 57, 70, 85, 101, 111, 187
    primary 111
Cardiac failure 143
    acute 23
    chronic 23
Cardiac involvement 29, 73
Cardiomegaly 85, 99, 248
    absence of 20
Cardiomyopathy 83, 111, 247
    hypertrophic 252
Cardiovascular disease 274
Cartilage matrix protein accumulates 300
Casts, absence of 245
Cauda equina tumor 341
Cavitatory disease 97
Cavity 90, 94, 188
Cefotaxime 61, 165, 183
Cellulitis, severe 215
Central cyanosis 8, 102, 106, 107
Central fever 177, 181
    causes of 182
Central nervous system
    infection, chronic 173
    irritation 363
    tumors 264

Cephalosporins 123
Cerebellar
    ataxia, progressive 348
    connection 305
    dysfunction 347
    involvement 312
    tumor 347, 348
Cerebellitis, postinfectious 347
Cerebellum 351
Cerebral
    cortical lesion 343
    function 303
    palsy
        ataxic 351
        dystonic 351, 352
Ceruloplasmin, serum 33
Cervical cord 343
Chemotherapeutic drugs 146
Cherry red spot 29
Chest
    examination 78
    pain 57, 83, 87, 89, 93
        acute onset of 89
    physical examination of 58
    retractions 58
    scan of 67
    signs 58
Cheyne-Stokes breathing 306
Child abuse 125
Chlamydia 298
Chloroma 154
Cholangitis, sclerosing 40
Cholecystitis 219
Cholestasis 163
    extrahepatic 53
    intrahepatic 51, 53
    laboratory evidence of 54
Cholestatic disorders 54
Cholesteatoma 305
Cholestyramine, use of 54
Chondrodysplasia 299
Chondrodystrophy 275
Choreoathetosis, form of 360
Chromosomal defects 254, 304
Chromosomal disorders 309
Churg-Strauss syndrome 193
Ciliary dyskinesia 58, 188
Cirrhosis 20, 40, 48
Clostridium difficile 298
Clot colic 243
Coagulation
    defect 115
    deficiency 132
    disorder 117, 125, 131
        congenital 117, 121

factor deficiency
  acquired 121
  congenital 125
  system, acquired disorder of 117
Cochlear damage, bilateral 312
Cochlear nerve 230
Cognitive disorder 316
Collagen vascular
  disease 62, 87, 89, 229
  disorders, majority of 171
Collapse 66
Coma 306
Complete blood count 234
  interpretation of 151
Congestion, acute severe 221
Connective tissue disorder,
  part of 117
Consolidation 66
Constipation 173
Constrictive pericarditis 20, 21
  diagnosis of 21
Convulsion
  focal 323
  generalized 203
  hypocalcemic 323
Copper, concentrations of 33
Cord compression 341
Corneal clouding 29
Coronary artery disease 196
Cortical function, normal 337
Cortical lesion 312
Corticospinal tracts 341
Cotrimoxazole 146
Cough 43, 57, 93, 157, 161, 183, 187, 235
  causes of severe 57
  mild 69
  persistent 59
  recurrent 57, 59
Cranial nerve 333
  palsy 212
Crohn's disease 171
Cushing's syndrome 272
Cutis laxa 288
Cyanosis 101, 105, 249
  pulmonary 107
  severe 101
Cyclosporine 128, 146
Cystadenomatoid malformation 66

Cystic fibrosis 58, 158, 161, 162, 188
  hallmark of 235
  typical of 163
Cysts
  congenital 90
  large 19
  ovarian 263
Cytochemistry 201
Cytomegalovirus 146, 153

D

Deafness 312
  complete 312
Deep-seated muscle abscesses 165
Deficient natural vasopressin 364
Dehydration fever 149
Dehydroepiandrosterone 268
Dementia 312
Dengue 15, 62, 150
  fever 62, 70
  illnesses 71
  shock syndrome 71
Dermatomyositis, juvenile 295
Descemet's membrane 33
Desmopressin 364
Destructive inflammatory
    pathology, acute 67
Dexamethasone 306
  suppression test 273
Diabetes
  insipidus 363, 364
  mellitus 43, 143, 274
    insulin dependent 41
Diabetic ketoacidosis 43, 65
  acute onset of 364
Diarrhea 234
  acute 227
  episodes of 187
Diarrheal episode 227
Diencephalic dysfunction 306
Diphtheria 215
Disseminated intravascular
    coagulation 117
Dizziness 329
Doll's eye movements 306
Drug fever 149, 177, 181
Duchenne's muscular dystrophy 112, 345
Dysmetria 351
Dysphagia 109

Dyspnea 83
Dystonia 347

E

Earache 195
Ebstein-Barr virus 153
  infection 178
Ecchymosis 15, 117, 118, 121, 127, 128, 131
Ecchymotic patches 117, 118
Echocardiography 252
Ectodermal dysplasia 163
Edema 3
  cerebral 306
  facial 71
  feet 23
  mild 239
  nutritional 23
  pulmonary 98
Ehlers-Danlos
  disorders 288
  syndrome 117
Electrolyte
  balance 364
  disturbances 112, 267
Electron microscopy 245
ELISA method 171
Embolism 335
  pulmonary 70, 77
Empyema 61, 62, 65, 66, 70, 89, 93
  bacterial 94
  subdural 211, 212
  tubercular 94
Encephalitis
  immune mediated 360
  viral 306, 355, 359
Encephalopathy 204, 211, 228
  acute 182
  diffuse 228
  infective 203
  metabolic 355
  subacute infective 205, 228
  symptoms of 173
Endocrine disorders
  complicated 269
  manifestation of 267
Endoscopic biliary drainage 54
Endoscopic retrograde cholan-
    giopancreatography 54

Index

Energy, excessive 274
Eosinophilic granulomas 290
Ependymoma 348
Epigastric pulsations 248
Epilepsy 357
Epstein-Barr virus 146
Erythrocyte sedimentation
    rate 234
Escherichia coli 298
Esophageal obstruction 109
Esophagitis 87
Esophagus 109
Estrogens, abnormal sources
    of 263
Expressive language 316
External genitalia
    masculinization of 268
    virilization of 268
Extracranial disease 191
Extrapyramidal system 347, 351
Extrapyramidal tracts 337

F

Fabry's disease 29
Face, puffiness of 19, 23
Facial
    asymmetry 143
    puffiness 70
    weakness 333
Failure to thrive 15, 47, 157,
        161, 324
Falciparum malaria 35, 36
Fallot's physiology 102
Fallot's tetralogy 102, 103, 251
Fanconi's anemia 117
Fanconi's syndrome 275
Febrile
    disease 192
    irritable 196
    seizures 357
Feeding 111, 343, 347
    difficulty 111, 247
Fever 57, 61, 65, 69, 87, 89, 93,
        127, 145, 149, 153, 165,
        169, 173, 177, 181, 183,
        187, 191, 195, 197, 199,
        203, 211, 215, 219, 227,
        233, 355
    biphasic 69

causes of 149
frequent 207
high 35, 161, 169, 187, 219
irregular 37
low 157
mild 44
non-infective 195
prolonged 223
recurrent 150, 157, 161
    episodes of 208
Fibromyalgia 284
Fibrosis
    intermittent 75
    pulmonary 41
Fingernails, base of 33
Finger-nose test 303
Fixed drug eruption 121
Flaccid paralysis 337
Florid hemolytic facies 140
Fluid 19, 66
    disturbances 267
    loss of 70
Friedreich's ataxia 353

G

G6PD deficiency 35, 135
Gait
    ataxic 305
    clumsiness of 351
    disturbances 304
    extrapyramidal 305
    high steppage 305
    spastic
        hemiplegic 304
        paraplegic 304
    waddling 305, 344
Galactosemia 3, 47
Gammaglobulin 41
Ganglia, basal 360
Gangliosidosis 29
Gangrene 284
Gastritis 87
    drug-induced 219
    severe 11
Gastroesophageal reflux
        disease 109
Gaucher's disease 8, 9, 144

Generalized epilepsy febrile
        seizure plus
        syndrome 356
Genetic defects 53
Genitals, ambiguity of 268
Glomerular disease 23, 243, 245
    diagnostic of 239
Glomerular pathology 239, 243
Glomerulonephritis 41
    chronic progressive 243
    recurrent 243, 244
Glossitis 136
Glucocorticoid 268
    deficiency 267, 268
Glycogen 3
    storage 29
        disease 29, 163
Gonadotropin 263
    releasing hormone 269
Gower sign 344
Granulomas 179
Granulomatous inflammation,
        evidence of 75
Graves' disease 41, 171
Gravity muscles 337
Gross motor 317
Growth
    charts 255
    hormone deficiency 253,
        254, 257
    spurt, normal 255
Gum bleeds 122

H

Head nodding 347
Headache 327, 329
    persistent 330
    recurrent 328
    syndrome, intermittent 329
Heart
    borders 88
    disease 335
        congenital 79, 83, 101, 106,
            111, 191, 247
        valvular 83
    enlarged 88
Heat fever 149, 177, 181
Hemarthrosis 132

Hematemesis 7
  episodes of 11
  recurrent 11
Hematological diseases 145, 146, 291
  primary 3, 128, 146
Hematological disorders 290
Hematological parameters rule 170
Hematology, clinical 115
Hematoma, subdural 324, 325
Hematuria
  extraglomerular 243, 245
  recurrent 239, 243
Hemiparesis 333, 336
  gradually progressive 331
  spastic 336
Hemiplegia
  acute 337
  sudden onset 361
Hemoconcentration 71
Hemoglobin, abnormal 105, 107
Hemoglobinopathy 105, 135
Hemoglobinuria 239
Hemogram 90
Hemolysis 115
  acute 36
  sudden 35
Hemolytic anemia 3, 33, 135, 136, 324
  feature of 39
Hemolytic facies 140, 141
Hemophilia 74, 290, 291, 297
  A 132
  B 132
  severe form of 117
Hemoptysis 97
Hemorrhage 115, 335, 336
Hemorrhagic disease, manifestation of 324
Hemosiderosis, pulmonary 97
Henoch-Schönlein purpura 290, 291, 335
Hepatic dysfunctions 118
Hepatic failure
  evidence of 32
  fulminant 32
Hepatic fibrosis, congenital 12, 13
Hepatic hydrothorax 16
Hepatic vein 1
  obstruction 20
Hepatitis 3, 31, 32, 35, 39, 44, 223
  A infection 44
  acute 31, 221
  amebic 219

autoimmune 39-41, 53, 171
chronic 39-41
neonatal 118, 119
severe 220
Hepatobiliary disease 2, 3
Hepatocellular failure, fulminant 31
Hepatocellular involvement, primary 36
Hepatocyte disease 1, 47
  groups of 49
Hepatocyte dysfunction, transient 13
Hepatojugular reflux 136
Hepatology, clinical 1
Hepatomegaly 9, 15, 18, 21, 22, 32
  mild 53
Hepatopulmonary syndrome 8
Hepatosplenomegaly 3, 28, 37, 140, 162, 179
  rules, absence of 212
Hepatotoxic drugs 31
Herniation 212
High fever 35, 161, 169
  acute onset of 61
Histiocytosis 153, 158, 177, 216
HIV encephalopathy 313
Hodgkin's lymphoma 169, 170, 216
Homocystinuria 335
Homovanillic acid, elevated 155
Hormones, extragonadal 268
Hydration, normalization of 364
Hydrocephalus 204, 205, 212, 229, 324
  acute 306
  congenital progressive 343
Hyperbilirubinemia, direct 49, 54
Hypercalciuria, idiopathic 241
Hypercoagulable state 284, 335
Hypergammaglobulinemia 41
Hyperimmunoglobulin D disorder 234
Hyperkalemia 112
Hypermobility syndrome 288
Hyperplasia, reticuloendothelial 27
Hyperreactive airway disease 235
Hypersensitivity 63, 93
Hypersplenism 122, 136
Hypertension 285

portal 1, 3, 7-9, 12, 48
pulmonary 248, 249
renoparenchymal 244
systemic 327
Hyperthyroidism 149, 177
Hypocalcemia 112
Hypokalemia 112
Hypoparathyroidism 163
Hypoperfusion 143
Hypophosphatemia, familial 275, 276
Hypothalamic dysfunction 182
Hypothetical model 62, 63
Hypothyroidism 27, 28, 163, 253, 257
  incomplete masculinization of acquired 271
Hypotonia 27, 304
  benign congenital 304
  generalized 316

I

Ibuprofen 298
Icterus 119
  mild 44
Idiopathic hypercalciuria 241
  classical symptom of 241
Idiopathic thrombocytopenic purpura 41, 117, 122, 123
Immune deficiency 58, 162, 188, 188
  congenital 158, 161
  diagnosis of 189
Immune reaction 44
Immunity 63
  cell-mediated 62
Immunochemistry 201
Immunocompromised host 61
Immunofluorescence 244, 245
Immunoglobulin A
  deficiency 188
  severe 189
  nephropathy 243, 244
Infections 19, 51, 145, 157, 181, 219
  acquired 47
  acute 192, 215

bacterial 62, 149, 153, 165, 225, 232
severe 221
viral 62, 149, 359
atypical bacterial 183
bacterial 165, 177, 231
chronic 53
congenital 27, 28, 47, 324
fungal 150, 157, 158, 162, 184
intracranial 195, 357
intrauterine 309
low grade 340
parasitic 150
persistent 211
recurrent 57, 161, 189, 211
  bacterial 58, 149, 157
  viral 58, 149, 233
severe bacterial 163
subacute 184
systemic 3
viral 43, 69, 149, 173, 223, 224, 229, 235
Infiltrative disorders 153, 177
Inflammation 339
acute severe 221
non-infective 149
Inflammatory disease 191, 196, 285
immune mediated 39
Inflammatory disorder 285, 300
Inflammatory pathology 327
Inhalation, wrong technique of 235
Injury, physical 118
Interstitial lung disease 57, 79, 106, 143, 187
evidence of 106
Intestinal colic 363
Intracellular metabolism, disruption of 306
Intracranial compartment 211
Intracranial contents, pressure-volume relationship of 306
Intracranial infection
primary 191
subacute 211
Intracranial pressure 211, 267, 306, 324
continuous monitoring of 306

Intracranial vascular malformation 335
Intradermal bleeds 123
Intrahepatic cholestasis
benign recurrent 54
progressive familial 51
Intravascular volume 72
Iron deficiency 140, 141
anemia 135, 141, 200
state 140
treatment of 141
Irritability 51, 173, 195, 199, 339, 363
Ischemia 284

J

Jaundice 2, 3, 15, 18, 43, 49, 51, 119, 223
absence of 221
acute onset of 31
acute severe 31
fluctuating 39
history of 135
mild 53
moderate 32
progressive 47
recurrent 53
severe 35
Joint
excessive mobility of 288
pain 73, 289, 293, 294
stiffness 299
swelling 131, 131
Juvenile idiopathic arthritis 297, 299
syndrome 297
systemic onset of 195

K

Kala-azar 3, 146, 177, 178
Karyotype 309
Kawasaki disease 112, 195, 196
diagnosis of 196
Kayser-Fleischer ring 32, 33, 40
Kidney disease 19
Klebsiella 189
drug-resistant 209
pneumonia 65

Knuckle pigmentation 272
Krabbe's disease 313
Kyphoscoliosis 291

L

Labyrinthitis, viral 305
Landau-Kleffner syndrome 230
Laurence-Moon-Biedl syndrome 271
Left coronary artery, anomalous origin of 111, 112
Left ventricular hypertrophy 85, 248
Leptospirosis 31, 35, 49, 178, 223
Lesions, regurgitant 247
Leukemia 3, 127, 135, 136, 144, 154, 169, 195, 216, 283, 287, 290, 291, 297, 324
acute 139
lymphatic 128
myeloid 128
Leukocytes 115
Leukocytosis, neurogenic 62, 165, 195, 196, 213, 231
Leukodystrophy, metachromatic 313
Leukopenia 170
Lipid storage disorders 3
Liver 48, 219
abscess 219, 220
pyogenic 220
biopsy 8, 13, 40, 119
cell
  destruction of 1
  failure 48
disease 16, 31, 117, 119
  chronic 7, 8, 12, 13, 23, 39, 40, 51
  hallmark of 2
  pre-existing chronic 31
  primary 3
  progressive chronic 7
enlarged 2, 27
enzymes, raised 119
fetal 33
function 13
  tests 48
neonatal 33
soft
  large 3
  small 3
span 2

Lobar 58
  distribution 58, 89
  emphysema, congenital 79, 111
Lordosis 305
Lower limbs 339, 341
  progressive deformity of 275
Lower motor neuron
    involvement 344
Lower respiratory infections
  recurrent 187
    bacterial 189
Lower respiratory tract 149
  infection, episodes of 109
Lump 15
Lung
  abscess 90, 94, 187
  cyst 58
  disease, interstitial 57, 79, 106, 143, 187
  function, decompensation of 187
  large areas of 187
Lymph node
  hard 216
  non-inflammatory enlargement of 215
  swellings 215
Lymphadenopathy, massive 216
Lymphohistiocytosis, hemophagocytic 146
Lymphoma 216
Lymphoreticular disorder 215

M

MacEwen's sign 332
Malaria 35, 37, 49, 139, 140, 150, 153, 161, 171, 178, 195, 208
  cerebral 355
  consistent features of 37
  recurrent 177
Malarial parasite 38
Malformation
  congenital 187, 323
  vascular 11
Malignancy 15, 19, 66, 144, 146, 149, 150, 153, 154, 177, 178, 181, 191, 217, 233, 290, 294, 332

  hematological 290
  intrathoracic 62
Malignant disorders 217
Malnutrition 163, 174
  chronic 258
  severe 208
Mannosidosis 29
Marfan's syndrome 288
Marrow
  aplasia 127
  disease 115
  failure 128
Massive hemorrhagic pleural effusion 67
Massive organomegaly 8, 19
Massive pleural effusion, signs of 66
McCune-Albright syndrome 264
Mediastinal mass 58
Mediastinum 91
Medulloblastoma 348
Melanocyte stimulation 267
Menarche
  onset of 257
  premature 265
Meningitis 149
  bacterial 173, 211, 212, 229, 355
  fungal 173, 204
  spinal 340
  subacute 203
  tuberculous 173, 175, 205, 211, 229, 355, 360
Menkes kinky hair disease 288
Mental retardation 29, 317
Metabolic disease 39, 112
Metabolic disorders 3, 49, 53, 300
  manifestation of 267
Metabolic disturbances 363
Metabolic tests 48
Metabolism, inborn error of 47, 359
Metallothionein 33
Metaphyseal dysplasias 276
Methemoglobinemia, acquired 105
Microabscesses, evidence of 178
Microcephaly 317
Midbrain, signs of 306
Midline cerebellar tumor 348
Migraine 328, 329
  juvenile forms of 329

Miller Fisher syndrome 347
Mimic hypermobility syndrome 288
Mineralocorticoid, deficiency of 267, 268
Minimal change nephrotic syndrome 24
Minimal intercostal retractions 80
Mitochondrial disorders 112
Mitral regurgitation 83, 84
  rheumatic 85
Mitral valve 112
  insufficiency increase 112
  prolapse 252
Morning stiffness 281
Motor regression 312
Motor unit, disorder of 351
Movements, involuntary 305, 351
Moyamoya disease 229, 335, 362
Mucolipidosis 29
Mucopolysaccharidosis 20, 253
  diagnosis of 28
Multiple cavities, causes of 163
Multiple epiphyseal dysplasia 300
Multiple large joint swellings, acute onset 297
Multisystem inflammatory disease, neonatal 234
Murmur 251
  functional 251
  innocent 251, 252
  mid-diastolic 98
Muscle
  atrophy of 341
  disuse, face of 288
  facial 344
  power 316
  tiredness 143
Muscular dystrophy 344
  diagnosis of 345
Muscular origin 283
Muscular weakness, element of 339
Musculoskeletal pain 285, 287
  syndromes 284
Myalgia 150
Myasthenia gravis 343
Myelodysplasia 127
Myelofibrosis 127
Myelofibrotic marrow disorders 144

Myeloid leukemia 154
Myelopathy, complicated 343
Myocardial disease 111
Myocardial dysfunction, transient 251
Myocardial infarction 77
Myocarditis, acute viral 65
Myocardium 112
   dysfunction of 111
Myoglobinuria 239
Myopathies, metabolic 344
Myositis 284

N

Nails, clubbing of 8, 107
Nasal discharge 187
Neck
   flexor muscles 344
   swelling 215
      bilateral 215
Necrotizing pneumonia 65
Neonatal hepatitis 118, 119
   diagnosis of 119
Nephritis, chronic 208
Nephropathies 24
Nephrotic syndrome 23, 25
Nerve conduction velocity normal 344
Nervous system, development of 303
Neuroblastoma 154, 290
Neurological disorder 111
   progressive 309
Neurological examination 303
Neurological lesion, diffuse 312
Neurology, clinical 303
Neuropathy 344
Niemann-Pick disease 29
Nodules
   pulmonary 75
   subcutaneous 281
Non-cirrhotic portal fibrosis 12, 13
   diagnosis of 13
Non-Hodgkin's lymphoma 170, 216
Noninfective disease 145
Noninfective inflammatory
   disorders 146
   pathology 184

Non-lobar non-pleural distribution 58
Nonrheumatic diseases 171
Nonsteroidal anti-inflammatory drugs, use of 232
Normocytic normochromic anemia 170, 213
Nutrition 316

O

Obesity 273
   idiopathic 271
   nutritional 271
Obstruction
   lymphatic 15, 19
   presinusoidal 12
Oculovestibular reflexes 306
Ocular muscles, external 344
Ocular myasthenia 311
Oculomotor apraxia 353
Oliguria 239
Ophthalmoplegia 311
Opioid antagonist 54
Organ dysfunction 118, 253
Organic defect 251
Organomegaly 7, 15
Osteomyelitis 165
   chronic recurrent multifocal 232
   tubercular 154
Osteopenia 207, 287
Osteopetrosis 144
Osteoporosis, development of 283
Otitis 305

P

Pain 111, 231, 299, 339, 363
   abdominal 195, 234
   cause of 195
   epigastric 87
   ischemic 339
   limb 283, 287
   musculoskeletal 285, 287
   neurogenic 284, 339
   severe abdominal 18, 219
   upper abdominal 219
Pallor 128
   severe 140
Palm, ventral surface of 115
Palmer grasp 303

Palpable spleen 3
Palpitations 83
Pancreas 219
Pancreatitis, acute 15, 219
Pancytopenia 146
Panhypopituitarism 163
Papilledema 332
Paracetamol 203
Paraplegia, spastic 343
Patent ductus arteriosus 248, 251
Peptic ulcer disease 11
Perforin deficiency 146
Periarticular structures 289
Pericardial effusion 66
Pericardial empyema 87
Pericardial involvement 73
Pericarditis 87
   constrictive 20, 21
   purulent 87
   pyogenic 65
Pericardium, level of 20
Perinatal period 101
Periodic fever syndrome 234
Peripheral blood smear examination 116
Peripheral pulmonic systolic murmur 252
Peritoneal cavity 19
Pertussis 157
Petechiae 122, 123
Pharyngitis 237
Phenytoin 128
Plantar grasp 303
Platelet 115, 122
   adequate 289
   count 116, 123
   disorder 115
      acquired 117, 122
      functional 122
   function
      defect, indicator of 133
      disorder 117, 122, 123
Pleural cavity 16
Pleural disease 43, 188
   immune mediated 44
Pleural distribution 58, 78, 90
Pleural effusion 43-45, 57, 58, 61, 65, 70, 71, 75, 90
   bilateral 71
   development of 89

Index

immune mediated 44
signs of 69
small 94
tubercular 95
typical 94
Pleuropneumonia 94
acute bacterial 94
low-grade infective 93
Pneumonia 57, 58, 65, 94, 149, 191, 237
acute bacterial 183, 191
basal 219
tubercular 94
Pneumothorax 43, 65, 70, 77, 78, 93
causes of 78
Poisoning 149
Polyangiitis, microscopic 75
Polyserositis 70
Pontine lesion 182
Portal hypertension 1, 3, 7-9, 12, 48
extrahepatic 11
feature of 13
presinusoidal 11
Portopulmonary syndrome 8
Precordial pulsations 111
Proteins
metabolism 47
serum 32
Proteinuria 244
Prothrombin
complex factor deficiency 132
time 32
Pseudohermaphrodite, male 268
Pseudoprecocity 268
Pseudotumor cerebri 327, 328
Psychosis, manifestation of 312
Puberty
central precocious 263
idiopathic precocious 264
normal 258
onset of 257
peripheral precocious 263
precocious 268
premature signs of 268
pseudoprecocious 263
true idiopathic precocious 264
Pubic hair 257
development 267

Pulmonary artery 111, 112
dilatation 248
Pulmonary capillary wedge pressure 83
Pulmonary disease 97, 106
Pulmonary hypertension 248, 249
development of 85, 251
symptoms of 83
Pulmonology, clinical 57
Purpura 115
absence of 170
fulminans 117
Pus, improper drainage of 61
Pyopericarditis, acute 219
Pyramidal fibers 343
Pyramidal pathways 337
Pyramidal tract 341
Pyrexia 149
Pyrizinamide 31
Pyrogenic response 149
Pyruvate kinase deficiency 135

Q

Quinine 123, 305

R

Radionuclide scan 105
Raised intracranial pressure 203, 205, 227, 228, 327, 331, 363
presence of 328
Rapidly progressive neck swelling 215
Reactive arthritis 289, 297, 298
specific syndromes of 289
Red cell aplasia 324
Reflex 303
abnormal persistence of 303
developmental 303
sympathetic osteodystrophy 284
Refractive error 330
Regurgitation, aortic 84
Renal failure 36
Renal tubular
acidosis 207, 275, 277, 299
disorder 48, 364
dysfunction 48
Replacement fluid, quantity of 133

Respiration, accessory muscles of 58
Respiratory disease 101, 111
primary 111
progressive 106
Respiratory distress 58, 61
acute 70
mild 44, 69
Respiratory dysfunction 162
Respiratory infection 183
recurrent 161
Respiratory problem 8
Respiratory system 44
Reticuloendothelial cell hyperplasia 178
Reticuloendothelial involvement 1
Retrocochlear pathology 312
Reye's syndrome 306
Rheumatic
carditis, acute 65
diseases 171
disorder, diagnosis of 281
fever, acute attack of 85
origin
mitral stenosis of 98
valvular heart disease of 83
valvular disease, diagnosis of 85
Rheumatoid
arthritis 281
factor, serum 281
Rheumatological disease 285, 300
pulmonary manifestations of 75
Rheumatological disorder 73, 75, 131, 146, 233
Rheumatology, clinical 281
Rickets 275
early 323
hypocalcemic variety of 275
non-nutritional 299
Rifampicin 31, 54
Right middle lobe emphysema 80, 81
Right ventricular hypertrophy 102, 248
Romberg sign 303
Root
involvement of 339
pains 341
Rule out fungal infection 174

S

Saccadic movements 353
Salicylates 305

Index

Salmonella 298
Sandhoff's disease 29
Sarcoidosis 153, 177
Scurvy 128, 207, 283, 290, 291, 363
Segmental parenchymal disease 90
Seizures 357, 361, 363
    prolonged 355
    rules 324
    symptomatic 308, 335
Sensory disturbances 341
Sensory motor neuropathy,
    hereditary 343
Sepsis 51, 117
Sequestration 66
Serology, viral 119
Serum ascitic albumin gradient 17
Serum sodium, gradual reduction
    of 364
Shigella 298
Shock 101
Short stature 291, 299
    familial 253, 258
    idiopathic 253, 258
Shoulder joint 289
Shunt, reversal of 249
Sialidosis 29
Sickle cell
    anemia 291
        diagnosis of 290
    disease 53, 74, 219, 229, 283,
        290, 335
        skeletal manifestations of 291
Sinusitis 58
Skeletal
    abnormalities 272
    disorder, primary 299
    dysplasias 253, 254
Skin, darkening of 268
Slowly progressive hypoxia,
    symptoms of 143
Soft systolic murmur, accidental
    detection of 251
Soft tissue 281, 291
Sonogram, abdominal 21
Space-occupying lesion 327, 340
    intracranial 204, 324, 348
    supra-tentorial 331, 332
Spasticity 312
Specific coagulation factors,
    deficiency of 132

Speech, delayed 319
Spherocytosis, hereditary 135
Spinal
    dysraphism 340
    muscular atrophy, juvenile 343
    tumors, clinical manifestations
        of 341
Splenomegaly 22, 140, 223
    mild 32
Staphylococcus epidermis 183, 184
Static neurological disorder 309
Status epilepticus 355
Stenosis
    aortic 251
    pulmonary 251
Steroids 146
    responsive nephrotic syndrome,
        management of 26
Stickler syndrome 288
Stomach 219
Storage disorder 8, 29, 47, 27, 144,
    178, 309
Strabismus, intermittent 311
Suck-rest-suck cycle 101, 247
Sudden infant death syndrome 237
Sulfur-rich copper-binding
    protein 33
Superficial bleed 115
Suprahepatic postsinusoidal
    venous obstruction 16
Sweat chlorides 163, 189
Swelling 73, 231, 281, 284
    spontaneous 132
    symmetrical 281
Syndromic disorder 309
Syphilis, congenital 363
Systemic disease 253, 257
Systemic inflammatory
    disease 150, 169
    disorder 165, 177, 181
        manifestation of 153
Systemic lupus
    diagnosis of 170
    erythematosus 166, 170
Systemic onset juvenile idiopathic
    arthritis 166, 167, 197,
        233
    diagnosis of 166
Systemic vasculitis 290
    part of 121

T

Tachypnea 58, 162
    silent 58
Tandem walking 303
T-cell leukemia 201
Tenderness 284
    severe 221
Tension pneumothorax 43
Testis, size of 268
Thalassemia major 135
Thelarche 257
    premature 265
Thrombasthenia 125
Thrombocytopenia 71, 128, 150
    immune mediated 122
    isolated 122
    megakaryocytic 117
Thrombophilic state 11
Thrombosis 284, 335
Thyroid function tests 309
Tics 305
Toe walking 312
Tonic neck response 303
Tonsillitis 58, 149
Tonsils 217
Toxic labyrinthitis 305
Toxoplasmosis 146, 153
Tracheoesophageal fistula 110
Tracheitis, bacterial 87
Trauma 62, 297, 335
True precocity 263, 269
Truncal dystonia 351
Tuberculin test 159
Tuberculosis 15, 20, 59, 65, 66,
    70, 89, 90, 93, 146, 153,
    157, 162, 169, 174, 177,
    178, 184, 188, 216, 225,
    229, 243
    clinical evidence of 294
    diagnosis of 158
    multidrug resistant 188
    mycobacterium 158
    pulmonary 315
Tubular proteinuria 23
Tumors
    adrenal 263
    extramedullary 341
    hypothalamic 182
    infratentorial 348

mediastinal 79
midline 327, 328
necrosis factor 234
ovarian 263
supra-tentorial 348
virilizing 268
Turner's syndrome 253, 271, 272
Typhoid 31, 49
    fever 35, 149, 150
    infection 31
Tyrosinemia 48
    diagnosis of 48

U

Ulcerative colitis 41
Ulcers, mouth 150
Umbilical sepsis, sequelae of 11
Upper respiratory
    infection 69
    symptoms 187
    tract 149
Urinary tract infection 208, 209, 243
Urolithiasis 243
Ursodeoxycholic acid 54

V

Vague arthralgia 150
Valproate 31
Valvular lesion, congenital 112
Vancomycin 61, 146
Vanillylmandelic acid 155
Vascular diseases 112
Vascular disorders 53, 117, 125
    acquired 121
    congenital 121

Vascular episode 227
Vascular lesion 229, 335
Vasculitis 204, 284, 290, 335, 361
    systemic 290
Vasculopathy 335
Vasogenic cerebral edema,
    management of 306
Vaso-occlusive crisis 283
Vena cava obstruction 1
    inferior 19
    superior 19
Venous obstruction 15, 16, 18-21
Venous sinus thrombosis 356
Ventricles, ependymal linings
    of 306
Ventricular enlargement 85
Ventricular septal defect 248, 251
    large 249
Ventriculoarterial connections,
    abnormal 101
Vertebral fracture 199
Vertigo 305
Vestibular dysfunction,
    peripheral 305
Vestibular nuclei, central
    abnormalities of 305
Viruses, hepatotropic 49
Visceral hematomas 121
Vision 317
    gradual diminution of 311
    impairment of 228, 230, 307
Visual pathways, anterior segment
    of 230
Vitamin
    B_{12} 141
    deficiency anemia 128,
    136, 137

D deficiency rickets 52
K deficiency 117, 118
Vitiligo 41
Voice, loss of 58, 215
Volvulus 267
Vomiting 173, 323, 327, 329
    cyclical 267
    intermittent non-bilious 87
    non-bilious 87
    recurrent 267, 269
von Willebrand's disease 122

W

Waddling gait 305, 344
Weakness
    generalized 143, 207
    pressure-volume relationship
    of 344
Wegener's granulomatosis 184, 192
Weight
    gain 271
    loss 39
Wheezing, frequent 235
Whooping cough 157
Wide pulse pressure 98, 99
William syndrome 288
Wilson's disease 3, 31-33, 39, 40
    laboratory tests of 32
Worsens hypoperfusion 112

Y

Yersinia 298

Z

ZN stain 174

EU GSPR Authorised Reprsentative
Logos Europe, 9 rue Nicolas Poussin
1700, La Rochelle, France
Phone: +33 (0) 6 67 93 73 78
E-mail: contact@logoseurope.eu

www.ingramcontent.com/pod-product-compliance
Ingram Content Group UK Ltd.
Pitfield, Milton Keynes, MK11 3LW, UK
UKHW060934280126
467427UK00003B/17